D1558661

SPEECH
IMPROVEMENT

SPEECH
IMPROVEMENT

MORTON J. GORDON

University of Hawaii
Kapiolani Community College

Prentice-Hall, Inc., Englewood Cliffs, New Jersey

Library of Congress Cataloging in Publication Data

GORDON, MORTON J
    Speech improvement.

    Includes bibliographical references.
    1. English language in the United States—
Pronunciation.   2. English language—Remedial English.
I. Title.
PE2815.G6   808.5   73–9845
ISBN   0–13–832386–0

© 1974 by PRENTICE-HALL, INC., *Englewood Cliffs, New Jersey*

Printed in the United States of America

10   9   8   7   6   5   4   3   2   1

PRENTICE-HALL INTERNATIONAL, INC., *London*
PRENTICE-HALL OF AUSTRALIA, PTY. LTD., *Sydney*
PRENTICE-HALL OF CANADA, LTD., *Toronto*
PRENTICE-HALL OF INDIA PRIVATE LIMITED, *New Delhi*
PRENTICE-HALL OF JAPAN, INC., *Tokyo*

To my wife Betty, and my children
Michael, Beth, David

Contents

part II
THE PRONUNCIATION
OF THE CONSONANT TARGETS
OF AMERICAN ENGLISH

part III
THE PRONUNCIATION
OF THE VOWEL AND DIPHTHONG TARGETS
OF AMERICAN ENGLISH

part IV
THE USE OF
STRESS AND INTONATION

Preface

TO THE TEACHER

I have planned *Speech Improvement* as a remedial speech textbook that will assist both native and nonnative speakers of English in overcoming various problems in articulation, rhythm, and intonation. The book is basically designed to be employed by a student who is enrolled in some type of remedial speech program—for example, a speech improvement course for native speakers, a course in spoken English for foreign students who are learning English as a second language, or a group speech therapy program for students with articulatory problems. Because the emphasis in the book is fundamentally practical, I have held the explanatory materials to a very simplistic level. The drill vocabulary has also been limited to a basic level, with much of it based on a third-grade reading ability.

The beginning of the textbook consists of a series of short background chapters which are required reading for all students. This material includes (1) an introductory chapter, (2) a unit that explains the remedial techniques and procedures employed throughout the book, (3) a chapter on the diagnostic step in speech improvement—particularly written for the beginning remedial speech instructor, and (4) a simplified chapter detailing the technical aspects of articulatory phonetics that are used to aid learning in the book. The heart of the book is a series of practice chapters containing drill materials for all the vowels, diphthongs, and consonants of American English—in addition to practice materials for English stress and intonation. Students are not assigned all these practice chapters but are held responsible only for the appropriate practice chapters that will teach them how to overcome their individual speech problems.

Because I strongly believe that the development of accurate listening skills are extremely important in a remedial speech program, I have included a variety of ear training exercises in the practice chapters. These include (1) drills aimed at developing aural recognition of the particular target being studied, (2) information regarding the nature of the more probable replacement errors associated with the target, and (3) aural discrimination tests to help the student recognize the difference between his incorrect usage and the study target. The practice section on production begins with simple exercises which become progressively more difficult as the student works his way through the chapter, and the section finally terminates in exercises aimed at helping the student learn to use his target accurately in conversation.

I have largely used pronunciations associated with General American speech in planning the practice materials. However, I have indicated in certain chapters the preferred Eastern and Southern American pronunciations of specific articulatory targets. The pronunciation targets have been illustrated with symbols taken from the International Phonetic Alphabet. Finally, I have included an articulation test and two copies of an evaluation form to facilitate your diagnosis of each student's problems.

SPEECH
IMPROVEMENT

part I

AN INTRODUCTION
TO SPEECH IMPROVEMENT

chapter one

A Few
Beginning Observations

1–1. INTRODUCTION

A. SPEECH COURSES

Speech improvement of one type or another is the goal of each of the wide variety of speech courses now available to the interested person. Some courses, such as *public speaking, group discussion*, and *argumentation and debate*, teach you the most effective ways of planning and organizing the content or message you wish to deliver to your listener. Other speech courses, such as *interpretative reading* and *storytelling*, are performance oriented and cultivate creativity in students. Courses in *semantics* cover a variety of matters, including learning to understand the language and looking at the relation of language symbols to emotions and attitudes. A course in *phonology* or *phonetics* includes scientific studies of English sounds, rhythm, intonation, and dialects. Finally, still other courses, such as *voice and diction* and *speech improvement*, are concerned with the fundamentals of oral delivery and teach you how to overcome various types of speech problems. The course you are about to start falls into the last category. You are going to learn in a practical manner how to skillfully and effectively control the mechanics of oral delivery in American English.

The fundamentals of oral delivery cover many related aspects of the act of oral communication, for example: (1) the articulation or pronunciation of the sounds of American English, (2) the use of stress to form the fundamental rhythm of American English, (3) the use of melody or intonation to form the fundamental melodic qualities of American English, (4) the amount of projection or volume the speaker uses in talking, (5) the degree of variety or expressiveness the speaker uses in talking, and (6) the degree of clarity or intelligibility the speaker uses in talking. The speaker with superior delivery is the one who skillfully integrates all these features of oral communication while transmitting his message. Obviously, the most effective overall communicator is the individual who combines a logical, well-thought-out message with highly skilled delivery.

The materials in this textbook emphasize the effective use of the articulatory, rhythmic, and melodic features of oral delivery. The book—and your course in speech improvement—are designed to offer you practical help in overcoming your basic problems in these areas. In an attempt to meet all your needs, I have provided practice materials for all the vowels, diphthongs, and consonants of American English—in addition to practice materials for English stress and melody.

It is helpful to remember that effective oral delivery is something that you will be able to use the rest of your life. A course in speech improvement is not like a course in history, psychology, or philosophy where you learn (1) a mass of information—much of which you forget when the course is over because you have no immediate need for it, and (2) a few general principles that stand you in good stead but that can serve only as general guidelines for daily living. Speech, however, is constant. We all talk every day of our lives, and effective oral delivery becomes a valuable asset that will help you in a variety of daily person-to-person contacts in any business or social situation.

B.   The Typical User of This Book

I have written this book for two kinds of students: (1) those of you who are native speakers of American English and who desire more effective use of your first language, and (2) those of you who are nonnative speakers of American English who want to improve your ability to speak American English as a second language. As a native speaker of American English, your problems in pronunciation, rhythm, and intonation evolve normally from faulty learning habits. As a nonnative speaker of American English, your problems in pronunciation, rhythm, and intonation typically stem from faulty learning habits that are related to specific differences between your first language and American English.

C.   Dialects

Before proceeding to the pronunciation guide in the next section, a few points should be noted about dialects and variations in pronunciation. Any form of speech that has distinctive characteristics may be called a *dialect*. These characteristics normally include similarities in such things as pronunciation, rhythm, intonation, vocabulary, and idiomatic usage. When people who live in a given geographical area speak essentially alike, they are said to speak the same dialect. If the dialect reflects the socially acceptable, habitual speech patterns of most individuals in that region, the dialect is considered to be a standard dialect. The United States has three such dialects: (1) *Eastern American* speech—this is generally considered to include eastern New England along with New York City and its surrounding areas, (2) *Southern American* speech—this is generally considered to include the Southern states from the Atlantic Ocean westward to Texas, and (3) *General American* speech—this is basically considered to include the remainder of the United States. Each of these dialects represents speech that is considered acceptable within its own area, and all three dialects are equally acceptable throughout the United States. Each dialect differs significantly from the others in certain aspects of spoken English.[1] For example, in General American speech the consonant /r/ as in fear is pronounced as /r/, but in Eastern and Southern American speech the pronunciation becomes /ə/ as in about. Some Southern American speech tends to employ much slower rhythm than either of the other two standard dialects. It should be noted, however, that there are many similarities among all three standard dialects. The standard pronunciations of many sounds are uniform throughout the United States (e.g., /s/ as in sap, /θ/ as in thought, and /f/ as in fun).

Dialects that reflect less socially acceptable speech patterns in a region are considered to be substandard. However, if somebody tells you that you speak substandard English, this does not mean that as a native speaker everything you say is incorrect. It simply indicates that certain of your specific speech characteristics are not acceptable, that is, that you mispronounce one or more English sounds. Of course, if you are a nonnative speaker who is learning English as a foreign language, your oral English will probably contain many more examples of unacceptable speech traits. In either instance, these substandardisms are the basic speech problems that this book and your course will help you to eliminate.

D. WHY BE CONCERNED ABOUT SUBSTANDARD SPEECH?

You might well ask, "What is so terrible if I employ some substandard English?" Consider momentarily a non-speech area. I am sure that all of you would agree that others tend to form opinions about us by observing the manner in which we dress. Smartly groomed, properly attired individuals are more likely to succeed vocationally and socially than persons who are poorly groomed

[1] It should be noted that boundary lines between standard dialects are quite fluid, and two dialects may frequently mix in fringe or border areas. It is interesting to note also that research indicates that ultimately the concept of three standard dialects will be replaced by the concept of smaller, standard regional speech areas. See A. J. Bronstein, *The Pronunciation of American English* (New York: Appleton-Century-Crofts, 1960), pp. 43–47.

and dressed. Our society expects us to conform to certain standards of dress and cleanliness. Slovenliness is not considered an attribute in our society. Although you may not realize it, people also tend to judge us by the manner in which we speak. Basically we are expected to speak acceptably. Unacceptable speech attracts negative attention to itself for a variety of reasons: (1) your incorrect speech is unfavorably conspicuous, (2) it interferes with effective oral communication—sometimes to the point of unintelligibility, (3) it is inappropriate to your present social or vocational situations. Your speech becomes a handicap. Just as the sloppily dressed applicant reduces his chances of being accepted at a job interview, so does the ineffective speaker reduce his chances of getting the desired position.

E. THE PRONUNCIATION GUIDE

I have largely used pronunciations associated with General American speech in planning this book, because this regional standard pronunciation appears to best describe the speech of the majority of Americans. Even in areas where General American is not spoken typically, there is frequent exposure to General American speech through the media of radio, television, and cinema. Thus General American speech is the most logical pronunciation guide to follow in a book of this type.

On the other hand, although I have employed General American as a pronunciation guide, I have indicated preferred Eastern and Southern American pronunciations in several chapters, e.g., the pronunciation of the consonant /r/ and the vowel /ɝ/ as in bird. Generally speaking, whenever there is a difference between the suggested pronunciation in this book and the preferred pronunciation of the majority of speakers in your community, always utilize your local pronunciation. The preceding statement also applies if you are a nonnative speaker of English. In actual practice, you are learning the dialect of American English that is spoken by your instructor, and presumably by the majority of Americans in the area around you. There is nothing wrong with your adapting the materials in this book to standard Eastern or Southern American if you happen to be attending school in one of these areas.

F. AN OVERVIEW OF TEACHING METHODS

Your course in speech improvement is designed to be a combination of individual and group instruction, and the textbook is designed to facilitate this approach. At the beginning of the course, your instructor will test your ability to use English pronunciation, rhythm, and intonation. The testing procedures used in this diagnostic step are discussed in detail in Chapter 3. The results of the test will determine the nature and extent of your individual speech improvement program. When your instructor has evaluated your test results, he will take time to discuss each of your problems with you. He will assign you the background materials in Chapters 2, 3 and 4 for classroom discussion, after which he will assign and hold you responsible *only* for those practice chapters that will help you overcome your specific speech problems. You will be allowed to work through the assigned practice units at your own rate of speed, but keep in mind that you want to complete your study of your speech problems by the end of the course. Your instructor will frequently evaluate your progress through the book.

The practice chapters in the book are normally divided into two major sections: (1) a section on listening, and (2) a section on practicing. The listening sections contain explanatory materials about the particular feature of speech improvement being covered in that chapter, and the nature of the more likely problems associated with that speech feature. There is also a series of aural recognition tests to help you learn to identify the problem. The practice section has a series of practice exercises that commence with simplified materials and progress to more difficult drills. The exercises generally require you to read various materials, such as word lists, phrases, sentences, and conversational patterns. The vocabulary in these drills has been simplified for you, and most of the words come from the following basic reading lists of American English words: (1) the first 1,000 words in the Thorndike list,[2] (2) the Gates list,[3] and (3) selected words from the *New Basic Readers* through Book 3/2.[4] In some instances, the vocabulary tends to be somewhat more difficult, primarily because the vocabulary for that particular sound is limited, and there are not enough basic words available. Whenever you are in doubt about either the pronunciation or the meaning of any word, always look the item up in a current standard American dictionary. From time to time as the course progresses, your instructor will plan periods of classroom practice in conversation. These assignments will allow you to carry your newly acquired speech skills from the preliminary reading drills into typical speaking situations.

During your class periods you will practice in several different ways: (1) with your instructor, (2) working alone with taped materials, (3) working with a partner, and (4) working as part of a group.

G. SUMMARY

Read over the following chapters in this part, because they will aid you in understanding and carrying out your particular speech improvement program. You will then be prepared to begin work in your first practice chapter.

[2]Reprinted by permission of the publisher from E. L. Thorndike and I. Lorge, *The Teacher's Word Book of 30,000 Words* (New York: Teachers College Press,© 1944 by Teachers College, Columbia University).

[3]Reprinted by permission of the publisher from A. I. Gates, *A Reading Vocabulary for the Primary Grades* (New York: Teachers College Press, © 1944 by Teachers College, Columbia University).

[4]*The New Basic Reading Series* (Glenview, Ill.: Scott, Foresman and Company, 1956).

chapter two

Learning About
Speech Improvement

2–1. THE IMPROVEMENT PROCESS

A. SKILLS AND HABITS

A **skill** may be defined as an activity that is carried out with great expertness; that is, you learn through much practice to skillfully coordinate a set of highly developed responses to certain stimuli in order to carry out a special skilled activity. Because skills are learned, it normally takes a long period of time to develop a fine degree of skill.

A **habit** may be defined as a way of performing an activity so frequently that it becomes automatic—to the point that it is often performed unconsciously. Thus an individual learns to develop a skill by expertly performing an activity in a specific manner—over and over again—until the activity becomes habitual and fully automatic. The degree of expertness developed depends upon the individual's ability to learn to consistently carry out the activity at a very high level of exactness. The extremely skilled individual rarely varies from a high level of skill that approaches perfection.

Examples of learned skilled activities are easy to find. Such varied activities as typing, playing the piano, playing pocket billiards, and playing golf all rely on the employment of skilled habitual responses. An expert pocket billiard player has learned to determine exactly where and how hard to strike his cue ball in order to make the cue ball travel across the table, hit the target ball, knock the target into the desired pocket, and then come to rest in perfect position for the next shot. The professional golf player has learned exactly how to hold a particular club for a given kind of shot. He knows exactly where he is going to strike the golf ball, and he knows exactly how to coordinate his bodily movements into a smooth rhythmical swing.

Speech is also considered to be a skilled activity. All of you who are reading this page are skilled, because you are able to speak a language—that is, you are able to integrate the skilled automatic responses required for talking. Speech is also a learned skill. You did not learn to talk the moment you were born. It took a number of years—perhaps as many as seven or eight if English is your first language—before you learned to pronounce all the sounds of English correctly and to use acceptable patterns of English stress and intonation. Thus there are very close similarities between learning to speak and such activities as typing, playing musical instruments, and participating in athletics.

B. THE DIFFICULTIES OF IMPROVEMENT

I frequently ask my students how much difficulty they think they will have in learning to overcome their speech problems, and also how much time they think they will need to complete their learning. My students frequently indicate that they believe that improvement will not be too difficult and that they will not need to practice very long. (What would your answers be if your instructor were to ask you these questions in class?) My students' answers are incorrect. They tend to underestimate the amount of time required for change, because the nature of their individual problems appears quite simple on the surface. Perhaps another look at related skilled activities will provide you with a better understanding of the degree of difficulty and the amount of time required for improvement. Keep in mind that we are talking about skilled activities that depend upon expert automatic responses for successful completion.

Let us begin by asking a question. How long does it take the billiard player to become an expert, or the golf player to be able to play a course in par (that is, to get around the golf course using the minimum number of required shots)? If you think about it for a few minutes, you will realize that a lot of time and effort is involved in either case. Proficiency in pocket billiards or golf does not come immediately, because learning to make new skilled responses is an extremely difficult procedure. The individual who is striving for improvement requires frequent and intensive practice sessions over a protracted period of time before he eliminates his less effectual habits and learns to substitute the improved set of responses that constitutes his goal. His rate of improvement depends upon several factors. How long has he been using his less effective responses? The longer he has performed the activity in a certain manner, the harder it will be for him to change his habits. Two related variables are (1) how long will it take the individual to learn to recognize his less effective responses? and (2) how long will it take him to learn to replace his inefficient responses with more skilled ones? Keep in mind that the remedial process is made more complicated by the fact that the old manner of activity is so automatic that it is probably performed unconsciously. In addition, the new skilled responses must also become automatic and unconscious. The golfer cannot stop and try to remember individual body movements in the middle of his swing during a game. The results of this approach can only be disaster!

Learning to overcome a basic speech problem, or problems, is just as difficult and time consuming as learning to correct a habitually inadequate golf swing, or learning to use the proper amount of English when hitting the cue ball in billiards. For example, if you are an eighteen-year-old native speaker of English, you have probably been pronouncing sounds in a certain manner for about ten years. The incorrect pronunciation is strongly habitual and most likely unconscious. You may find it very difficult to learn to recognize this firmly rooted mispronunciation, and then to learn to use the correct pronunciation. Your ultimate goal is not just learning to pronounce a different sound in a few words, but, like the golfer, you are interested in how well you perform during the "game." In this instance the "game" is consistently accurate usage of the new sound in all phases of speaking.

If you are a nonnative speaker of English, you will encounter all the previously described problems. However, the problems will tend to be more difficult to solve. Your problems in English pronunciation, rhythm, and melody equal the difference between English and your native language. Because these differences are frequently radical ones, learning to speak oral English as a second language is much more difficult than learning to improve your ability to speak your own language. For instance, certain English sounds do not appear in your language; they simply do not exist for you. Other English sounds appear in your language, but they appear in somewhat different form. Learning to recognize the difference between English and non-English sounds is extremely difficult. Learning to replace non-English pronunciations with English pronunciations in conversational situations is also extremely difficult.

It should be clear by now that overcoming speech problems is not a simple process, and that you must be willing to exert a lot of effort if you are going to learn to utilize your oral delivery more effectively. Let us now consider how you will spend your time practicing to overcome your speech problems outside class.

C.   THE AMOUNT AND TYPE OF PRACTICE TIME

Having noted that proficiency in any skilled activity requires much time and practice before the new skilled responses become automatic and unconscious, the next question to consider is the amount of time you should devote to oral practice each week outside class. My students frequently ask me whether they should concentrate their practice into a few lengthy practice sessions, or whether they should split up their practice into a larger number of shorter periods. Which approach do you think is most effective? Educators who have studied methods of developing skills agree that the best way to improve a skilled activity is to practice frequently. Let us say that you have decided that you can spend 100 minutes a week practicing to overcome your speech problems. You have a choice of two 50-minute practice sessions on Tuesday and Friday, or five 20-minute practice sessions Monday through Friday. The most effective program is the one that requires you to practice for five 20-minute periods per week. The reason is simple. The more frequently you practice, the less likely you are to forget what you learned during the previous practice period. You may well learn more in 50 minutes on Tuesday than in 20 minutes, but by the time Friday rolls around and you practice again, you will probably have forgotten much of what you learned on Tuesday. On the other hand, the learning achieved on Monday is quite likely to be relatively fresh in your mind on Tuesday, and Tuesday's learning will be fresh on Wednesday, and so it will go through the week.

There is no prescription for the exact number of days and the amount of time you should practice, except that your practice should be frequent. Some problems are more difficult to overcome than others, and some students learn more rapidly than others. As a general rule you should spend more time if you are a nonnative speaker than if you are a native speaker. When your instructor discusses your speech problems with you, he will help you plan a practice program that seems most effective for you.

The next question to consider is where you should carry out your practice. The essential requirement is your ability to concentrate on the problem at hand, which means you want to work some place that is reasonably quiet and free from distractions. Much of your early practice will involve training yourself to evaluate or monitor your speech. Noise from radios, television sets, lawn mowers, and people talking is distracting. The noise also masks or blots out the sound of your voice, making it impossible to accurately evaluate your speech. So pick a quiet room at home, or an empty classroom at school, a quiet spot outside on your campus, or even the back seat of your car if you drive to school.

Whenever possible, practice with somebody else. There are definite advantages to working with another person (e.g., a classmate, a friend, or somebody at home). Quite often you will find that a second person can evaluate your speech more accurately than you can, especially when you are beginning your improvement program. More will be said about this aspect of oral practice later in the chapter.

D. YOUR MOTIVATION FOR IMPROVEMENT

I think that I can say—without reservation—that your motivation is the single most important factor in determining how much improvement you will make. This is true regardless of whether you are a native speaker improving your first language or a nonnative speaker improving your ability to speak English as a second language. You must have a sincere desire to learn; that is, you must be able to see that skilled oral delivery will lead you to successful and satisfying school, business, and social relationships. Unless you can see your improvement program in this light, you are not likely to learn very much during your course, and you will most likely remember little or nothing a few months after your course is completed. If you are a nonnative speaker of English, motivation takes on added meaning. You must be willing to use English frequently, because you cannot learn to speak English by practicing your own language. Nonnative speakers who come to the United States to learn English as a foreign language frequently spend much of their time talking to friends who come from their own country. On campus they congregate in small ethnic groups and speak their own languages. Off campus they spend most of their time speaking their own languages with family and friends. Since you are already highly skilled in your first language, there is no need to constantly continue practicing it. Instead, it is imperative that you spend your time practicing English conversation and that you listen to English on television, on the radio, at the movies, and so on. The nonnative speaker who learns the most English when he comes to the United States is the one who is alone—he does not know anybody from his country and he cannot spend his time using his native language. He is forced to speak English, or end up never talking to anybody.

2–2. PHASE I OF THE IMPROVEMENT PROCESS: LEARNING TO LISTEN

We are now ready to examine some of the details of the actual speech improvement learning process. Carefully study the following fundamental concepts about aural listening, presented first through our continuing comparison between the athlete and the speech student.

A. THE NECESSITY OF ERROR RECOGNITION FOR THE ATHLETE

The athlete who wishes to improve his game by learning to employ new skilled responses must be able to relate the comments of his coach to his particular difficulties. Before he can alter his performance—that is, before he can eliminate his less effective habits and substitute a more skilled set of responses—he must learn to recognize the difference between his habitually faulty technique and the improved technique suggested by his coach. When the golf pro tells a pupil that he needs less body sway in his swing or that he is raising his head while swinging the golf club at the ball, the pupil must learn to observe carefully the differences between the acceptable and the unacceptable techniques. To achieve this learning, the pupil makes use of a wide range of sensory channels for purposes of evaluating or monitoring his practice. These senses include the following: (1) the *sense of touch* or the related sensation of pressure—for example, the pupil utilizes these senses in learning how to hold his golf club with the proper amount of pressure in the correct part of his hands; (2) the *sense of kinesthesis* which involves an awareness or feeling of muscle tension and bodily movement—for example, the pupil makes use of this sense to become conscious of the movement associated with raising his head as he swings at the ball, or he employs kinesthesia to learn about the proper amount of bodily tension required for a correct swing; (3) the *sense of sight*—for example, the pupil uses vision to observe demonstrations of correct procedures by the pro; and (4) the *sense of hearing*—for example, the pupil must be able to hear what the pro is telling him. Unless the golf player employs these various sensory aids to detect the basic differences between the correct and incorrect swings while he is practicing, he is quite likely to retain his habitually ineffective swing. At best, he might occasionally improve his swing by accident. It is quite likely that the pupil who fails to make the necessary distinctions between swings may practice for hours without realizing that he is practicing improperly. Thus real progress comes only when the player swings, recognizes exactly what went wrong, and alters his swing with the next attempt. Continued recognition of this type results eventually in the eradication of the improper swing.

B.   EAR TRAINING

The circumstances in speech improvement are identical. Like the athlete, the first thing you must do is to recognize the difference between your particular ineffective way of speaking and a more skilled manner of delivery. You must also learn to utilize the same sensory channels in order to help bring about the desired learning. There will be no real progress unless you learn to identify the exact nature of your problem. Trying to improve without this knowledge would be like attempting to thread a needle while standing in a totally darkened room.

The most important sense channel for you during the beginning portion of your speech improvement program is hearing. The term given to the general recognition procedure is *ear training* in order to emphasize that the learning techniques are essentially *aural*. Two terms associated with ear training throughout the textbook are *target* and *replacement*. The term "target" is used to refer to the particular feature of speech improvement that is being studied. The term "replacement" is used to identify the particular problem you have in using the target. Since most of the practice chapters are devoted to the pronunciation of English sounds, a "target" most frequently refers to the sound that you are learning to pronounce. The "replacement" most frequently describes your particular way of mispronouncing the target. Thus your target might be the consonant /θ/ as in **th**ought, while your replacement might be the consonant /t/ as in **t**ie or the /f/ as in **f**un. This means that your pronunciation of the word **thought** might become either **taught** or **fought**, depending upon which replacement you are habitually using. In the chapters on stress and intonation, the terms "target" and "replacement" refer to correct and incorrect ways of using stress and melody. Most of the examples used to illustrate the ideas presented in the following sections of this chapter are based on prounciation. Keep in mind, however, that all the ideas discussed may be adapted to other features of delivery.

Your primary objective in ear training is to learn through intensive listening to recognize the difference between the aural image of your target and the aural image of your replacement. This difference between two auditory images is referred to in the book as *discrimination*. You must learn to establish the target and the replacement sounds as concrete images in your mind while you are listening to the speech of others in a variety of different spoken exercises. The untrained listener is rarely aware of individual sounds while listening to a stream of conversation. For him, language is a mixture of unidentified sounds which flow rapidly out of a speaker's mouth. You, as a student of speech improvement, cannot be an untrained listener! It is imperative for you to be able to break down the mass of sounds you hear coming from a speaker's mouth; it is imperative for you to be able to break up familiar words into sound particles so that you can focus your attention on the particular sounds you are learning about. You must become so skilled at aural discrimination that you can tell immediately the difference between your target and your replacement, whether the key sound appears in a simple word or is buried in the middle of a complex sentence. *Remember: Accurate listening skills lead to accurate pronunciation skills.*

2–3. APPLYING EAR TRAINING TO THE PRACTICE MATERIALS

Let us now relate the basic ideas on aural listening to some practice materials for ear training. To simplify my explanations about applying the previously developed basic concepts to the practice chapters, I am going to use Chapter 5 to illustrate the practice procedures and exercises. Chapter 5 deals with the pronunciation of the target /θ/, and for demonstration purposes let us assume that /θ/ is one of your pronunciation targets. All the practice chapters for pronunciation follow essentially the same format, differing only in certain particular types of practice drills. Thus each chapter contains three basic sections: (1) ear training, (2) beginning oral drill, and (3) conversation. The chapters on stress and intonation also follow basically the same outline. You will find it easier to understand the organization of the demonstration practice chapter if you first read the explanatory comments in this unit, and then immediately relate these comments to the corresponding material in Chapter 5.

A. A FEW REMINDERS ABOUT EAR TRAINING PRACTICE

The first major section in the practice chapter deals with ear training. The first phase of ear training involves the recognition of your target, and in Chapter 5, Section 5–1 there are two test drills for recognizing /θ/. Before looking at the exercises, however, it is necessary to say a few additional things about ear training practice.

Ear training exercises are primarily planned for use in class, although there are suggestions for review outside class. Whenever you begin a chapter, your instructor will always assign the ear training materials first. A typical practice chapter starts with test exercises that help you learn to recognize your target in words and sentences, and ends with test drills that help you learn to discriminate between your target and your replacement. Your instructor will either do the drills with you or ask you to listen to them on tape. If the drills are taped, instructions for each taped exercise will precede the drill on tape. If your instructor feels that you require extra ear training help, he will ask you to repeat some of the exercises in class either with him or with a partner. Remember that the most important sense channel in ear training is hearing and that ear training drills are designed for listening. Although listening tests are found in the practice chapters or in Appendix 1, *never* look at them while you are carrying out the exercise. Furthermore, *never* look at your instructor's mouth, because sometimes you may get a visual clue as to what sound he is pronouncing. Simply concentrate solely and intently on your instructor's speech—shut your eyes if it helps your concentration. If you have difficulty, follow the suggestions given for reviewing the ear training drills outside of class, using somebody at school or at home to assist you. Make certain that your helper knows the exact difference between your target and your replacement before he helps you with discrimination drills. Your ear training practice will be carried out most effectively if you observe carefully all the preceding suggestions.

B.   Ear Training Exercises for the /θ/ Target

Now let us look at the two test exercises in Chap. 5, 5–1. The objective in both tests is to learn to recognize the aural image of the /θ/ target. The exercise in Chap. 5, 5–1B requires you to listen to a list of words containing /θ/ and to decide whether you heard the target at the beginning, in the middle, or at the end of the word. The exercise in Chap. 5, 5–1C requires you to listen to some sentences and to determine which words in each sentence contain /θ/. In both drills you are asked to write down your answer, and then to check them when the answers are read to you at the end of the test. If you have difficulty recognizing and separating the aural image of /θ/ from the other sounds in the tests, your instructor will help you by pronouncing just the target. He will say /θ/ alone until you become thoroughly familiar with it. Then he will let you attempt the tests again.

C.   Discrimination Exercises Between /θ/ and the Various Replacements

When you have satisfactorily learned to recognize the target, you are ready to move into the second phase of your ear training—learning to discriminate between the aural image of /θ/ and the aural image of your particular replacement. This material is found in Chap. 5, 5–2.

Chap. 5, 5–2A is a list of the more probable replacements for the /θ/ target. Three replacements are shown for /θ/: /t/, /s/, and /f/. Your instructor will tell you which replacement you are employing in your speech. If you are not using one of the listed replacements, your instructor will describe for you the specific nature of your particular replacement.

Three test exercises are provided to help you learn to discriminate between /θ/ and each of the common replacements. Your instructor will only carry out with you that portion of the exercise that compares /θ/ with your particular replacement. If, for example, your replacement is /t/, there is no need to learn to discriminate between /s/ and /θ/ or /f/ and /θ/, since you do not substitute /s/ or /f/ for the target. Learning to discriminate between /θ/ and these other consonants is simply a waste of your time. In the event that you are not using one of the listed replacements, your instructor will provide you with appropriate discrimination tests.

The exercise in Chap. 5, 5–2B requires you to recognize the difference between nearly identical pairs of words. You will observe that in all three parts of the exercise, the words in Column 1 contain /θ/, while the words in Column 2 contain a replacement. Pairs that differ in only one sound—such as **thank-tank**, **thumb-sum**, and **thought-fought**—are called *minimal pairs*. Minimal pairs are frequently very difficult to separate, and this type of drill is extremely effective in teaching you how to discriminate between a target and your replacement. Your instructor will select at random some of the words containing /θ/ and some of the words containing your replacement. He will read them to you slowly in the beginning, and then with increasing speed. Listen carefully to determine which sound he is pronouncing. Sometimes he may repeat the same word two or three times in a row. Do not be fooled! Record exactly what you think he said. The general instructions for the drill are similar to the earlier ear training exercises, and your instructor will go over them with you in class. In the event that you have difficulty learning to discriminate between /θ/ and your target, this is a particularly valuable drill to ask somebody to help you with outside class. Read carefully the instructions in Chap. 5, 5–2B for extra practice.

The exercise in Chap. 5, 5–2C is similar to the one in Chap. 5, 5–2B, except that the paired words are placed in identical sentences. This discrimination test will be harder than the preceding drill. Your instructor will go over the directions with you in class.

The exercise in Chap. 5, 5–2D is the final drill in the discrimination section. The objective in this drill is to permit you to listen to a list of familiar /θ/ words, and see if you can discriminate between the correct pronunciation with /θ/ and the incorrect pronunciation with your habitual replacement. Your instructor will select some words from the various practice lists within the chapter and vary his pronunciation while reading the words to you. If your replacement is /t/, he might pronounce the first two words in the exercise in Section 5–4B with /θ/

e.g., "thumb, thigh," and then say the third word with your replacement e.g., "timble." The general instructions are similar to the earlier drills, and your instructor will go over them with you in class. This is also an excellent exercise for additional discrimination practice outside class. Explain the directions to your helper, and ask him to read you some of the words from the exercises in Chapter 5, Sections 5–4B, D and E.

2–4. PHASE II OF THE IMPROVEMENT PROCESS: BEGINNING ORAL DRILL

Carefully study the following fundamental concepts about beginning oral practice. Keep in mind the earlier comments about the amount and type of practice time. Although you are starting the practice phase of your improvement program, the employment of skilled listening habits continues to be of primary importance. Up to now you have concentrated on listening for the target and the replacement in the speech of another person, but from this point on you must begin listening to your own speech. There is a definite need for constant self-evaluation of your speech throughout all your practice drills. You must make certain that you are using your target and not your replacement. In the beginning, you may find self-evaluation more difficult than evaluating the speech of a second person. It is at this point that you can begin making effective use of the other sense channels to help you sharpen your aural discrimination capabilities.

For example, the potential target /θ/ requires contact between the tongue tip and the backs of the upper front teeth. The /f/ replacement requires contact between the biting edges of the upper front teeth and the lower lip, while the /t/ replacement requires contact between the tongue tip and the gum area just above the upper front teeth. There are definite differences in the sensation of touch between /f/ and /θ/ and /t/ and /θ/, and your awareness of these differences as you pronounce the target can aid you considerably in evaluating your pronunciation of /θ/. All these sounds are also highly visual, and you can employ your sense of sight to further check your pronunciation of /θ/ by observing your practice before a mirror. The sense of kinesthesis can help you check the pronunciation of other potential targets. The vowel /i/ as in bead requires strong tensing of the tongue muscles, and you can attempt to feel this tension while practicing the pronunciation of /i/. If you find it difficult to become aware of the muscular tension, you can employ pressure and touch by placing your thumb under the fleshy part of your chin and trying to feel the tongue muscles pressing against your finger. Thus, whenever feasible, try to employ as many senses as you can. Making use of a multisensory approach will make it easier for you to learn to listen accurately to your own speech. It will help to further fix your target and replacement in your mind as concrete images, and it will focus your attention on the specific way you are pronouncing your target in the beginning stages of your pronunciation practice.

One additional point needs to be mentioned. When practicing a target, it is not enough just to recognize that you have used your replacement. *Do not stop there*. You must reinforce your learning by attempting to correct yourself immediately after you have recognized the replacement. This step will be elaborated on during our discussion of the various types of oral practice procedures and exercises later in this chapter.

A.   THE ROLE OF IMITATION AND PLACEMENT IN ORAL PRACTICE

There are two basic practice tools which may be used to help you overcome your speech problems—*imitation* and *placement*. Imitation is the method by which we have all learned to speak our native languages, and imitation is the best method of teaching you speech improvement. This is true whether you are a native speaker or a nonnative speaker of English. Whenever your instructor practices with you or asks you to listen to him on tape, listen carefully to his pronunciation and imitate him as accurately as possible. Whenever feasible, listen to other speakers around you who are skilled in the use of your target and imitate their speech. However, sometimes imitation is not sufficient. You may find that you simply cannot pronounce a target correctly, no matter how many times your instructor demonstrates the pronunciation for you. This is particularly true if you are a nonnative speaker of English who is trying to learn the pronunciation of an English sound that does not appear in your language. When imitation fails, your instructor will turn to placement. Placement means that your instructor will try to teach you the pronunciation of the target through explanation and demonstration. The multisensory approach described above becomes absolutely vital to the student who is having difficulty and requires placement assistance in order to start pronouncing his target correctly. If you are one of these individuals, your instructor will explain in detail just how the sound is formed, and he will demonstrate the pronunciation of the target many times while simultaneously calling your attention to the appropriate sensory channels. Let us look again at /θ/ as a target. Your instructor will talk to you about the contact between the tongue tip and the backs of the upper front teeth as mentioned earlier. He may also mention an alternate placement and suggest that you try placing your tongue tip between your upper and lower front teeth. He will teach you that the contact between the tongue and the teeth is very light or loose, and that this loose contact is essential to the pronunciation of /θ/, because a certain amount of breath must be blown smoothly out of the mouth while saying the target. He will teach you to feel this escaping breath by placing your hand close to his mouth while he pronounces /θ/. He will also show you how to see the escaping breath, by holding a piece of facial tissue in front of his mouth while he pronounces the target. The smoothly escaping air will cause the tissue to blow steadily. Your instructor may also follow the same step-by-step illustrations and show you exactly how you are pronouncing your replacement so that you know the exact mechanical differences between the two sounds. When you are ready, you will begin trying to pronounce /θ/, making use of vision, touch, and pressure—in addition to hearing—as you again begin attempting to imitate your instructor's pronunciation of /θ/.

2–5. APPLYING THE FUNDAMENTALS OF BEGINNING ORAL DRILL TO THE PRACTICE MATERIALS

Let us now relate the basic ideas on beginning oral practice to the appropriate drill materials in Chapter V. Before examining these materials, a few added observations are in order about oral practice procedures.

A. ORAL PRACTICE PROCEDURES IN THE CLASSROOM

The practice exercises in this section begin with simple materials and become progressively more difficult as you proceed through the chapter. Practice begins with the pronunciation of the isolated target—the target alone—and progresses through various oral reading drills until you complete the unit by practicing the target in structured beginning conversation. Although these practice drills are planned sequentially, do not consider the arrangement unalterable. If you find one particular exercise very difficult, skip over it and proceed to the next drill. You can attempt the more difficult exercise a second time at a later date when you have attained better control over the target.

The practice exercises may be done in several ways, and your instructor will select one or more of the following methods of doing the drills in class: (1) your instructor will do the exercises with you, (2) he will ask you to listen to them on tape, (3) he will ask you to do the drills with one or more partners in your class, and/or (4) he will ask you to practice alone. Let us examine each of these methods individually. Note the emphasis on self-evaluation and follow-up correction as needed, and keep in mind the comments in Section 2-2A about the value of employing all appropriate sense channels.

1. Practicing with Your Instructor

When your instructor practices with you during class, listen carefully to his pronunciation and imitate him as accurately as you can. Your instructor will ask you to evaluate each practice item immediately after saying it, by telling him whether you used the target or your replacement. If you use the replacement, your instructor will ask you to repeat the material until you are able to use the target correctly. If you find the exercise difficult and frequently employ your replacement, your instructor will give you whatever help is required and ask you to repeat the material by yourself. He will recheck your progress at a later time. Your instructor will periodically evaluate your progress through all your assigned chapters.

2. Practicing with Taped Materials

If you work from taped lessons, listen carefully to the recorded exercises, and imitate the speaker as accurately as you can. Check each exercise as you complete it, and re-record any particular portions where you detect your replacement. If you find yourself using replacements frequently, redo all the drills—several times if necessary—until you are consistently employing the target correctly throughout the lesson. When you have completed a taped lesson to your satisfaction, tell your instructor, and he will check the taped materials and evaluate your progress.

3. Practicing with One or More Partners

The following procedure is suggested when you are practicing with one or more partners. (This is an excellent technique, especially when you are beginning your pronunciation practice, because other listeners can frequently detect your mistakes more accurately than you can.) Your instructor will either pair you off with a partner or ask you to join a small group of other students. Let us assume that you are part of a small group. When your turn comes to practice, tell your audience what target you are learning, describe your replacement, and then read one of your exercises from the practice chapter. As you complete each part of the drill (e.g., a word, a phrase, a sentence), tell your audience whether you think you employed your replacement or the target. See if they agree with your evaluation. If they do not, assume that your self-monitoring was faulty, and try the drill again. Also repeat the exercise if you used the target correctly, but evaluated your speech improperly and told your audience that you said the replacement. Once again, successful learning depends upon your ability to make accurate judgments between target and replacement. You must become a trained listener! When you employ your replacement, *know* that you used it. When you employ your target, *know* that also. Finally, listen carefully to the other members of the group when it is their turn to speak. Practice in evaluating their targets will further improve your ability to listen accurately to your own speech.

4. Practicing Alone

You are most likely to make a mistake and not hear it when you are practicing alone, since you do not have your instructor, a recording, or a partner to help you. Listen with particular care for examples of your replacement, and carry out the following procedures in evaluating yourself. Assume that you are practicing a list of words. Say a word. Next make one quick silent decision. You either used the target, or you used the replacement. If you decide that it was the replacement, say the word over again—just once—and repeat the evaluation procedure. Keep doing this until you are satisfied that you heard your target. Follow this procedure with all the drills. The constant monitoring procedure helps you keep your attention focused on your target and your replacement, and this routine is significantly more effective than simply sitting and reading exercises to yourself one after the other.

B.   ORAL PRACTICE PROCEDURES OUTSIDE CLASS

Earlier in the chapter we discussed the amount and type of nonclassroom practice time that is required for an effective speech improvement program. Obviously the way you practice outside the classroom is equally as important as the practice techniques you employ inside the classroom. When you practice alone, or with a partner from class, follow the suggestions given in the preceding section for this kind of practice. If you ask a friend or somebody at home to check your speech progress, make sure that you explain the exact difference between your target and your replacement before starting to practice.

C.   PRONOUNCING ISOLATED /θ/

Now let us turn to the practice exercises for /θ/ and examine them. The exercise in Chap. 5, 5–4A requires you to pronounce an isolated target. If you cannot pronounce isolated /θ/ correctly, your instructor will go over the comments about producing /θ/ through placement and simultaneously demonstrate the correct articulatory techniques for you.

D.   PRONOUNCING /θ/ IN FAMILIAR WORDS

The exercise in Chap. 5, 5–4B requires you to pronounce /θ/ in a list of familiar words. You will notice that the words are placed in three lists marked as follows: *Beginning*, *Middle*, and *End*. The use of this arrangement requires a few words of explanation.

Sounds are typically said to be distributed in three possible positions within words: (1) at the beginning—or initially, (2) in the middle—or medially, and (3) at the end—or finally. Some sounds appear in all three positions (e.g., /θ/); other sounds appear in two positions; and one vowel /ʊ/ as in **pull** appears only in one position. The position of the sound within a word has practical implications for oral practice. Sometimes, for no obvious reason, you may find it much easier to pronounce a sound in one particular position. When you find this to be true, always start your oral practice with words containing the sound in the easier position. If you are a nonnative speaker of English, the relationship between ease of pronunciation and the position of the sound within the word is also important, although for more predictable reasons. Sound distribution varies from language to language. For example, let us pretend that /θ/ occurs in your language—but only at the beginning and middle of words. Let us also assume that English /θ/ and your /θ/ are similar. You will probably have little difficulty in pronouncing /θ/ when it is in the beginning and middle of English words, but you will most likely have trouble saying /θ/ at the end of English words. If your instructor finds that you have this kind of distribution problem, he will ask you to begin practicing /θ/ in the easier positions in order to focus your attention on the actual act of saying /θ/. Then he will ask you to try learning to pronounce /θ/ in the more difficult final position.

You can readily see that sound distribution within a word can be an important learning factor. Whether you are a native or a nonnative speaker, each time you begin practicing a new target in words, it will be worth your while to check and see if you can pronounce the target more easily in some particular position. This search will be of particular importance if your target is especially difficult and if you began your pronunciation practice through a combination of placement and imitation. You will frequently find that distribution is a key factor in this instance in helping you start to learn the target in familiar words.

E.   Pronouncing Word Pairs Containing /θ/ and a Replacement

The exercise in Chap. 5, 5–4C requires you to read some of the words from the paired lists in the earlier discrimination tests. Do only word pairs from the lists that contain /θ/ and your replacement. The objective in this drill is to see if you can rapidly—but correctly—move from either target to replacement or replacement to target when the key sounds are in minimal pairs. The pronunciation of the target in this drill will be more difficult than in the preceding drill because of the closeness of /θ/ and your replacement.

F.   Pronouncing Familiar Words
Containing /θ/ and a Replacement

The exercise in Chap. 5, 5–4D is similar to the preceding drill. It will be more difficult, because your replacement precedes the target in each practice word (e.g., **teeth, south,** and **fourth**).

G.   Pronouncing Familiar Words Containing
Frequent /θ/ Consonant Clusters

The exercise in Chap. 5, 5–4E requires you to pronounce /θ/ in typical /θ/ consonant clusters (e.g., **thr**ill and hea**lth**). You may wish to examine at this point the brief definition of a consonant cluster found in Chap. 4, 4–4E. Frequently the most difficult pronunciation of a consonant target in a single word occurs when it is combined with one or more other consonants in a cluster. The pronunciation of a consonant within a cluster is usually identical to the pronunciation of the consonant outside the cluster.

H.   PRONOUNCING /θ/ IN PHRASES

The exercise in Chap. 5, 5–4F gives you an opportunity to practice /θ/ when several words are joined together in a phrase. The pronunciation of a target becomes much more difficult when you progress from the single word to a sequence of words. If you are practicing alone, perhaps the best initial approach to this exercise is to go over each key /θ/ word in the phrase first, make certain that you are saying it correctly, and then put the phrase together. Self-evaluation will become more difficult, because you are listening for your target in a series of words rather than in just a single word.

I.   PROUNOUNCING /θ/ IN SENTENCES

The exercise in Chap. 5, 5–4G gives you a chance to practice /θ/ in still longer language segments. This exercise is similar to the preceding drill and should be practiced accordingly. Self-evaluation will become increasingly harder, because you have more language to keep track of.

J.   PRONOUNCING /θ/ IN BEGINNING CONVERSATION

The exercise in Chap. 5, 5–4H is the final drill in the section on beginning oral practice, and it provides you with an opportunity to practice the target in structured conversation. You will notice when you read the instructions that the exercise is carried out in two ways: (1) by yourself, and (2) with a helper. This combined approach permits you to commence the drill by acquiring practice through oral reading, as you have been doing thus far, and then allows you to move from the reading into structured conversation. The first phase of the exercise requires you to complete each of the conversational sentences or starter patterns in Chap. 5, 5–4H, with words which allow you to say the sentences so that they make sense. For example, the second practice pattern reads: "Are you **through** eating the _____ ?" The key practice word for /θ/ is printed in bold-face type. You can list various completion items such as **pie**, **fruit**, **steak**, or **rice**. All these words enable you to read the starter pattern in a sensible way. Your first objective is to read the pattern in a conversational manner, pronouncing the key /θ/ word correctly. You should be able to accomplish this with each of your different completion words. Your second—and most important objective—is to continue the conversational approach when another person is reading you only the completion items. You want to be able to look at your helper, listen for the completion word he has selected, and then talk to him by saying the entire pattern in a realistic conversational manner. Naturally, the pronunciation of the key /θ/ word must continue to be correct. If necessary, memorize the patterns before you begin your second phase of the exercise. Your ability to respond automatically during the second phase with a correctly pronounced /θ/ or to catch any replacements that you might use and correct them is a certain indication of your growing ability to use /θ/ as a habitual automatic response.

2–6. CONVERSATION PRACTICE: THE FINAL PHASE OF IMPROVEMENT

This aspect of your speech improvement program is undoubtedly the most important phase of the entire learning sequence. Learning to pronounce your target automatically while you are talking more or less spontaneously is the final and most important part of your training. This final phase of learning is absolutely essential. Unless you can learn to use your target accurately in conversation, all you can claim is that you have learned to improve your oral delivery while reading aloud. Of course, this is better than using your target inaccurately while reading aloud. However, it is neither very practical nor sufficient, since we do not go around reading aloud to others. Thus you cannot say that you have actually mastered your target until you have developed enough control over your speech problem so that you can readily recognize the difference between your target and your replacement and are capable of a reasonable degree of fluent, accurate, and automatic usage of the target throughout any conversational situation you choose to enter. The more fluent you become in the use of your target, the more proficient and effective is the oral delivery of your conversation.

A distinction must be made at this point between the native speaker and the nonnative speaker. The goal of accurate conversational fluency just discussed is intended primarily for the native speaker. If you are a nonnative speaker, you cannot expect to achieve the same level of accuracy in your second language. I frequently tell my foreign students that if I were learning to speak their languages, I could never learn to speak them as well as they do. Actually, nobody should expect you to speak English as fluently as the native speaker, and your listeners will be tolerant of mistakes in your oral English. A reasonable goal for you is speech which contains a minimum number of replacements so that your oral language is quickly and easily intelligible. Beyond this level, the closer you can come to the speech of the native speaker, the better.

2–7. PRACTICE MATERIALS FOR CONVERSATION

The third major section in Chapter 5 contains suggested activities for learning to pronounce the target automatically while you are talking more or less spontaneously. Conversation practice is normally organized in two ways: (1) a drill requiring you to use the target in actual spontaneous conversation, and (2) a variety of oral activities organized by your instructor during periods of classroom conversation.

A.   CARRYING /θ/ INTO SPONTANEOUS DAILY CONVERSATION

The exercise in Chap. 5, 5–5A explains how you can begin practicing your target during normal conversation, starting with key words containing the target and expanding to all words in your particular vocabulary containing /θ/. The objectives in this drill are basically these: (1) organize a list of key /θ/ words that you use frequently during your everyday oral language, and (2) evaluate your pronunciation of these key words as you utter them during normal conversation, taking time to correct yourself whenever you hear your replacement instead of the target. The exercise is vital, because it furnishes you with a specific method of starting to check your ability to use the target correctly during spontaneous conversation when you are simultaneously concentrating on the "how" and "what" of speaking. The "how" in this instance pertains to how successfully you are controlling your pronunciation of /θ/, while the "what" equals your message. Let us say, for example, that one of your key /θ/ words is **three**. During the course of a conversation you have occasion to say: "I am taking tree courses this summer." You recognize that during your message you used your /t/ replacement in the word **three,** so you stop your conversation and repeat the statement: "I am taking three courses this summer." If you still hear yourself saying "tree," repeat the message again. Self-evaluation and correction become exceedingly difficult under these circumstances. However, no matter how complex your message may be, you must continue keeping track of your oral delivery. It is one thing to spot a mispronounced sound when it is in a single word, or even in a lengthy sentence, but it is much more complicated to recognize and correct your replacement when it is buried in the midst of some ideas you are presenting to one or more listeners. Successful completion of this exercise is another indication that you are developing /θ/ as an automatic response.

The directions for this drill are self-explanatory. Read them over carefully. Pay particular attention to the suggestions about correcting yourself only in comfortable situations, and about organizing daily practice periods. Your instructor will indicate whether or not he wants you to use a notebook to keep track of your progress. He will also check your selected list of key words to make sure that it is suitable. If you have any questions, your instructor will go over them with you.

B.   GENERAL CLASSROOM EXERCISES IN SPEAKING

The conversation activities planned by your instructor will cover a variety of different assignments, and each activity will be discussed fully in class before you carry it out. The class exercises will generally start with speaking activities requiring a certain amount of outside preparation—for example, persuasive talking, informative talking, demonstration talking, and talks about controversial issues followed by classroom conversational discussion. Later in the course you

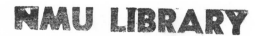

will be given assignments which require little or no preparation, such as role playing and impromptu talking. The planned speeches will be delivered extemporaneously. This means that you will give the talk using notes which you have organized in outline form, rather than writing out the entire speech and reading it to the class. Such speaking activities furnish you with another check on your ability to use the target correctly in a conversational situation when you are simultaneously concentrating on the "how" and "what" of speaking. You will find the beginning classroom talks easier, because the time allowed for planning will permit you to develop a better idea of what you want to say. Good control over your message will make self-evaluation simpler and result in better use of your target. The assignments on role playing and impromptu speaking involve spontaneous talking, and these speaking situations approximate the conversational situations that occur outside class. These talks will be much more difficult, because you will frequently be struggling to figure out what you want to say. As a result you may make more mistakes, since you will find it harder to keep track of your target. Finally, the entire process becomes more complex as the course moves along. Some of you, especially nonnative speakers of English, are going to learn many targets while you are taking your course in speech improvement. Eventually you will end up having to keep track of a number of targets during your conversation practice.

Your instructor will try to maintain a relaxed and informal atmosphere during the classroom speaking situations. You will normally give your talks in a group discussion type situation, either sitting around a large table or sitting in a circle in the middle of the classroom. Your instructor will give you your choice of sitting or standing when it is your turn to speak, depending upon whatever makes you feel most comfortable. If possible, he will allow you to volunteer to talk when you are ready, rather than follow a more arbitrary method, such as speaking in alphabetical order.

The conversation assignments will enable you to practice all the various aspects of oral delivery. Conversing as a member of a group forces you to employ adequate projection and vitality, to speak expressively, and to employ consistent visual or eye contact so that each listener in your audience feels that you are talking directly to him. You will need to consider all these features of oral communication in addition to the effective use of pronunciation, stress, and intonation. During your sessions of conversation practice, your instructor will encourage oral group evaluations of each speaker. Use these occasions to offer constructive criticisms of your peers, commenting on their strong points as well as on their weaknesses in oral delivery.

2–8. SOME GENERAL OBSERVATIONS ABOUT SPELLING

We have seen that each practice chapter contains three major sections: (1) ear training, (2) beginning oral drill, and (3) conversation. Each unit on pronunciation also contains some brief basic information about the relationship between the pronunciation of the target and English spelling. Because these materials are typically brief, you may be tempted to skip over them casually. This would be a mistake! Take time to examine the comments, because an understanding of the types of spellings involved will help you learn the target more efficiently. Some students make frequent mistakes, simply because they are deceived by the spelling.

A. THE RELATIONSHIP BETWEEN YOUR PRONUNCIATION TARGET AND ENGLISH SPELLING

You will find out very quickly in your course in speech improvement that the relationship in English between spelling symbols and pronunciation is extremely unreliable, and that you cannot use spelling as a reliable guide to correct English pronunciation. Turn to page 55. You will observe that the most frequent spelling for /θ/ is **th** as in (**th**ought). If you turn to page 64 you will note that **th** is also the most frequent spelling for /ð/ as in (**th**em). The existence of more than one pronunciation for the same spelling is just one example of the irregularities you will discover in English between spelling and pronunciation. More will be said about this in Chapter 4. Whenever you start a new pronunciation chapter, look over the section on common spelling, and make certain that you are aware of the more frequent spellings for your target.

B. GENERAL PRONUNCIATION PROBLEMS AND SPELLING

There will be numerous occasions when you have trouble pronouncing words that are not found within a practice chapter and that do not contain any of your targets. The following suggestions are helpful in these instances. Buy yourself a small notebook to keep track of these special words. If you find a word outside class that you cannot pronounce, look it up in a standard American dictionary, and write down the word in your notebook, using the phonetic symbols explained in Chapter 4. Check your pronunciation with your instructor in class and memorize the correct pronunciation. When you locate an unknown word during class, show it to your instructor. He will write the word in phonetic symbols, say it for you several times, and ask you to list the word in your notebook and memorize it.

If you are a student who is taking a vocational program, you will probably come across many technical terms that are frequently employed in your future profession. This special vocabulary—often referred to as *jargon*—will be extremely important to you, and you want to be able to pronounce it accurately, check each word in a dictionary, and then consult with your instructor about those words you still cannot say. I remember one Japanese woman—a naturalized American citizen for whom English was a second language—who brought me a list of over 100 technical terms that were needed in her particular allied health program. We sat down after class, and I taped all the words on her cassette machine; we then practiced them frequently throughout the semester.

One final word to the nonnative speaker. Purchase a standard *American* dictionary. If you cannot afford a hard-cover edition, buy one of the many pocket editions that are available. Many of my foreign students use English language dictionaries that they bought at home. The entries in each of these dictionaries make use of both English and the student's particular native language. These dictionaries tend to be inadequate when it comes to standard American pronunciation, and frequently my students are misled regarding common meanings of English words and current idiomatic usage.

chapter three

The Diagnostic Step
in Speech Improvement

The purpose of this chapter is twofold: (1) to offer the instructor some suggestions about the diagnostic step, particularly the instructor who has some knowledge of theory but not a great deal of experience in teaching speech improvement, and (2) to acquaint the student with the diagnostic procedures the instructor will probably employ in determining the nature and extent of the student's speech problems.

I. THE DIAGNOSTIC STEP:
LOCATING THE PROBLEM

I have found that the best way to gather information about the exact nature of a student's speech problems is to sample his speaking ability in two ways: (1) ask him to read a series of test sentences designed to furnish information on the pronunciation of specific sounds, and (2) ask the student to deliver a short conversational speech. This combination of activities normally provides me with an accurate profile of the student's speaking ability.

A.   THE ARTICULATION TEST SENTENCES

I have provided the instructor with a series of test sentences which are found in Appendix 2. Each sentence tests for the pronunciation of one of the sounds covered in a practice chapter. I have also included in Appendix 3, two copies of an evaluation form—one for your records and one to be filled out and returned to the student for his use. You will notice that space is provided on the evaluation form for comments on each of the tested sounds, along with room for information on stress, intonation, and clarity.

Remedial speech teachers tend to classify pronunciation problems in four specific ways, and to record their comments in some concise method of note-taking. The four common classifications are (1) substitution, (2) distortion, (3) omission, and (4) addition. I shall explain each classification and indicate a simple form of note-taking. However, there are many ways of recording your comments, and you may well decide to devise your own recording procedures. The classification system and the accompanying shorthand notations will give you a concise method of readily describing a student's pronunciation problems while he is reading the test sentences.

A substitution occurs when the student replaces the tested sound with another clearly recognizable sound; for example, he substitutes /t/ for /θ/. I would note this in the following manner in the space next to the /θ/ target on the evaluation form:

$$/θ/ - t/θ\text{\underline{\hspace{2cm}}}$$

The diagonal line between the two symbols indicates that /t/ was pronounced instead of /θ/. The substitution is the most frequent type of pronunciation problem you will come across. Substitutions involving the same target do not normally vary in the speech of a given speaker. If he uses /t/ for /θ/, you are not likely to hear /f/ for /θ/ or /s/ for /θ/. However, do not consider this statement to be inviolable. This is particularly true with nonnative speakers of English in whom language differences may produce multiple substitutions of a target.

A distortion occurs when the student replaces the tested sound with a sound that is not clearly discernable: it may resemble a combination of two sounds, or in the case of a nonnative speaker it may actually be a non-English sound that you cannot quite recognize. Let us return to the example of /t/ for /θ/. Instead of clearly replacing /θ/ with /t/, the student may use a pronunciation that resembles a mixture of /t/ and /θ/. I would note this in the following manner next to /θ/ on the evaluation sheet:

$$/θ/ - \text{dst. } /t/\text{\underline{\hspace{2cm}}}$$

Distortions involving the same target sounds tend to vary from speaker to speaker, and it pays to observe carefully the exact nature of the distortion. For instance, one student might begin his pronunciation with /θ/ and finish his articulation with something that resembles /t/. Another student may reverse the procedure and start his pronunciation with /t/ and finish his articulation with a sound resembling /θ/. It is further possible for one student to employ both distortions on different occasions.

An omission occurs when the student eliminates the tested sound; for example, he omits the final /t/ in post. I would note this problem in the following manner next to the /t/ target on the evaluation form:

$$/t/ - \text{ⓣ fnl.} \underline{\hspace{2cm}}$$

An addition occurs when the student adds an extra sound to the word. Thus in words like **good** and **would** some students add the vowel /ə/ after the final /d/. These words then become /gudə/ and /wudə/. I would note this problem in the following manner next to the /d/ target on the evaluation sheet:

$$/d/ - \text{ad. fnl.} /ə/ \underline{\hspace{1.5cm}}$$

As the student reads each test sentence, try to determine in what particular way—or ways—the tested sound is being mispronounced. Keep track of the total number of mispronounced targets in each test sentence in order to check for consistency of occurrence. Students who have a specific sound problem such as /t/ for /θ/ do not mispronounce /θ/ just once; they mispronounce the target with varying degrees of frequency in different /θ/ words. The more frequently a given student mispronounces /θ/, the more consistent his replacement is said to be. There is a fairly reliable relationship between replacement consistency on a given target and difficulty of correction. The more recurrent the replacement, the more severe the problem, and the more difficulty the student will have in altering his pronunciation. Thus error consistency becomes a useful diagnostic tool in planning a student's overall speech improvement program. I use a system of checks; for example, √ √ √ equals three errors on a particular target in a test sentence.

B.   EVALUATING STRESS AND MELODY

While the student is reading the sentences, you may also begin forming some opinions about his use of stress and melody. If so, jot them down in the appropriate section at the bottom of the evaluation form. The chapters on stress and intonation contain complete explanations of the fundamentals of English stress and melody, and the diagnostic terms employed on the evaluation form reflect the content of these chapters. One word of caution is necessary. Some speakers read aloud poorly, because they do not always recognize the vocabulary. If the student appears to be having difficulty recognizing the words in the test sentences, withhold your judgment as to his use of English rhythm and melody until he has completed the conversation portion of the test.

C. PRONUNCIATION AND SPELLING

A few words should be said here about the fundamental difference between the complex sound problems described in Chapter 2 and the more generalized pronunciation problems that arise when a student mispronounces words, simply because he does not know how to say them. We have already learned that some students mispronounce words, because they are deceived by the spelling rather than because they cannot pronounce some specific sound. Pronunciation problems that are inherently rooted in a particular sound are much more difficult to correct than a pronunciation problem that occurs because the student is confused by spelling. Normally the latter type of problem exists only in a single word, rather than in a group of words containing the same problem sound.[1] Once the student hears the correct pronunciation, he is usually able to memorize the word, regardless of how badly he has been mispronouncing it. While testing, make certain that you know which errors are related to the sound you are testing, and which errors are caused by confusions due to spelling.

D. CONVERSATION AS A MEANS OF TESTING

The second part of my diagnostic evaluation is a short conversation or talk. I like to have my students carry out this assignment for several reasons: (1) conversation is a better gauge of the student's ability to use stress and intonation; (2) pronouncing the targets in the key words in the test sentences is less difficult than pronouncing the same targets during conversation—consequently, some problems may be overlooked during the reading of the test sentences; and (3) conversation provides clues to the student's use of general intelligibility during message delivery.

I ask my students to come to class prepared to speak for two minutes on a subject that is thoroughly familiar to them, one that they can discuss with little or no preparation. I have found through past experience that too much preparation results in speech that does not reflect the student's typical oral delivery with complete accuracy. Extreme care in preparation—that is, close memorizing or writing out the talk word for word—may even obscure some of the student's problems during conversation. Since my diagnostic objective at this juncture is not how perfectly my student can perform, but rather some insight into his typical conversational speaking ability, it becomes imperative that the student's first talk reflect as closely as possible his habitual, everyday conversational use of pronunciation, stress, and melody. Otherwise, my initial diagnosis will not be totally valid.

---

[1] There are two notable exceptions to this. The /ə/ as in about and the /ɚ/ as in paper are represented by a wide variety of spellings. This causes some students to use replacements which are suggested by the varied spellings. In these instances the pronunciation problems are considered basically sound problems, because the students mispronounce /ə/ and /ɚ/ in many words containing those sounds.

Easily discussed topics that my students frequently choose include (1) their family, (2) their hobbies, (3) current and past job experiences, (4) high school experiences, and (5) comparisons of high school and college (e.g., teaching, grading, social activities, and sports). My nonnative speakers often speak about such additional things as (1) life in their country, (2) differences between their country and Hawaii (e.g., education, food, transportation, and customs), and (3) their initial impressions of life in the United States. I allow my students to write down some brief reference notes for use while they are talking, but they are cautioned against memorizing their speeches or writing them down in their entirety. I tell them that I prefer that they give their conversations without any prior oral practice at home. Sometimes a speech turns out to be too short, and I feel a need for additional samples of the student's conversation. In this instance, I ask the student questions about his topic and invite the other members of the class to question the speaker.

During the speech I check for additional examples of pronunciation problems, evaluate stress and melody, and make the appropriate notations on my evaluation sheet. I also find it valuable to check further for error consistency. Finally, I evaluate for clarity, trying to determine if any factor or factors are causing the student to be unintelligible at times. Some factors contributing to poor clarity include (1) mispronunciation of a certain sound or a combination of certain sounds, (2) the use of extremely rapid and choppy rhythm, (3) inadequate projection, (4) slurred or slushy speech due to lax articulation, and (5) use of a clenched or tight jaw which leads the speaker to converse with his lips and jaws barely parted.

Do not consider the test battery to completely reflect the student's total speech profile. Frequently you will discover additional problems as the course progresses and as you learn more about the student's speaking ability. Sometimes I am not certain about the nature of a particular problem after the testing is over, and I indicate this uncertainty with a question mark at the proper place on the evaluation sheet: ? Later in the course I recheck this area by in-depth testing.

E. IMPLEMENTING THE TEST BATTERY

I usually give my students just one day to decide what they wish to talk about—to make certain that planning is held to a minimum. For the same reason, the students are told not to practice reading the test sentences, because too much practice may lead to an invalid evaluation, and this in turn may prevent me from giving them the maximum amount of aid during the course. When the students come to class, I ask them to read the sentences first and then to give their conversations. I collect all their evaluation forms before the testing begins. I tell the students that I will return a completed copy of the form to them at a later date. At that point I will take time to explain my comments to each of them before they start their practice programs, indicating among other things which problems appear most severe, which problems should be tackled early in the improvement program, and so forth.

A relaxed and informal atmosphere makes for a better testing situation—just as it makes for a better teaching situation—and I attempt to encourage this type of atmosphere. Many students in a speech improvement class are uncomfortable, or even fearful, of having to stand up in front of the entire class and speak. For this reason, I let my students sit in a circle and give them a choice of either sitting or standing by their chairs when they are tested. Students also tend to be more relaxed if they are able to choose the time when they speak. I ask students to volunteer rather than follow some prearranged ordering. If nobody wants to volunteer to be the first speaker, they talk in alphabetical order. However, I tell them that any one of them may alter this procedure and volunteer to talk if he decides that he is ready before his scheduled turn. If you are a beginning speech improvement instructor, you might wish to consider the possibility of tape recording the test performances. The advantages of being able to check and recheck each student's responses are obvious.

II.   THE DIAGNOSTIC STEP: EVALUATING THE PROBLEM

A.   GETTING YOUR STUDENTS STARTED

Deciding how to organize the mass of information that you have recorded on the evaluation form can pose a genuine problem, especially if you are a beginning teacher of speech improvement. Most students will have more than one target to study, and the question of how to best organize the various problems into a meaningful sequence of lessons is important. Nobody can offer you a recipe, but there are certain factors you can take into consideration which will enable you to provide each student with an effective program. Some of these factors are itemized below. They are not listed in order of importance, and the applicability of any one criterion will vary from student to student. Go over your test results with these points in mind:

1.   Do any of the student's problems appear to affect his intelligibility and thus interfere with his ability to communicate verbally?

2.   Which replacements appear most frequently? Which replacements appear least frequently? We have already learned that a frequent replacement is more severe and thus more difficult to alter. Keep in mind that a frequently recurring replacement is likely to color an individual's manner of conversation and become particularly noticeable to his listener.

3.   Which problem can the student correct most easily through imitation? The more easily the student can imitate your pronunciation of a target, the less difficulty he should have learning to pronounce the target. Conversely, the less easily the student can imitate your pronunciation of the same target, the more difficulty he should have learning to pronounce it. If the student requires help with placement, the target becomes still more difficult for him to learn.

4. If the problem is one of pronunciation, it becomes desirable to consider visibility and kinesthesis. Sounds that are readily seen and felt are much easier to correct than sounds which are not readily seen and felt.

If your student is a nonnative speaker of English, there are additional complicating factors caused by the differences between the student's first language and English. A general rule of thumb may be observed: a sound that occurs in English—but not in your student's first language—is normally very difficult to learn. A sound that occurs in both languages—but with substantial differences—tends to be less difficult. A sound that occurs in both languages—but with only slight deviations—tends to be still easier to learn. Of course, you may well state: "I don't understand the differences between English and the different languages spoken by my students." Neither do I all of the time. Let me elaborate this point.

Over the years I have had repeated experiences with students from certain geographical locations. I have come to recognize and understand the nature of the more common speech problems exhibited by these students when they start learning English as a foreign language. From time to time a student from an area totally unfamiliar to me enrolls in one of my classes. As I therefore know nothing about the linguistic composition of his native language, a comparison between his language and English becomes very difficult for me. And, although during testing I invariably discover some similarities between his language and mine, ultimately it becomes necessary for me to sit down with this student and ask him about those features of his language that I do not understand. Suppose that I need some information about the pronunciation of English /p/ as in **p**ea in order to assist the student with his pronunciation of English /p/. I ask him if /p/ appears in his language. If /p/ does not occur in his language, I ask him to pronounce a few English words containing /p/ and try to analyze what he is doing when he attempts to pronounce English /p/. Once I have figured out exactly what characterizes his pronunciation, I explain to him how English /p/ is formed, detail what he is doing, and proceed from there. If it turns out that /p/ does occur in his language, I ask him to pronounce several words in his language containing /p/ while I listen carefully for differences between his /p/ and English /p/. Once I have determined the important differences between the two consonants, I explain to him the differences between his pronunciation and my pronunciation, outline what he is doing, and proceed from there. I do not expect my student to be a completely reliable informant, since he is essentially an untrained listener, but I almost always find that he is able to offer some constructive insights into his own language.

If you are short on practical teaching experience with nonnative speakers of English, I strongly urge you to sit down with your student and follow the procedures I mentioned above. In addition, tape-record your speech samples and play them back repeatedly until you have figured out to the best of your ability exactly what problems your student is having with his target. Sometimes you will also come across a native speaker with a puzzling problem, and it will be necessary to observe the same procedures.

B. SUMMARY

To summarize, always remember that students are human beings, and human beings are all different! In going over the preceding points and attempting to determine what appears most relevant (and should therefore come first or at least early in the student's program), keep in mind the added factor of personal needs. Take, for example, students *A* and *B*. Both students frequently mispronounce the same sound. The overall test profiles of both students reveal that this mispronunciation is the most striking feature of their speech problems, and it would appear that this target is a logical place to begin both practice programs. The basic data shows that mispronunciation of the sound contributes strongly to unintelligibility in the speech of both students, and that neither student is able to imitate the target with ease. The consistency of the misarticulation, plus the inability to imitate the correct pronunciation of the target easily, indicates that the sound will be difficult for both students to learn.

It turns out that student *A* has a job, and that he is having trouble being understood at the office and on the telephone. His lack of clarity is coming from his mispronunciation of the same sound target that caused a lack of intelligibility during the speech test. Student *A*'s immediate need is intelligible oral communication, and he strongly desires to start remedial practice with the harder target. Student *B*, on the other hand, wishes to begin his program with another sound— one that he mispronounces much less frequently and can imitate easily. Student *B* is afraid that the first sound is too difficult for him. Student *B* reveals himself to be an insecure individual who appears to require some quick success in speech improvement in order to build up his self-confidence and improve his motivation. Since a quick successful experience is more important to *B* than improved clarity at this point in his program, student *B* begins his speech work with the easier target of his choice.

chapter four

A Technical Look
at Speech Improvement

4–1. INTRODUCTION

The study of speech improvement may easily become complex and confusing to the student, because there are numerous technical terms which may be used to explain the process of speech production. The use of technical terminology has been held to a minimum in this book, and only those terms that are absolutely necessary are included. This chapter contains simplified explanations of the technical jargon used in those chapters devoted to the pronunciation of the sounds of American English. The technical terminology that pertains to stress and melody is included in Part IV.

4–2. THE USE OF SYMBOLS

A. THE INTERNATIONAL PHONETIC ALPHABET

You have already come across several symbols while reading through the first three chapters. This graphic symbol system is used throughout the book to illustrate the various vowels, diphthongs, and consonants presented in the practice chapters. The symbols are based on the phonetic marking system that is known as the International Phonetic Alphabet (I.P.A.). You may justifiably ask why a phonetic system was selected instead of one of the diacritic systems from a recent edition of a standard American dictionary. A phonetic system is more concise, because it lets each symbol stand for only one sound. This one-for-one representation is usually not a feature of current diacritic systems in that some dictionaries use more than one diacritical mark for the same sound, or they employ a variation of one diacritical mark for completely different sounds. Dictionaries also differ somewhat in their choices of diacritical marks.

Let us examine further the value of the one-symbol-for-one-sound feature of a phonetic system. This aspect is very important, because you already know that the relationship in English between symbols and the pronunciation of sounds is notably inconsistent. While English spelling has been slow to change during the past few centuries, our pronunciation of English has been—and still is—in a state of constant change. Consequently, oral English has undergone such numerous transformations that today there is frequently no consistent relationship between the current pronunciation of a word and its current spelling. Examples of this inconsistency are easily supplied. You are probably aware of words with dissimilar spellings but identical pronunciations; for example, the vowel /i/ as in (see) is heard as the sound of the bold face letters in all the following words: seize, seed, key, east, field, be, and policeman. Conversely, you probably know also of words with similar spellings but widely different pronunciations; for example, the pronunciation of the letters ough is quite different in through, cough, though, and rough. The g's in German and gate, the c's in cost and cider, and the s's in cubs and cups all stand for multiple sounds. You probably know of letters which, in certain words, no longer represent a sound, for example, the l in calm and balmy, the b in dumb, and the t in often. With this kind of spelling irregularity in English, you can readily see the need for a graphic system that assigns a single symbol to each sound in the language.

The I.P.A. was selected, because it appears to be the most widely known and used phonetic system for symbolizing sounds. The I.P.A. is listed for you in Figure 1. To simplify the system for you, each symbol is identified with a key word, and several diacritical equivalents are also shown. To further clarify the symbols, whenever a symbol is shown for the first time in a practies chapter, a key word is used to illustrate the symbol. Note that the key words accompanying each symbol are useful only if the key word is pronounced correctly in accordance with the accompanying symbol. The symbols will always appear within two diagonal marks, /   /.

4–3.   THE TOOLS OF PRONUNCIATION

A few brief words of explanation are necessary about the anatomical structures of the human body that are directly involved in the production of

FIGURE   1

The International Phonetic Alphabet

The following symbols comprise the I.P.A. as it is used in this textbook. The diacritical marks are taken from current standard American dictionaries.

I.P.A. Consonants		Diacritical Marks
/θ/	thought	th
/ð/	them	~~th~~, t͟h
/f/	fun	f
/v/	vine	v
/l/	lap	l
/r/	rap	r
/s/	sap	s
/z/	zip	z
/ʃ/	ship	sh
/ʒ/	measure	zh
/tʃ/	chip	ch
/dʒ/	juice	j
/p/	pie	p
/b/	buy	b
/t/	tie	t
/d/	die	d
/k/	key	k
/g/	got	g
/n/	not	n
/ŋ/	thing	ŋ, ng
/m/	me	m
/j/	yellow	y
/w/	we	w
/ʍ/	wheat	hw
/h/	how	h

I.P.A. Vowels		Diacritical Marks
/i/	bead	ē
/ɪ/	bid	i, ĭ
/e/[1]	cave	ā
/ɜ/	bed	e, ĕ
/ae/	bad	a, ă
/a/[2]	ask	ă, â

[1]This vowel may be pronounced as either a single vowel /e/ or as the diphthong /eɪ/. Because the diphthongal form is heard more commonly in American English, I have used the diphthongal glide symbol /eɪ/ in Chapter 32.

[2]This vowel is not typically heard in American English as a single vowel except in Eastern New England and New York City. It is typically heard in American English as the first sound in the diphthongs /aɪ/ and /aʊ/.

FIGURE   1   (Cont.)

I.P.A. Vowels		Diacrical Marks
/u/	pool	ü, o͞o
/ʊ/	pull	u̇, o͝o
/o/³	post	ō
/ɔ/	call	ȯ, ô
/ɑ/	father	ä, ŏ
/ʌ/	rub	ə, ŭ
/ə/	about	ə
/ɝ/	bird	ər, û
/ɜ/⁴	bird	ər, û
/ɚ/	paper	ər

I.P.A. Diphthongs⁵		Diacritical Marks
/aɪ/	ride	ī
/aʊ/	out	au̇, ou
/ɔɪ/	boy	ȯi, oi

speech. These structures are closely associated with the actual shaping and forming of speech sounds, and they are literally the tools that you employ to produce speech. If your instructor needs to teach you the pronunciation of a target through placement, his explanation and demonstration will involve the bodily structures discussed in this section.

A.   ARTICULATORS AND POINTS OF ARTICULATION

In the technical terminology of speech, the anatomical structures involved in speaking are either called *articulators* or *points of articulation*. Articulators tend to be movable and the principal ones are (1) the lips, (2) the tongue, (3) the soft palate, and (4) the lower teeth and lower jaw. Points of articulation tend to be immovable. The principal fixed reference points are (1) the upper teeth, (2) the upper gum ridge, and (3) the hard palate. Since most of the principal

---

[3] This vowel may be pronounced as either a single vowel /o/ or as the diphthong /oʊ/. Because the diphthongal form is heard more commonly in American English, I have used the diphthongal glide symbol /oʊ/ in Chapter 37. It should be noted that the single vowels /o/ and /e/ do occur regularly in some languages, and the native speakers of these languages will need to learn the diphthongal glides /eɪ/ and /oʊ/.

[4] The vowel /ɜ/ is similar to /ɝ/. /ɜ/ is standard in Eastern and Southern American speech, while /ɝ/ is standard in General American speech. A more detailed explanation of the differences is found in Chapter 42.

[5] Although other diphthongs are heard in American English, the standard ones most commonly spoken in the United States are /aɪ/, /aʊ/, and /ɔɪ/—plus the two frequently heard diphthongal forms described in footnotes 1 and 3—/eɪ/ and /oʊ/. See C. M. Wise, *Applied Phonetics* (Englewood Cliffs, N. J.: Prentice-Hall, Inc., 1957), p. 96. In this textbook these diphthongs are considered to be the five standard diphthongs of General American speech.

articulators and the points of articulation are fairly familiar to you, only a few additional comments are needed concerning them. Supplement your reading by looking over the speech mechanism shown in Figure 2 and then examining the inside of your own mouth with the aid of a mirror and a flashlight.

1. The Tongue

To facilitate certain sound descriptions, the *tongue* is commonly divided into four sections. These sections are (1) the *tip*, which is the forwardmost part of the tongue, (2) the *blade*, which is the area just behind the tip, (3) the *middle*, which is the area just behind the blade, and (4) the *back*, which is the area nearest the throat. Frequently the tip and blade are referred to as the *front* of the tongue.

2. The Upper Gum Ridge

The *upper gum ridge*—also known as the *upper tooth ridge*—marks the forward beginning of the roof of the mouth. This point of articulation forms an arch above and behind the upper front teeth, and the arched ridge extends in both directions toward the sides of the mouth. The part of the area most important for speech is located in the center of the arch, just above and behind the central front teeth. You can easily feel your upper gum ridge by sliding your tongue tip up the backs of your front teeth until you reach the gum line at the base of the teeth. The gum ridge juts toward the back of the mouth and is characterized by vein-like ridges.

3. The Hard Palate

The *hard palate* is located directly behind the upper gum ridge and joins the gum ridge. This portion of the roof of the mouth is distinguished by a hard smooth surface which rises to the roof's highest point and then slopes down to the soft palate.

4. The Soft Palate

The *soft palate* is located directly behind the hard palate and joins it. This articulator is characterized by a somewhat soft and spongy surface. The soft palate completes the downward slope started by the hard palate and ends in a small fleshy globe called the *uvula*. The soft palate is the only movable portion of the roof of the mouth. During the pronunciation of nasal consonants (e.g., /m/, /n/, and /ŋ/), the soft palate has a lowering and fronting movement, which forces the air to pass above the soft palate and out through the nasal passages. During the pronunciation of all other English sounds, the soft palate has a rising and backing movement, which tends to block the nasal passages. This blockage forces the escaping breath stream to pass under the soft palate into the mouth and then out between the lips.

FIGURE 2

The Speech Mechanism

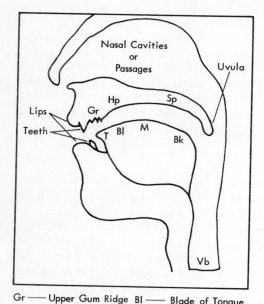

Gr —— Upper Gum Ridge Bl —— Blade of Tongue

Hp —— Hard Palate M —— Middle of Tongue

Sp —— Soft Palate Bk —— Back of Tongue

T —— Tongue Tip Vb —— Vocal Bands

5. The Vocal Bands

The *vocal bands* are located within the *larynx* or "Adam's apple." The chief function of the larynx is to produce tone through the vibratory movements of the vocal bands. Vocal band movement depends to a large extent upon a supply of energy from the lungs. This energy takes the form of escaping breath, and it is this escaping breath that is transformed into sound and ultimately into speech. There is no vocal band movement when the bands are relaxed and far apart. When you are not talking, the escaping air from your lungs moves quietly between your vocal bands, through an area called the *glottis*, and eventually passes out of your body. When the bands are tense and brought closely together, the air passing between them causes the bands to vibrate and produce tone. English sounds that include vocal band vibration as part of their pronunciations are called *voiced* sounds. This feature is also referred to as *voicing*. Included in this category are all vowels, all diphthongs, and fifteen consonants. English sounds that do not include vocal band vibration as part of their pronunciation are called *voiceless* sounds. Only ten sounds fall into this category, and they are all consonants. Although these consonants are produced without vocal tones or sound, a certain amount of noise accompanies their pronunciation. This noise is caused largely by the breath as it escapes from the mouth. The difference between a voiced and voiceless sound is easily demonstrated. Place your fingers on your larynx and pronunce the vowel /i/. You should be able to feel the vibrations produced by the movements of the vocal bands while you are pronouncing /i/ in your mouth. Keeping your fingers on your larynx, switch to a voiceless consonant such as /s/ or /f/. You will no longer feel the vibrations while you are saying these consonants. Repeat the same procedure by placing your hands over your ears. When you pronounce /i/ you should be able to hear the vocal bands vibrating while you are forming /i/ in your mouth. When you pronounce /s/ or /f/, all you will hear is the noise caused by the breath escaping from your mouth.

Whether or not a consonant is voiced or voiceless is very important, because the presence or absence of voicing is the principal means of distinguishing between nine pairs of English consonants. These pairs—sometimes referred to as *cognates*—are listed below for you. If you are a nonnative speaker of English, you particularly need to be aware of the voiced members of these pairs, because many of these voiced consonants may not appear at all in your language. Your language may only contain the voiceless members, and you may mispronounce the voiced English cognates by unvoicing; for example, you may use the voiceless /s/ in place of the voiced /z/, the voiceless /f/ in place of the voiced /v/, and so on. Sometimes distribution may create a partial voicing problem, and you may substitute a voiceless consonant for a voiced consonant in one particular position. If you have a general pronunciation problem caused by your tendency to unvoice English consonants, your instructor will discuss this list with you.

Voiced Consonants		Voiceless Consonants	
/ð/	them	/θ/	thought
/v/	vine	/f/	fun
/z/	zip	/s/	sap
/ʃ/	ship	/ʒ/	measure
/dʒ/	juice	/tʃ/	chip
/b/	buy	/p/	pie
/d/	die	/t/	tie
/g/	got	/k/	key
/w/	we	/ʍ/	wheat

4–4. GENERAL TERMINOLOGY

A few additional terms that are used in the book need to be defined at this point.

A.   VOWEL

A *vowel* is generally defined in one of two ways: (1) the outgoing breath stream escapes freely without blockage or constriction; or (2) a vowel is the most prominent sound within a syllable and acts as the center of the syllable.

B.   DIPHTHONG

A *diphthong* consists of a sequence of two vowel sounds which are pronounced together within the confines of a single syllable. The two vowels must appear within the same syllable, because two vowels that appear next to each other—but occur in adjacent syllables—are not considered to be diphthongal. Thus neither the vowels /i/ nor /ə/ as in (id*i*ot), nor the vowels /i/ and /ae/ as in (r*e*act), are considered diphthongs, because they appear in separate syllables. However, the two adjacent vowels occurring in such words as **high**, **out**, and **boy** all appear within a single syllable and constitute the English diphthongs /aɪ/, /aʊ/, and /ɔɪ/.[6] Diphthongs are characterized by a smooth, continuous gliding movement of the articulators as the speaker moves from the first vowel to the second one. The articulators normally involved include (1) the lips, (2) the tongue, and (3) the lower jaw.

C.   CONSONANT

A *consonant* is generally defined in one of two ways: (1) the outgoing breath is either blocked completely or it is constricted in some manner; or (2) a consonant generally occurs before or after a vowel at the margin of a syllable.

D.   SYLLABLE

You can see from the preceding definitions of a vowel, a diphthong, and a consonant that sounds and syllables are closely related. Every *syllable* normally contains one of the following: (1) a vowel alone: /i/; (2) a diphthong alone: /aɪ/; (3) a combination of a vowel or a diphthong and one or more consonants: /θi/, /iθs/, and /zis/. Thus words are composed of speech sounds which in turn are organized into syllables.

E.   CONSONANT CLUSTERS

Besides appearing as single sounds, certain consonants typically combine with other consonants that are directly next to them to form closely articulated sequences of sounds. Such combinations are called *consonant clusters*. The more

[6]Note the comments in footnotes 1 and 3 in this chapter regarding the diphthongs /eɪ/ and /oʊ/. The explanatory comments about the formation of diphthongs also applies to /eɪ/ and /oʊ/.

important English consonant clusters occur at the beginnings and at the ends of words. Typical clusters appearing at the beginnings of words include /st/ as in **st**ove /pr/ as in **pr**ice, and /kl/ as in **cl**ear. Characteristic clusters appearing at the ends of words include /nd/ as in le**nd**, /lts/as in be**lts**, and /ps/ as in ma**ps**. If you are a nonnative speaker of English, you may have extra difficulties in pronouncing English consonant clusters, because many English clusters may not appear in your language.

F.   FACTORS AFFECTING VOWEL PRONUNCIATION

The pronunciation of vowels is largely determined by three factors: (1) muscle tension, (2) tongue position, and (3) lip position. The sections on placement in the vowel practice chapters contain comments, where appropriate, about these factors. The suggestions are based on the following discussion and on Figure 3. You may find it helpful to review these comments and Figure 3 when you actually begin the oral practice exercises for a given vowel, especially if you require help from your instructor with vowel formation.

FIGURE 3

The Relative Location and Relative Degree of Tongue Arching for Vowels

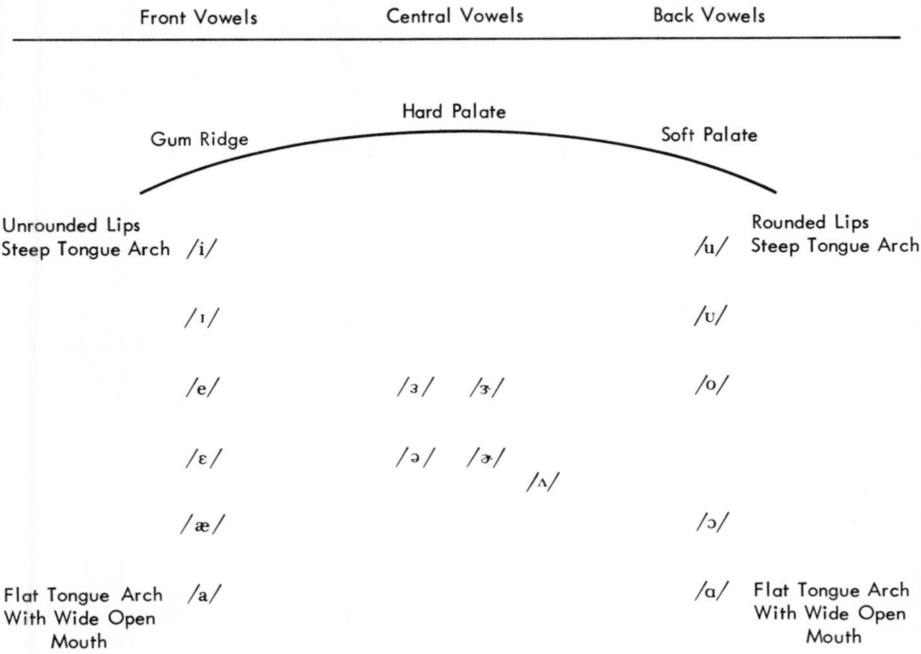

1. Muscular Tension

Vowels are pronounced with varying degrees of tenseness, and this tension is caused largely by the muscles of the tongue. Vowels such as /i/ and /u/ are pronounced with a strongly tensed tongue, while vowels such as /ɪ/ and /ʊ/ are pronounced with a much more relaxed tongue.

2. Tongue Position

Some part of the tongue is normally arched or elevated during vowel pronunciation, and the degree of arching varies from vowel to vowel. When you pronounce the following vowels, the front part of your tongue is arched—mainly the blade area: /i/, /ɪ/, /e/, /ɛ/, /ae/, and /a/. These vowels are frequently referred to as *front* vowels. The tongue arch is steep and close to the front of the hard palate for /i/. The mouth opening is very small. The arch flattens, the tongue blade drops lower in the mouth, the lower jaw drops, and the mouth opens progressively wider as you pronounce the remaining vowels in the series. By the time you reach /ae/ and /a/, there is little tongue arching, the tongue is low in the mouth, and the mouth is open wide (see Figure 3).[7]

When you pronounce the following set of vowels, the back part of your tongue is arched: /u/, /ʊ/, /o/, /ɔ/, and /ɑ/. These vowels are frequently referred to as *back* vowels. The tongue arch is steep and close to the soft palate for /u/. The mouth opening is very small. The arch flattens, the back of the tongue drops lower in the mouth, the lower jaw drops, and the mouth opens progressively more widely as you pronounce the remaining vowels in the series. By the time you reach /ɑ/, there is little tongue arching, the tongue is low in the mouth, and the mouth is open wide (see Figure 3).

When you pronounce this final set of vowels, the middle of the tongue is arched: /ɜ/, /ɝ/, /ə/, /ɚ/, and /ʌ/. These vowels are frequently referred to as *central* vowels. The degree of arching is the same for all these sounds and is in the area of the hard palate (see Figure 3).[8]

The location of the tongue arch and the amount of arching is very important, because if you change the arch sufficiently, you will end up pronouncing a different vowel. Unfortunately it is difficult to place your tongue in the correct position for many vowels, because you cannot see what you are doing, and because the difference in position between close vowels is slight (e.g., between /i/ and /ɪ/). Your instructor will demonstrate the pronunciation of the front and back vowels for you. Observe carefully how his lower jaw descends and his mouth opens wider as he moves from the higher to lower vowels in a given series.

---

[7]There is some tendency for the tongue arch to move slightly back into the mouth as the arch flattens with each successively lower vowel position. My students find that these backing differences are generally hard to see and feel, and consequently of little help in pronouncing front vowels.

[8]The fact that /ʌ/ is slightly farther back in the mouth than the other central vowels is of little remedial value.

3. Lip Position

The last major factor involves changes in the relative position of the lips. Vowels are considered as either generally *round* or generally *unround*. Front vowels are classified as unround, although there is a marked contrast between the lip positions for higher and lower front vowels. The narrow slit-like appearance of the lips for /i/ and /ɪ/ differs considerably from the more or less unround position adopted for /ae/ and /a/. Back vowels are classified as round, although there is a definite variation between the very round /u/ and the less rounded /ɔ/. However, the lowest back vowel, /ɑ/, is not considered round. It is pronounced with the lips basically in the same relatively unround lip positions of /ae/ and /a/. Central vowels are usually classified as unround.

Your instructor will demonstrate the pronunciation of the front and back vowels again. Observe carefully how the position of his lips varies from vowel to vowel in each series. The use of an incorrect lip position can easily alter vowel quality. Listen to what happens when your instructor pronounces /i/ with rounded lips and /u/ with unrounded lips. Observe how the change in lip position creates definite vowel distortion. Finally, it should be noted that lip positions of identical vowels may vary slightly from speaker to speaker.

G.   Diphthong Pronunciation

We have noted that diphthongs are characterized by gliding movements of the lips, tongue, and lower jaw. Now that we have studied vowel pronunciation, we can return to diphthongs and discuss their articulatory movements more clearly. Remember that the movements are smooth and continuous, that the articulators function simultaneously, and that the transition from the first vowel into the second vowel is heard as a gradual blending of the two sounds. The tongue movements, or glides, are illustrated schematically for you in Figure 4. Take /aʊ/ for example. The arrow from /a/ to /ʊ/ indicates the approximate path of the tongue during the pronunciation of the diphthong. When you pronounce /aʊ/, your tongue glides upward and backward starting from the low front position for /a/ and ending in the higher back position for /ʊ/. Simultaneously your lips are gradually closing from the unrounded position for /a/ to the rounded position for /ʊ/. In conjunction with your tongue and lips, your lower jaw is also gliding up as your mouth progressively closes to the /ʊ/ position. Your instructor will demonstrate the pronunciation of /aʊ/ and the other diphthongs for you. Study Figure 4, and observe your instructor's pronunciation carefully.

H.   Factors Affecting Consonant Pronunciation

The pronunciation of consonants is mainly determined by two interrelated factors: (1) the manner of articulation, and (2) the place of articulation. The

FIGURE 4
The Relative Positions and Movements of Diphthongs

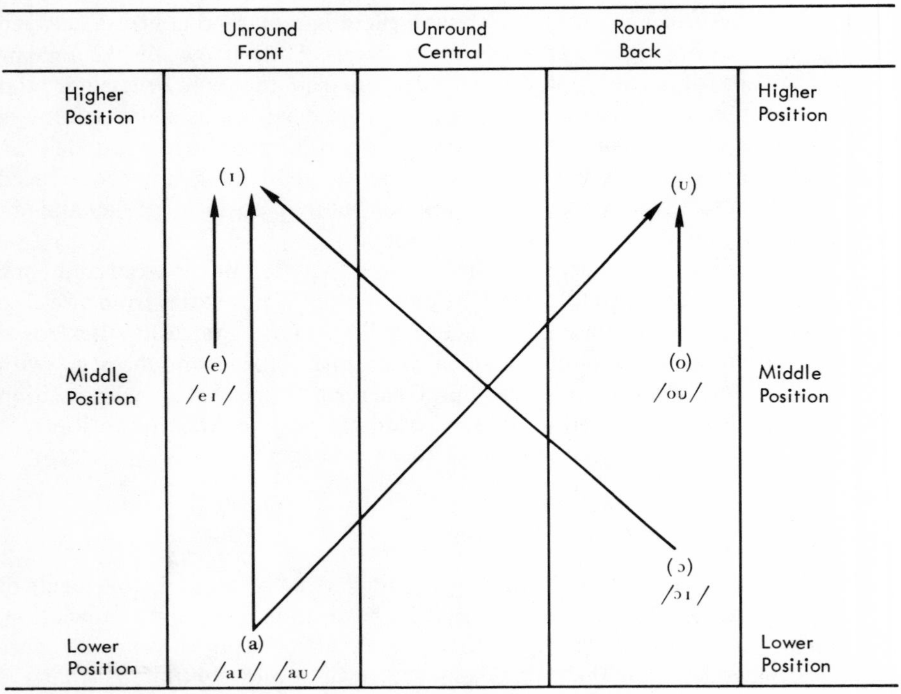

	Unround Front	Unround Central	Round Back	
Higher Position	(ɪ)		(ʊ)	Higher Position
Middle Position	(e) /eɪ/		(o) /oʊ/	Middle Position
			(ɔ) /ɔɪ/	
Lower Position	(a) /aɪ/ /aʊ/			Lower Position

sections on placement in the consonant practice chapters contain comments about these factors. The suggestions are based on the following discussion and on Figure 5. You may find it helpful to review these comments and Figure 5 when you actually begin the oral practice exercises for a given consonant, especially if you require help from your instructor with consonant formation.

1.   The Manner of Articulation

We have already said that consonants are characteristically formed by modifying the outgoing breath stream in one of two fundamental ways: (1) the breath is blocked completely, or (2) the breath is constricted or partially shut off in some particular way. Consonants that are formed because the speech mechanism has completely blocked the breath stream are spoken quickly with short duration and are called *stop* sounds. Consonants that are typically articulated by breath stream constriction tend to have longer duration and are conveniently classified according to the specific way the speech mechanism restricts the outgoing breath. The terms used to describe the nature of these sounds are *nasal*,

FIGURE 5
The Consonant Chart

Manner of Articulation

Place of Articulation	STOPS Voiceless	STOPS Voiced	NASALS Voiced	FRICATIVES Voiceless	FRICATIVES Voiced	AFFRICATES Voiceless	AFFRICATES Voiced	LATERAL Voiced	GLIDES Voiced	GLIDES Voiceless
Both Lips	/p/	/b/	/m/						/w/	/ʍ/
Lip & Teeth				/f/	/v/					
Tongue & Teeth				/θ/	/ð/					
Tongue & Upper Gumridge	/t/	/d/	/n/	/s/	/z/			/l/		
Tongue, Upper Gumridge & Hard Palate				/ʃ/	/ʒ/	/tʃ/	/dʒ/		/r/	
Tongue & Hard Palate									/j/	
Tongue & Soft Palate	/k/	/g/	/ŋ/						/w/	/ʍ/
Glottis				/h/						

49

fricative, affricate, glide, and *lateral.* The respective categories for the consonants are listed in Figure 5 along with information about voicing.

Some explanatory comments are now necessary regarding the specific ways that the different consonants are produced.

(a).   STOPS: /p/, /b/, /t/, /d/, /k/, /g/

These sounds, which are also called *plosives,* are typically articulated in three stages: (1) the breath stream is blocked completely at some point, (2) the air in the mouth is compressed behind the stoppage point and a small amount of air pressure builds up, and (3) the blocked air is released suddenly and the compressed breath stream is exploded out of the mouth. The explosion of the voiceless stops, /p/, /t/, and /k/, is also characterized by a strong explosive puff of air that is known as *aspiration.* The degree of aspiration varies widely according to distribution. Voiced stops are essentially unaspirated.

(b).   NASALS: /m/, /n/, /ŋ/

Nasal consonants occur when the soft palate is lowered and fronted. They acquire their distinctive nasal quality when the escaping breath stream is forced above the soft palate and out through the nasal cavities or passages.

(c).   FRICATIVES: /f/, /v/, /θ/, /ð/, /s/, /z/, /ʃ/, /ʒ/, /h/

Fricatives are formed when the breath stream is forced under pressure between two closely placed articulators, or between a closely placed articulator and a point of articulation. These areas of extreme constriction are all formed in the mouth with the single exception of /h/, which is formed at the glottis. The outgoing breath in all instances escapes with a noticeable noisy or friction-like quality. This quality is particularly evident with voiceless fricatives, although a certain amount of local frictional quality is also heard with the pronunciation of voiced fricatives.

(d).   AFFRICATES: /tʃ/, /dʒ/

An affricate is a sound that combines the qualities of a stop and a fricative. It is formed by initially placing the articulators in a stop position, compressing the breath and allowing the air pressure to build up, and then completing the consonant by releasing the breath with a distinct fricative quality.

(e).   GLIDE: /r/, /w/, /ʍ/, /j/

These sounds occur as the tongue modifies the escaping breath stream by moving from one position to another. The tongue starts from an initial position and quickly glides into the position of the following vowel. The quality of the consonant becomes clear *only* as the tongue moves into position for the following vowel.

(f).   LATERAL: /l/

The only lateral consonant in English is /l/. Lateral escape of the breath stream occurs when the air is forced out of the mouth around one or both sides of the tongue.

2. *The Place of Articulation*

Obviously articulators and points of articulation are extremely important factors in consonant production. The following major articulators and articulatory points are employed to further describe the consonants in Figure 5: *both lips, lip and teeth, tongue and teeth, tongue and upper gum ridge, tongue, upper gum ridge, and hard palate, tongue and hard palate, tongue and soft palate, and glottis.*

Your instructor will demonstrate the pronunciation of some of the more visible sounds for you. Study Figure 5, and observe your instructor's pronunciation carefully.

part II

THE PRONUNCIATION
OF THE
CONSONANT TARGETS
OF
AMERICAN ENGLISH

chapter five

The Consonant Target /θ/ (thought)

COMMON SPELLING FOR /θ/

The most frequent spelling is found in the word **th**ought.

5–1. EAR TRAINING FOR THE /θ/ TARGET

A. A FEW REMINDERS ABOUT EAR TRAINING

The following test exercises will help you learn to recognize your /θ/ target. If this is the first practice chapter assigned to you by your instructor, you may wish to review the discussion about listening practice in Chap. 2, 2–2B to 2–3C.

B. RECOGNIZING /θ/ IN WORDS

You will hear a list of words containing /θ/. After listening to each word, write *B* if you heard /θ/ at the beginning of the word, *M* if you heard /θ/ in the middle, and *E* if you heard /θ/ at the end of the word. The answers will be read

to you at the end of the drill. This exercise is found in Appendix 1. If you have difficulty recognizing the target, you may find it worthwhile to review the test with somebody outside class.

C.   RECOGNIZING /θ/ IN SENTENCES

You will listen to a series of sentences containing a number of /θ/ words. Each sentence will be read several times. Try to locate the /θ/ words in each sentence, and write them down. The /θ/ words in each test sentence will be read to you at the end of the drill. The sentences appear later in the chapter in Section 5–4G. If you have difficulty recognizing the target, you may find it worthwhile to review the test with somebody outside class.

5–2.   DISCRIMINATING BETWEEN /θ/ AND THE VARIOUS REPLACEMENTS

A.   PROBABLE TYPES OF REPLACEMENT

The following exercises will help you learn to compare /θ/ with your replacement. You are probably substituting one of the following common replacements for /θ/: (1) /t/ as in (taught), (2) /s/ as in (sought), or (3) /f/ as in (fought). Your instructor will tell you which replacement you are using. If you are not employing one of the more common replacements, your teacher will tell you exactly how you are mispronouncing /θ/ and provide you with some discrimination drills.

B.   PAIRED LISTS OF WORDS

The words in the following paired lists are identical, except that the words in Column 1 contain the target, and the words in Column 2 contain one of the replacements. When your instructor carries out this exercise with you, he will select some of the words from the columns containing /θ/ and your replacement, mix them up, and then read them to you. Each time you hear a word, write *T* for target or *R* for replacement. The words will be read slowly at the beginning of the exercise and with increasing speed later in the drill. The answers will be read to you at the end of the test. If you are asked to listen to the taped version of the test, listen *only* to the drill that compares /θ/ with your particular replacement. Write *T* for target and *R* for replacement, and listen to the answers at the end of the test.

If you have difficulty recognizing the difference between the target and your replacement, you may find it worthwhile to review the drill with somebody outside class. In this event, have your helper select words at random from the two appropriate lists, and see if you can tell if your helper has said a word containing the target or the replacement. You should not have to spend a lot of time trying to decide which sound you have heard. The more rapidly you can identify accurately the difference between the target and your replacement, the more effectively you have mastered the difference between the two sounds.

1.	**Column 1** /θ/	**Column 2** /t/	**2.**	**Column 1** /θ/	**Column 2** /s/	**3.**	**Column 1** /θ/	**Column 2** /f/
	thank	tank		thumb	sum		thought	fought
	thorn	torn		thought	sought		thin	fin
	through	true		thank	sank		think	fink
	three	tree		thin	sin		thread	Fred
	thin	tin		thick	sick		three	free
	path	pat		thing	sing			
	both	boat		think	sink			
	bath	bat		bath	bass			
				mouth	mouse			
				path	pass			
				faith	face			
				fourth	force			

C. PAIRED SENTENCES

The following paired sentences are identical except that the final word in the first sentence contains the target, and the final word in the second sentence contains one of the replacements. When your instructor does this exercise with you, he will select some of the sentences containing /θ/ or your replacement, mix them up, and then read them to you. Write *T* when you hear the target and *R* when you hear the replacement. The answers will be read to you at the end of the test. If you are asked to listen to the taped version of the test, listen *only* to the drill that compares /θ/ with your particular replacement. Write *T* or *R* and listen to the answers at the end of the test. This drill may be reviewed outside class in the manner described in Section 5–2B.

/θ/ – /t/	/θ/ – /f/	/θ/ – /s/
1. I think it's thin. I think it's tin.	1. I think it's thread. I think it's Fred.	1. It was very thick. It was very sick.
2. Did you get a bath? Did you get a bat?	2. Are you three? Are you free?	2. Did he think? Did he sink?
3. Are you through? Are you true?	3. They went and thought. They went and fought.	3. I want a bath. I want a bass.
4. It looks like a three. It looks like a tree.		4. It's near his mouth. It's near his mouse.
		5. I saw the path. I saw the pass.

D.   Listening for Replacements in Familiar /θ/ Words

You will hear a list of familiar words containing /θ/. Sometimes the words will be pronounced correctly with /θ/; other times the words will be said incorrectly with your replacement. Write *T* for target and *R* for replacement. The answers will be read to you at the end of the test. If you are asked to listen to the taped version of the test, listen *only* to the drill that compares the target with your particular replacement. Write *T* or *R*, and listen to the answers at the end of the test. The materials for this exercise will be taken from the word lists that are found further on in the chapter.

5–3.   A FEW REMINDERS ABOUT ORAL PRACTICE PROCEDURES

If this is the first practice chapter assigned to you by your instructor, you may first wish to review the comments about beginning oral practice in Chap. 2, 2–4. Before you actually begin practicing each individual pronunciation drill, you may also desire to review the supplementary explanations about the exercise in Chap. 2, 2–5.

5–4.   THE PRONUNCIATION OF /θ/

A.   Pronouncing Isolated /θ/

In the event that you cannot pronounce /θ/ through imitation alone, your instructor will help you with the following suggestions about placement. Should placement be required, you should review the definition of a fricative in Chap. 4, 4-4H and the description of /θ/ in Figure 5 in Chapter 4.

1. The Position of the Tongue

The position of the tongue is clearly visible when you pronounce /θ/, and if you use a small mirror, you should easily see what you are doing. Remember that there are two ways of positioning your tongue: (1) lightly press your tongue tip against the back of your upper front teeth, or (2) lightly press your tongue tip between your upper and lower front teeth. Use the position that is easiest for you, and be sure to concentrate on the loose contact between your tongue tip and your teeth.

2. The Escaping Breath

After you have placed your tongue in one of the correct positions, blow some breath out of your mouth in a smooth steady stream. The definitely noisy or friction-like quality of the escaping breath is /θ/. If you are unable to accomplish this, your instructor will teach you to feel this escaping breath by placing your hand close to his mouth while he pronounces /θ/. He will also show you how to observe the escaping air by holding a piece of facial tissue in front of his mouth while he pronounces the target. The smoothly escaping breath will cause the tissue to blow steadily. Continue trying to produce the target. Note that if you press your tongue too tightly against your teeth, you may either say /t/ or a distorted /θ/; if you fail to touch your teeth with your tongue, you may say /s/. In the event you touch your upper teeth to your lower lip, you will probably produce /f/.

B. PRONOUNCING /θ/ IN FAMILIAR WORDS

Pronounce each of the following words carefully. If you are either practicing with your instructor or listening to the exercise on tape, imitate your speech model as accurately as possible.

Beginning	Middle	End
1. thumb	1. nothing	1. path
2. thigh	2. anything	2. cloth
3. thimble	3. plaything	3. breath
4. thunder	4. everything	4. earth
5. Thursday	5. author	5. north
6. thank	6. birthday	6. both
7. third		7. mouth
8. thousand		8. bath
9. thing		9. underneath
10. thorn		
11. thick		
12. thin		
13. thirsty		

C. PRONOUNCING WORD PAIRS
CONTAINING /θ/ AND A REPLACEMENT

Select some of the words from the paired lists in Section 5–2B containing /θ/ and your replacement. Read one pair of words at a time, pronouncing the word with the target first (e.g., **thank–tank**). Make sure that you are saying /θ/ first and /t/ second. Reverse the procedure and pronounce the replacement word first and the target word second, making certain that you are using /t/ first and /θ/ second. Try to develop speed and accuracy as you do the drill. If you are either practicing with your instructor or listening to the exercise on tape, imitate your speech model as accurately as possible. If you are listening to the taped exercise, listen *only* to the drill that compares the target with your particular replacement. You will find this exercise more difficult than the word list in Section 5-4B because of the closeness of target and replacement.

D. PRONOUNCING FAMILIAR WORDS CONTAINING /θ/ AND A REPLACEMENT

This drill is similar to the preceding exercise except that your replacement precedes the target in each word. Pronounce each of the words carefully. If you are either practicing with your instructor or listening to the exercise on tape, imitate your speech model as accurately as possible. If you are listening to the taped exercise, listen *only* to the drill that compares your target with your particular replacement. You will find this exercise more difficult than the preceding one, because your replacement precedes the target in each practice word.

/t/ – /θ/	/s/ – /θ/	/f/ – /θ/
1. teeth	1. south	1. fourth
2. tooth	2. something	2. faith
3. toothpaste	3. southwest	
4. toothpowder	4. blacksmith	
5. toothache		
6. toothpick		
7. twentieth		

E. PRONOUNCING FAMILIAR WORDS CONTAINING FREQUENT /θ/ CONSONANT CLUSTERS

You may find this exercise the most difficult of all the drills dealing with the pronunciation of /θ/ in single words. It is often much more difficult to pronounce a consonant target when it is combined with another consonant in a cluster. Pronounce each of the words carefully. If you are either practicing with your instructor or listening to the drill on tape, imitate your speech model as accurately as possible.

/θr/	/lθ/	/ŋθ/	/nθ/
1. thrill	1. health	1. length	1. eleventh
2. through	2. wealth	2. strength	2. ninth
3. throw			3. tenth
4. three			4. fourteenth
5. threw			5. fifteenth
6. thread			6. seventh
7. throat			
8. throughout			

F. PRONOUNCING /θ/ IN PHRASES

Pronounce each of the phrases carefully. If you mispronounce a word, say it over again several times and then repeat the entire phrase. If you are

either practicing with your instructor or listening to the exercise on tape, imitate your speech model as accurately as possible.

1. a **birthday** on **Thursday** at **three**
2. a **thousand thirsty panthers**
3. **nothing worth** seeing in the **north** or **south**
4. a **mouthful** of Turkey on **Thanksgiving**
5. the child's **thick thumb** in his **mouth**

G.   PRONOUNCING /θ/ IN SENTENCES

Pronounce each of the sentences carefully. If you use a replacement, say the word over again several times and then repeat the entire sentence. If you are either practicing with your instructor or listening to the exercise on tape, imitate your speech model as accurately as possible.

1. **Thank** you for giving me a **third thick** slice of steak.
2. He **thought** he saw **three** boys in the **thunderstorm.**
3. I **think Arthur** is coming to my **birthday** party on **Thursday.**
4. The **thimble** was on the floor **underneath** the **cloth** and the **thread.**
5. The **thief** opened his **mouth** to speak, but the **thin** policeman wouldn't let him say **anything.**
6. **Something** happened to one of the **three** fillings in his **mouth,** and he got a **toothache.**

H.   PRONOUNCING /θ/ IN BEGINNING CONVERSATION

This exercise gives you an opportunity to begin using some of your previously learned /θ/ words in beginning conversation. Complete the starter patterns that are listed below by finding from five to ten words that you can substitute meaningfully in the blanks for each pattern. Where possible, fill in the blanks with target words from your practice lists; however, the completion words **do not** have to contain the target. Write the words on a sheet of paper, and then practice each pattern, using the different completion words that you have selected for the pattern. Make sure that you are saying /θ/ and not your replacement. When you are satisfied that you are reading the patterns conversationally without any replacements, you are ready to practice with somebody else. During class your instructor may ask you to practice the exercise with him, or he may ask you to do it with another student. Outside of class you may wish to practice with a friend or somebody at home.

Choose a pattern and ask your helper to begin saying the completion words. Each time your partner says a word, you repeat the pattern completing it with the word selected from your list. Pretend that you are actually talking to somebody. Look directly at your helper's face, listen for the completion word, and then ask the question or complete the statement as realistically as possible. The drill should move along smoothly and rapidly in the manner of good conversation. Keep checking to make certain that you are not using your replacement. The exercise may be expanded by asking your helper to think of additional words which may be used to complete the patterns.

1. "Did you **thank** him for the _____ on Thursday?"
2. "Are you **through** eating the _____?"
3. "Do you have **three** _____?"
4. "When I'm **thirsty** I like to drink _____."
5. "Did you find Ann's _____ on the **path**?"
6. "I **think** I want a _____ on my next **birthday**."
7. "I **thought** my **math** class last **month** was _____."

5–5.   CONVERSATION PRACTICE

So far you have learned how to pronounce your target by reading various kinds of exercises which contain /θ/ words. Now you are ready to move into the final and most important part of your training program—learning to pronounce /θ/ automatically while you are talking more or less spontaneously. If this is the first practice chapter assigned to you by your instructor, you may wish to review the introductory comments on conversation practice in Chap. 2, 2–6, 2–7. Before you actually begin preparing the exercise in Section 5–5A, you may desire to review the supplementary comments about the exercise in Chap. 2, 2–7A.

A.   CARRYING /θ/ INTO SPONTANEOUS DAILY CONVERSATION

Prepare a list of from five to ten key words containing /θ/ that you use frequently while talking. Practice the list and make sure that you are using /θ/ correctly. Then begin keeping track of how often you are employing the words on your list, and each time you hear yourself pronounce one of the key words, ask yourself whether you used /θ/ or your replacement. If you hear yourself use the replacement in the key word, repeat the word immediately and reevaluate your pronunciation. The importance of verbally correcting yourself has been stressed previously. However, one additional word needs to be mentioned regarding conversation practice. There is a time and a place for everything. I do not think that it is advisable for you to correct yourself aloud if this will embarrass you because of the nature of the conversation or the situation. Correct yourself aloud only when you are comfortable in the conversation or the situation. Your instructor may ask you to keep track of your progress by reporting your practice in a small notebook. One simple way of doing this is to write one word on a page, and use a *T* to indicate a successful pronunciation and an *R* to indicate an unsuccessful pronunciation. Total the number of *T*'s and *R*'s at the end of the day, and you will know how well you did with each word. If you do not find many examples of the key words at the end of the day, go out of your way and deliberately use the words. For example, let us say that you have included the word "thank" on your list because you often say "thank you" to people. Become superpolite for practice purposes, and say "thank you" as frequently as possible.

It is important to carry out this kind of practice as frequently as possible every day. However, even with the best of intentions most students find it impossible to constantly keep track of pronunciation while talking to others. If you find that you keep forgetting to listen for the key words, try setting up some definite practice periods each day. Some students find it easiest to listen for their key words during meals. Others listen while reciting in class and still others during coffee breaks. Occasionally students who spend a lot of time commuting between home and school every day tell me that they use some of this time for key word practice. Whatever you do, find two or three 10-minute blocks of time during the day when you can simultaneously concentrate on the "how" and "what" of speaking. Your conversation practice will be even more helpful if you can get one of your friends or a member of your family to help you. Tell them what key words you are practicing in conversation, make certain that they know the exact difference between /θ/ and your replacement, and ask them to correct you during your conversational practice periods. If it will not make you overly tense about your pronunciation, ask them to correct you more frequently. The more frequently you are reminded about having used your replacement, the more rapidly you will learn to use /θ/ in conversation. Eventually you want to begin listening for /θ/ in all words in your particular vocabulary that contain this target.

B.   General Classroom Exercises in Speaking

Your instructor will plan a series of classroom conversation activities, and each assignment will be discussed fully in class before you carry it out. When your instructor announces the first speaking activity, you may wish to review the introductory comments on classroom speaking in Chap. 2, 2–7B.

chapter six

The Consonant Target
/ð/ (**th**em)

COMMON SPELLINGS FOR /ð/

The most frequent spelling is found in the word **th**em.

6–1. EAR TRAINING FOR THE /ð/ TARGET

A. A FEW REMINDERS ABOUT EAR TRAINING

The following test exercises will help you learn to recognize your /ð/ target. If this is the first practice chapter assigned to you by your instructor, you may wish to review the discussion about listening practice in Chap. 2, 2–2B to 2–3C.

B. RECOGNIZING /ð/ IN WORDS

You will hear a list of words containing /ð/. After listening to each word, write *B* if you heard /ð/ at the beginning of the word, *M* if you heard /ð/ in the middle, and *E* if you heard /ð/ at the end. The answers will be read

to you at the end of the drill. This exercise is found in Appendix 1. If you have difficulty recognizing the target, you may find it worthwhile to review the test with somebody outside class.

C. RECOGNIZING /ð/ IN SENTENCES

You will listen to a series of sentences containing a number of /ð/ words. Each sentence will be read several times. Try to locate the /ð/ words in each sentence, and write them down. The /ð/ words in each test sentence will be read to you at the end of the drill. The sentences appear later in the chapter in Section 6–4F. If you have difficulty recognizing the target, you may find it worthwhile to review the test with somebody outside class.

6–2. DISCRIMINATING BETWEEN /ð/ AND THE VARIOUS REPLACEMENTS

A. PROBABLE TYPES OF REPLACEMENT

The following exercises will help you learn to compare /ð/ with your replacement. You are probably substituting one of the following common replacements for /ð/: (1) /d/ as in **d**ie, (2) /z/ as in **z**ip, (3) /θ/ as in **th**ought, or (4) /v/ as in **v**ine. Your instructor will tell you which replacement you are using. If you are not employing one of the more common replacements, your teacher will tell you exactly how you are mispronouncing /ð/ and provide you with some discrimination drills.

B. PAIRED LISTS OF WORDS

The words in the following paired lists are identical, except that the words in Column 1 contain the target, and the words in Column 2 contain one of the replacements. Complete instructions for this type of exercise are given in Chap. 5, 5–2B.

1. Column 1 /ð/	Column 2 /d/	2. Column 1 /ð/	Column 2 /z/
there	dare	breathe	breeze
though	doe	teethe	tease
they	day	clothe	close
than	Dan	writhe	rise
those	doze		
then	den		
lather	ladder		
father	fodder		
lathe	laid		
breathe	breed		

3. Column 1 /ð/	Column 2 /θ/	4. Column 1 /ð/	Column 2 /v/
mouth (verb)	mouth (noun)	than	van
teethe	teeth	that	vat
either	ether	leather	lever

C. Paired Sentences

The following paired sentences are identical except that the key word in the first sentence contains /ð/, and the key word in the second sentence contains one of the replacements. Complete instructions for this type of exercise are given in Chap. 5, 5–2C.

/ð/ – /d/	/ð/ – /z/
1. Will it breathe?	1. Will he clothe it?
Will it breed?	Will he close it?
2. Is it they?	2. Will it writhe?
Is it day?	Will it rise?
3. It's my father.	
It's my fodder.	
4. I see the lather.	
I see the ladder.	

D. Listening for Replacements in Familiar /ð/ Words

You will hear a list of words containing /ð/. Sometimes the words will be pronounced correctly with /ð/; other times the words will be said incorrectly with your replacement. Complete instructions for this type of exercise are found in Chap. 5, 5–2D.

6–3. A FEW REMINDERS ABOUT ORAL PRACTICE PROCEDURES

If this is the first practice chapter assigned to you by your instructor, you may wish to review the comments about beginning oral practice in Chap. 2, 2–4. Before you actually begin practicing each individual pronunciation drill, you may also desire to review the supplementary explanations about the exercise in Chap. 2, 2–5.

6–4. THE PRONUNCIATION OF /ð/

A. Pronouncing Isolated /ð/

In the event that you cannot pronounce /ð/ through imitation alone, your instructor will help you with the following suggestions about placement. Should placement be required, you should review the definition of a fricative in Chap. 4, 4–4H and the description of /ð/ in Figure 5 in Chap. 4.

1. The Position of the Tongue

The position of the tongue is clearly visible when you pronounce /ð/, and if you use a small mirror you should easily see what you are doing. Remember that there are two ways of positioning your tongue: (1) lightly press your tongue tip against the back of your upper front teeth, and (2) lightly press your tongue tip between your upper and lower front teeth. Use the position that is easiest for you, and be sure to concentrate on the loose contact between your tongue tip and your teeth.

2. The Escaping Breath

After you have placed your tongue in one of the correct positions, blow some breath out of your mouth in a smooth steady stream. This consonant is voiced and has a moderately friction-like quality. You must be certain that your vocal bands are vibrating as you blow the breath out of your mouth. Check for the vibration of the bands by placing your fingers on your larynx as you pronounce /ð/. If you are unable to feel the vibration from your own larynx, your instructor will place your fingers on his larynx and say /ð/. Keep practicing until you can feel the vibration from your own larynx while pronouncing /ð/. When that happens you can double-check your pronunciation of /ð/ by placing your hands over your ears while saying the target. You should be able to hear the vibration. If your tongue is placed in the correct position, and you do not feel or hear the vibration, you are pronouncing /θ/ rather than /ð/. The primary difference between /θ/ and /ð/ is voicing. Finally, if you press your tongue too tightly against your teeth, you may either say /d/ or a distorted /ð/; if you fail to touch your teeth with your tongue, you may say /z/; and if you touch your upper teeth to your lower lip, you will probably pronounce /v/.

B.   Pronouncing /ð/ in Familiar Words

Pronounce each of the following words carefully. If you are either practicing with your instructor or listening to the exercise on tape, imitate your speech model as accurately as possible.

Beginning	Middle		End[1]
1. than	1. bother	4. father	1. breathe
2. that	2. breathing	5. mother	2. smooth
3. the	3. either	6. brother	3. with

[1]If you are having difficulty pronouncing final /ð/, read footnote 3 in Chapter 8, and adapt the comments to the pronunciation of final voiced /ð/.

Beginning	Middle	
4. their	7. grandmother	15. smoothly
5. them	8. grandfather	16. weather
6. there	9. feather	17. lather
7. these	10. leather	18. gather
8. they	11. neither	19. northern
9. this	12. other	20. southern
10. those	13. another	21. clothing
11. though	14. rather	

C. PRONOUNCING WORD PAIRS CONTAINING /ð/ AND A REPLACEMENT

Select some of the words from the paired lists in Section 6–2B containing /ð/ and your replacement. Read one pair of words at a time, pronouncing the word with the target first (e.g., **there–dare**). Make sure that you are saying /ð/ first and /d/ second. Reverse the procedure, and pronounce the replacement word first and the target word second, making certain that you use /d/ first and /ð/ second. Try to develop speed and accuracy as you do the drill. If you are either practicing with your instructor or listening to the exercise on tape, imitate your speech model as accurately as possible. If you are listening to the taped exercise, listen *only* to the drill that compares the target with your particular replacement. You will find this exercise more difficult than the word list in Section 6–4B because of the closeness of target and replacement.

D. PRONOUNCING /ð/ IN PHRASES

Pronounce each of the phrases carefully. If you mispronounce a word, say it over again several times, and then repeat the entire phrase. If you are either practicing with your instructor or listening to the exercise on tape, imitate your speech model as accurately as possible.

1. **bother** to **gather them**
2. a **smooth** red **feather**
3. did **that with lather**
4. **breathe with the weatherman**
5. **although they're southern**
6. gave **those** to **their brother**
7. one of **those** over **there**

E. PRONOUNCING SHORT PHRASES CONTAINING /ð/ AND A REPLACEMENT

This drill is similar to the exercise in Section 6–4C, except that your replacement precedes the target in each phrase. Pronounce each of the phrases carefully. If you are either practicing with your instructor or listening to the exercise on tape, imitate your speech model as accurately as possible. If you are listening to the taped exercise, listen *only* to the drill that compares your target with your particular replacement. Although these phrases are shorter than those in the preceding drill, you may find this exercise more difficult, because your replacement directly precedes /ð/ in each phrase.

/d/ – /ð/	/z/ – /ð/	/θ/ – /ð/	/v/ – /ð/
1. paid them	1. buys them	1. bath there	1. gave them
2. add that	2. edges that	2. both that rather	2. leave that
3. good though	3. goes there	3. math they took	3. drive those
4. crowd there	4. was this	4. underneath them	4. save these
5. ride the bike	5. washes there	5. month this is	5. love this
6. need these	6. cleans these		6. serve these
7. made this	7. dries those		7. dive there
8. weed those			

F.   PRONOUNCING /ð/ IN SENTENCES

Pronounce each of the sentences carefully. If you use a replacement, say the word over again several times, and then repeat the entire sentence. If you are either practicing with your instructor or listening to the exercise on tape, imitate your speech model as accurately as possible.

1. **Neither father** nor **mother** were **bothered** by **the weather.**
2. **Grandfather** gave **them another** pair of **leather** gloves.
3. **They** decided **that they'd rather** try **the other** road.
4. **Their brother** didn't want to **bother either** of **the** teachers.
5. **They** didn't know **whether** or not it was safe to ride on **the smooth** tire.

G.   PRONOUNCING /ð/ IN BEGINNING CONVERSATION

This exercise gives you an opportunity to begin using some of your previously learned /ð/ words in beginning conversation. Complete instructions for this type of drill are given in Chap. 5, 5-4H. Read the instructions, and adapt them to practice with /ð/.

1. "Did **they** find **their** _____?"
2. "Did you **bother** to get the _____?"
3. "Can you buy **another** _____ for **their mother**?"
4. "Can you bring **this** _____ to **them**?"
5. "Does **Father** want **these** _____?"
6. "Did you see **them** at **the** _____?"

7. "Will you give **this** to your _____?"

8. "Do **they** want **that** _____?"

9. "Do you like **those** _____?"

10. "Do you have **their** _____?"

6-5. CONVERSATION PRACTICE

So far you have learned how to pronounce your target by reading various kinds of exercises which contain /ð/ words. Now you are ready to move into the final and most important part of your training program—learning to pronounce /ð/ automatically while you are talking more or less spontaneously. If this is the first practice chapter assigned to you by your instructor, you may wish to review the introductory comments on conversation practice in Chap. 2, 2–6 to 2–7.

A. CARRYING /ð/ INTO SPONTANEOUS DAILY CONVERSATION

This exercise requires you to use /ð/ in daily conversation, starting with key words and expanding to all the /ð/ words in your particular vocabulary. Complete instructions for this type of drill are given in Chap. 5, 5–5A, and there are some supplementary comments about the exercise in Chap. 2, 2–7A.

B. GENERAL CLASSROOM EXERCISES IN SPEAKING

Your instructor will plan a series of classroom conversation activities, and each assignment will be discussed fully in class before you carry it out. When your instructor announces the first speaking activity, you may wish to review the introductory comments on classroom speaking in Chap. 2, 2–7B.

chapter seven

The Consonant Target
/f/ (fun)

COMMON SPELLINGS FOR /f/

The most frequent spelling is found in the word **fun**; less frequent spellings include **puff**, **nephew**, and **laugh**.

7–1. EAR TRAINING FOR THE /f/ TARGET

A. A FEW REMINDERS ABOUT EAR TRAINING

The following test exercises will help you learn to recognize your /f/ target. If this is the first practice chapter assigned to you by your instructor, you may wish to review the discussion about listening practice in Chap. 2, 2-2B to 2-3C.

B. RECOGNIZING /f/ IN WORDS

You will hear a list of words containing /f/. After listening to each word, write *B* if you heard /f/ at the beginning of the word, *M* if you heard /f/ in the middle, and *E* if you heard /f/ at the end of the word. The answers will be read to you at the end of the drill. This exercise is found in Appendix 1. If you have difficulty recognizing the target, you may find it worthwhile to review the test with somebody outside class.

C.   RECOGNIZING /f/ IN SENTENCES

You will listen to a series of sentences containing a number of /f/ words. Each sentence will be read several times. Try to locate the /f/ words in each sentence, and write them down. The /f/ words in each test sentence will be read to you at the end of the drill. The sentences appear later in the chapter in Section 7-4G. If you have difficulty recognizing the target, you may find it worthwhile to review the test with somebody outside class.

7–2.   DISCRIMINATING BETWEEN /f/ AND THE VARIOUS REPLACEMENTS

A.   PROBABLE TYPES OF REPLACEMENT

The following exercises will help you learn to compare /f/ with your replacement. You are probably substituting one of the following common replacements for /f/: (1) /p/ as in **p**ie, (2) /θ/ as in **th**ought, (3) /t/ as in **t**ie, or (4) a fricative /p/, which is symbolized by /ᵽ/. This sound is formed when you tense your lips moderately, hold them very close together, and then blow breath steadily out of your mouth through the slit-like opening between your lips. The friction-like quality of the escaping breath is /ᵽ/. Your instructor will tell you which replacement you are using. If you are not employing one of the more common replacements, your teacher will tell you exactly how you are mispronouncing /f/ and provide you with some discrimination drills.

B.   PAIRED LISTS OF WORDS

The words in the following paired lists are identical, except that the words in Column 1 contain the target, and the words in Column 2 contain one of the replacements. Complete instructions for this type of exercise are given in Chap. 5, 5-2B.

1. Column 1	Column 2	2. Column 1	Column 2	3. Column 1	Column 2
/f/	/p/[1]	/f/	/θ/	/f/	/t/
fat	pat	fought	thought	fell	tell
feel	peel	fink	think	fill	till
fill	pill	Fred	thread	fail	tail
fine	pine	free	three	fan	tan
fig	pig			fear	tear
fool	pool			fold	told

[1]If your replacement is /ᵽ/, your instructor will carry out this drill with you by changing the /f/–/p/ pairs to /f/–/ᵽ/ pairs.

1. Column 1	Column 2	2. Column 1	Column 2	3. Column 1	Column 2
/f/	/p/[1]	/f/	/θ/	/f/	/t/
found	pound			off	ought
fan	pan			roof	root
fast	past			if	it
field	peeled			knife	night
faint	paint			half	hat
puffy	puppy			life	light
leafing	leaping				
chief	cheap				
calf	cap				
leaf	leap				

C.   PAIRED SENTENCES

The following paired sentences are identical, except that the final word in the first sentence contains /f/, and the final word in the second sentence contains one of the replacements. Complete instructions for this type of exercise are given in Chap. 5, 5-2C.

/f/ – /p/[2]

1. I think it's fine.
   I think it's pine.
2. He bought a fig.
   He bought a pig.
3. I see the fan.
   I see the pan.
4. He bought a small calf.
   He bought a small cap.

/f/ – /θ/

1. I think it's Fred.
   I think it's thread.
2. Are you free?
   Are you three?
3. They went and fought.
   They went and thought.

/f/ – /t/

1. Is it fall?
   Is it tall?
2. I see a fool.
   I see a tool.
3. Is it far?
   Is it tar?
4. He's a chief.
   He's a cheat.
5. Look at the roof.
   Look at the root.

D.   LISTENING FOR REPLACEMENTS IN FAMILIAR /f/ WORDS

You will hear a list of words containing /f/. Sometimes the words will be pronounced correctly with /f/; other times the words will be said incorrectly with your replacement. Complete instructions for this type of drill are found in Chap. 5, 5-2D.

7–3.   A FEW REMINDERS ABOUT ORAL PRACTICE PROCEDURES

If this is the first practice chapter assigned to you by your instructor, you may wish to review the comments about beginning oral practice in Chap. 2, 2-4.

[2]If your replacement is /p̶/, your instructor will carry out this drill with you by changing the /f/–/p/ pairs to /f/–/p̶/ pairs.

Before you actually begin practicing each individual pronunciation drill, you may also desire to review the supplementary explanations about the exercise in Chap. 2, 2-5.

7–4. THE PRONUNCIATION OF /f/

A. PRONOUNCING ISOLATED /f/

In the event that you cannot pronounce /f/ through imitation alone, your instructor will help you with the following suggestions about placement. Should placement be required, you should review the definition of a fricative in Chap. 4, 4-4H and the description of /f/ in Figure 5 in Chap. 4.

1. The Position of the Upper Teeth and the Lower Lip

Lightly press your upper front teeth against your lower lip. This position is clearly visible when you pronounce /f/, and if you use a small mirror, you should not have any difficulty seeing what you are doing. The replacement /p/ is made by pressing the two lips firmly together. If you are not careful, sometimes you may press your lips together after placing your teeth on your lower lip. This may cause you to say /p/ or a distorted /f/. We noted earlier that /p̶/ is pronounced with the lips very close together. If you begin pronouncing /f/ with correct lip and teeth contact, and then part your lips, you may either say /p̶/ or a distorted /f/. If your tongue tip touches your upper gum ridge you may pronounce /t/; if your tongue tip is between your upper and lower front teeth, or just touching your upper back teeth, you may pronounce /θ/.

2. The Escaping Breath

When your teeth are lightly biting your lower lip, begin blowing some breath out of your mouth in a smooth steady stream. The definitely noisy or friction-like quality of the escaping breath is the voiceless consonant /f/.

B. PRONOUNCING /f/ IN FAMILIAR WORDS

Pronounce each of the following words carefully. If you are either practicing with your instructor or listening to the exercise on tape, imitate your speech model as accurately as possible.

Beginning		Middle	End
1. firm	5. feel	1. office	1. rough
2. fellow	6. find	2. sofa	2. off
3. far	7. for	3. afraid	3. if
4. fell	8. follow	4. affair	4. leaf

Beginning		Middle	End
9. funny	15. fence	5. awful	5. life
10. fool	16. fond	6. cheerful	6. roof
11. fail	17. face	7. useful	7. chief
12. fear	18. farmer	8. suffer	8. giraffe
13. favor	19. fire	9. halfway	9. calf
14. fall	20. finger	10. difference	10. handkerchief
		11. careful	
		12. after	

C.   PRONOUNCING WORD PAIRS CONTAINING /f/ AND A REPLACEMENT

Select some of the words from the paired lists in Section 7-2B containing /f/ and your replacement. Read one pair of words at a time, pronouncing the word with the target first (e.g., **fat**–**pat**). Make sure that you are saying /f/ first and /p/ second. Reverse the procedure and pronounce the replacement word first and the target word second, making certain that you use /p/ first and /f/ second. Try to develop speed and accuracy as you do the drill. If you are either practicing with your instructor or listening to the exercise on tape, imitate your speech model as accurately as possible. If you are listening to the taped exercise, listen *only* to the drill that compares the target with your particular replacement. You will find this drill more difficult than the word list in Section 7-4B because of the closeness of target and replacement.

D.   PRONOUNCING FAMILIAR WORDS CONTAINING FREQUENT /f/ CONSONANT CLUSTERS

You may find this exercise the most difficult of all the drills dealing with the pronunciation of /f/ in single words. It is often much more difficult to pronounce a consonant target when it is combined with another consonant in a cluster. Pronounce each of the words carefully. If you are either practicing with your instructor or listening to the drill on tape, imitate your speech model as accurately as possible.

/fl/	/fr/	/lf/	/fs/	/ft/
1. flag	1. Friday	1. shelf	1. chef's	1. soft
2. flood	2. French	2. herself	2. chief's	2. left
3. fly	3. frost	3. himself	3. thief's	3. gift
4. flower	4. french toast	4. yourself	4. giraffes	4. sniffed
5. floor	5. frog	5. myself	5. laughs	5. lift
6. flames	6. frown	6. itself		6. swift
7. flash	7. from			
8. flew	8. friendly			
9. flat	9. fresh			
10. float	10. free			

E. Pronouncing /f/ in Phrases

Pronounce each of the phrases carefully. If you mispronounce a word, say it over again several times, and then repeat the entire phrase. If you are either practicing with your instructor or listening to the drill on tape, imitate your speech model as accurately as possible.

1. **finally** a **wonderful phonograph**
2. **four** or **five** pieces of **French** toast
3. **offer enough fresh flowers**

4. **safe from** the **swift flood**
5. **sniffng** the **chef's famous coffee**

F. Pronouncing Short Phrases Containing /f/ and a Replacement

This drill is similar to the exercise in Section 7-4C, except that your replacement precedes the target in each phrase. Pronounce each of the phrases carefully. If you are either practicing with your instructor or listening to the exercise on tape, imitate your speech model as accurately as possible. If you are listening to the taped exercise, listen *only* to the drill that compares your target with your particular replacement. Although these phrases are shorter than those in the preceding drill, you may find this exercise more difficult, because your replacement directly precedes /f/ in each phrase.

/p/ – /f/	/θ/ – /f/	/t/ – /f/
1. stop fishing	1. seventh field	1. get fixed
2. drop four	2. eighth finger	2. wet fur
3. ripe figs	3. ninth fish	3. right feeling
4. cheap fish	4. tenth faucet	4. bright fence
5. escape fast	5. tooth filled	5. polite friends
6. leap far	6. both feet	6. eight fellows
7. cap for me	7. south fence	7. white fish
8. hope fell	8. bath full	8. great favor
9. cup filled	9. sixth farmer	9. wheat farmer
10. on top finally	10. mouth fell open	

G. Pronouncing /f/ in Sentences

Pronounce each of the sentences carefully. If you use a replacement, say the word over again several times, and then repeat the entire sentence. If you are either practicing with your instructor or listening to the exercise on tape, imitate your speech model as accurately as possible.

1. Her **nephew offered** to **fix** the **fan before Fay telephoned** the **factory**.
2. The **laughing fisherman found** his cup, but not his **knife** or **fork**.
3. The **surface** of the ground was **frozen before February** was **half** over.

4. My **grandfather** kept **stuffing himself full** of Mike's **wonderful fried fish.**

5. They **cheerfully** gave a **handful** of peanuts to the **elephant after** it had **performed** the trick.

H.   Pronouncing /f/ in Beginning Conversation

This exercise gives you an opportunity to begin using some of your previously learned /f/ words in beginning conversation. Complete instructions for this type of drill are given in Chap. 4, 4-4H. Read the instructions, and adapt them to practice with /f/.

1. "Is the _____ at the **office**?"

2. "Will you **telephone** him about the _____?"

3. "Can you **finish fixing** the _____ **after breakfast**?"

4. "Please buy me **four** or **five** pounds of _____."

5. "Did you **forget** the _____?"

6. "Were you **laughing** when you saw the _____?"

7. "Do me a **favor** and **find** my _____."

8. "Did you **find** some **fresh** _____ at the market?"

7–5.   CONVERSATION PRACTICE

So far you have learned how to pronounce your target by reading various kinds of exercises which contain /f/ words. Now you are ready to move into the final and most important part of your training program—learning to pronounce /f/ automatically while you are talking more or less spontaneously. If this is the first practice chapter assigned to you by your instructor, you may wish to review the introductory comments on conversation practice in Chap. 2, 2-6 to 2-7.

A.   Carrying /f/ into Spontaneous Daily Conversation

This exercise requires you to use /f/ in daily conversation, starting with key words and expanding to all the /f/ words in your particular vocabulary. Complete instructions for this type of drill are given in Chap. 5, 5-5A, and there are some supplementary comments about the exercise in Chap. 2, 2-7A.

B.   General Classroom Exercises in Speaking

Your instructor will plan a series of classroom conversation activities, and each assignment will be discussed fully in class before you carry it out. When your instructor announces the first speaking activity, you may wish to review the introductory comments on classroom speaking in Chap. 2, 2-7B.

chapter eight

The Consonant Target
/v/ (**vine**)

COMMON SPELLINGS FOR /v/

The most frequent spelling is found in the word vine; a less frequent spelling is found in the word of.

8–1. EAR TRAINING FOR THE /v/ TARGET

A. A FEW REMINDERS ABOUT EAR TRAINING

The following test exercises will help you learn to recognize your /v/ target. If this is the first practice chapter assigned to you by your instructor, you may wish to review the discussion about listening practice in Chap. 2, 2-2B to 2-3C.

B. RECOGNIZING /v/ IN WORDS

You will hear a list of words containing /v/. After listening to each word, write *B* if you heard /f/ at the beginning of the word, *M* if you heard /v/ in the middle, and *E* if you heard /v/ at the end of the word. The answers will be read to you at the end of the drill. This exercise is found in Appendix 1. If you have difficulty recognizing the target, you may find it worthwhile to review the test with somebody outside class.

C.   RECOGNIZING /v/ IN SENTENCES

You will listen to a series of sentences containing a number of /v/ words. Each sentence will be read several times. Try to locate the /v/ words in each sentence, and write them down. The /v/ words in each test sentence will be read to you at the end of the drill. The sentences appear later in the chapter in Section 7-4G. If you have difficulty recognizing the target, you may find it worthwhile to review the test with somebody outside class.

8–2.   DISCRIMINATING BETWEEN /v/ AND THE VARIOUS REPLACEMENTS

A.   PROBABLE TYPES OF REPLACEMENT

The following exercises will help you learn to compare /v/ with your replacement. You are probably substituting one of the following common replacements for /v/: (1) /b/ as in **buy**, (2) /w/ as in **we**, (3) /f/ as in **fun**, (4) a fricative /b/, which is symbolized by /ƀ/. This sound is formed when you tense your lips moderately, hold them very close together, and then blow voiced breath steadily out of your mouth through the slit-like opening between your lips. Your instructor will tell you which replacement you are using. If you are not employing one of the more common replacements, your teacher will tell you exactly how you are mispronouncing /v/ and provide you with some discrimination drills.

B.   PAIRED LISTS OF WORDS

The words in the following paired lists are identical, except that the words in Column 1 contain the target, and the words in Column 2 contain one of the replacements. Complete instructions for this type of exercise are given in Chap. 5, 5-2B.

1. Column 1 /v/	Column 2 /b/[1]	2. Column 1 /v/	Column 2 /w/	3. Column 1 /v/	Column 2 /f/
van	ban	vine	wine	vat	fat
very	bury	vent	went	veal	feel
vest	best	vest	west	van	fan
veil	bail	verse	worse	vast	fast
vote	boat	veil	wail	veil	fail
vent	bent	vary	wary	view	few
calve	cab	vend	wend	vine	fine

[1]If your replacement is /ƀ/, your instructor will carry out this drill with you by changing the /v/–/b/ pairs to /v/–/ƀ/ pairs.

1. Column 1 /v/	Column 2 /b/[1]	2. Column 1 /v/	Column 2 /w/	3. Column 1 /v/	Column 2 /f/
rove	robe			divine	define
dove	dub			rival	rifle
				service	surface
				invest	infest
				leave	leaf
				have	half
				save	safe
				serve	surf

C. PAIRED SENTENCES

The following paired sentences are identical except that the final word in the first sentence contains /v/, and the final word in the second sentence contains one of the replacements. Complete instructions for this type of exercise are given in Chap. 5, 5-2C.

/v/ – /b/[2]

1. He knows about the van.
   He knows about the ban.
2. He needs the veil.
   He needs the bail.
3. Did you get the vote?
   Did you get the boat?
4. He has some new calves.
   He has some new cabs.

/v/ – /w/

1. Give me the vine.
   Give me the wine.
2. Is it verse?
   Is it worse?
3. It's in the vest.
   It's in the west.

/v/ – /f/

1. Did you see the vat?
   Did you see the fat?
2. He got a vine.
   He got a fine.
3. She saw the moving van.
   She saw the moving fan.
4. It was too vast.
   It was too fast.
5. He has a rival.
   He has a rifle.
6. It was a smooth service.
   It was a smooth surface.
7. He wants to serve.
   He wants to surf.

D. LISTENING FOR REPLACEMENTS IN FAMILIAR /v/ WORDS

You will hear a list of words containing /v/. Sometimes the words will be pronounced correctly with /v/; other times the words will be said incorrectly with your replacement. Complete instructions for this type of drill are found in Chap. 5, 5-2D.

[2]If your replacement is /b/, your instructor will carry out this drill with you by changing the /v/–/b/ pairs to /v/–/b/ pairs.

8–3.   A FEW REMINDERS ABOUT ORAL PRACTICE PROCEDURES

If this is the first practice chapter assigned to you by your instructor, you may wish to review the comments about beginning oral practice in Chap. 2, 2-4. Before you actually begin practicing each individual pronunciation drill, you may also desire to review the supplementary explanations about the exercise given in Chap. 2, 2-5.

8–4.   THE PRONUNCIATION OF /v/

A.   PRONOUNCING ISOLATED /v/

In the event that you cannot pronounce /v/ through imitation alone, your instructor will help you with the following suggestions about placement. Should placement be required, you should review the definition of a fricative in Chap. 4, 4-4H and the description of /v/ in Figure 5 in Chap. 4.

1.   The Position of the Upper Teeth and the Lower Lip

Lightly press your upper front teeth against your lower lip. This position is clearly visible when you pronounce /v/, and if you use a small mirror, you should not have any difficulty seeing what you are doing. The replacement /b/ is made by pressing the two lips firmly together. If you are not careful, sometimes you may press your lips together after placing your teeth on your lower lip. This may cause you to say /b/ or a distorted /v/. We noted earlier that /b̶/ is pronounced with the lips very close together. If you begin pronouncing /v/ with correct lip and teeth contact, and then part your lips, you may either pronounce /b̶/ or a distorted /v/. The pronunciation of the /w/ replacement includes the rounding of the lips. Avoid lip rounding while pronouncing /v/.

2.   The Escaping Breath

When your teeth are lightly biting your lower lip, begin blowing some breath out of your mouth in a smooth steady stream. This consonant is voiced and has a moderately friction-like quality. You must be certain that your vocal bands are vibrating as you blow the breath out of your mouth. Check for the vibration of the bands by placing your fingers on your larynx as you pronounce /v/. If you are unable to feel the vibration from your own larynx, your instructor will place your fingers on his larynx and say /v/. Keep practicing until you can feel the vibration from your own larynx while pronouncing /v/. When that happens, you can double-check your pronunciation of the target by placing your hands over your ears while saying /v/. You should be able to hear the vibration. If you are using the correct lip and teeth position for /v/, and you do not feel or hear the vibration of the bands, you are pronouncing /f/ rather than /v/. The primary difference between /f/ and /v/ is voicing.

B.   PRONOUNCING /v/ IN FAMILIAR WORDS

Pronounce each of the following words carefully. If you are either practicing with your instructor or listening to the exercise on tape, imitate your speech model as accurately as possible.

Beginning	Middle	End [3]
1. Valentine	1. seventeen	1. alive
2. voting	2. waving	2. arrive
3. very	3. travel	3. dive
4. vine	4. heavy	4. give
5. visit	5. advance	5. have
6. voice	6. clever	6. love
7. various	7. divide	7. serve
8. value	8. even	8. gave
9. violin	9. however	9. leave
10. vaseline	10. heaven	10. drive
11. Vermont	11. never	11. save
12. valley	12. several	12. cave
	13. living room	13. grave
	14. ever	14. expensive

C.   PRONOUNCING WORD PAIRS CONTAINING /v/ AND A REPLACEMENT

Select some of the words from the paired lists in Section 8-2B containing /v/ and your replacement. Read one pair of words at a time, pronouncing the word with the target first (e.g., **very–bury**). Make sure that you are saying /v/ first and /b/ second. Reverse the procedure and pronounce the replacement word first and the target word second, making certain that you use /b/ first and /v/ second. Try to develop speed and accuracy as you do the drill. If you are either practicing with your instructor or listening to the exercise on tape, imitate your speech model as accurately as possible. If you are listening to the taped exercise, listen only to the drill that compares the target with your particular replacement. You will find this drill more difficult than the word list in Section 8-4B because of the closeness of target and replacement.

[3] We noted in Chapter 3 that some students, especially nonnative speakers of English, might have trouble pronouncing certain voiced consonants. These students have a tendency to mispronounce the voiced consonant by unvoicing it. If you are finding the pronunciation of /v/ difficult because you are constantly unvoicing it, the following suggestion will help your pronunciation of final /v/. English vowels tend to be longer when they precede final voiced consonants; for example, the /eɪ/ in **save** is longer than the /eɪ/ in **safe**, and the /i/ in **leave** is longer than the /i/ in **leaf**. This feature is best observed in words of one syllable, because stressed vowels tend to be longer than unstressed vowels in English. Start practicing final /v/ with one-syllable words, and concentrate on prolonging the vowel. With adequate vowel length the pronunciation of final /v/ will become easier for you. If you continue to have difficulty, deliberately exaggerate the vowel length until you can establish final /v/. Then return to practicing the words with normal vowel length.

D. PRONOUNCING FAMILIAR WORDS
   CONTAINING FREQUENT /v/ CONSONANT CLUSTERS

You may find this exercise the most difficult of all the drills dealing with the pronunciation of /v/ in single words. It is often much more difficult to pronounce a consonant target when it is combined with another consonant in a cluster. Pronounce each of the words carefully. If you are either practicing with your instructor or listening to the drill on tape, imitate your speech model as accurately as possible.

/vd/	/vz/
1. arrived	1. receives
2. loved	2. saves
3. moved	3. hives
4. served	4. drives
5. dived	5. gloves
6. waved	6. leaves
	7. knives

E. PRONOUNCING /v/ IN PHRASES

Pronounce each of the phrases carefully. If you mispronounce a word, say it over again several times, and then repeat the entire phrase. If you are either practicing with your instructor of listening to the drill on tape, imitate your speech model as accurately as possible.

1. **drove seventy** miles to the **river**
2. **volley** ball in the **evening**
3. **deliver** the **vinegar** and **vanilla**
4. **sleeve of** the **velvet vest**
5. **provide** a **screwdriver** for the **television** set

F. PRONOUNCING SHORT PHRASES CONTAINING /v/ AND A REPLACEMENT

This drill is similar to the exercise in Section 8-4C, except that your replacement precedes the target in each phrase. Pronounce each of the phrases carefully. If you are either practicing with your instructor or listening to the exercise on tape, imitate your speech model as accurately as possible. If you are listening to the taped exercise, listen *only* to the drill that compares your target with your particular replacement. Although these phrases are shorter than those in the preceding drill, you may find this exercise more difficult, because your replacement directly precedes /v/ in each phrase.

/f/ – /v/

1. rough voting
2. chief visiting
3. sniff various things
4. half value
5. off very much
6. leaf vegetables
7. safe valley
8. enough viewing

/b/ – /v/

1. club Vermont
2. rub vaseline on
3. grab votes
4. Bob visited
5. scrub vests

G. PRONOUNCING /v/ IN SENTENCES

Pronounce each of the sentences carefully. If you use a replacement, say the word over again several times and then repeat the entire sentence. If you are either practicing with your instructor or listening to the exercise on tape, imitate your speech model as accurately as possible.

1. They **gave everyone** a **lovely silver vegetable** dish.
2. **David** was **invited** to spend from **five** to **seven** days **of** his **vacation** camping at the **cove.**
3. The banks of the **river** in the **valley** were **alive** with **violets** and **clover.**
4. The **eleven** boys from **Virginia** were **shivering** because it was **very** cold in the **cave** that **November.**
5. The **vice-president arrived** and **discovered** that the **expensive self-service elevator** wasn't working.

H. PRONOUNCING /v/ IN BEGINNING CONVERSATION

This exercise gives you an opportunity to begin using some of your previously learned /v/ words in beginning conversation. Complete instructions for this type of drill are given in Chap. 5, 5-4H. Read the instructions and adapt them to practice with /v/.

1. "Did you **give** him the _____ ?"
2. "Do you **have** the _____ ?"
3. "Is the _____ **very expensive**?"
4. "Are you **serving** _____ for dinner?"
5. "Can you **deliver** the _____ ?"
6. "Did the _____ **arrive**?"
7. "Did you **receive** the _____ ?"
8. "Did you buy **seven** _____ ?"
9. "Are you going to _____ on your **vacation**?"

8–5.   CONVERSATION PRACTICE

So far you have learned how to pronounce your target by reading various kinds of exercises which contain /v/ words. Now you are ready to move into the final and most important part of your training program—learning to pronounce /v/ automatically while you are talking more or less spontaneously. If this is the first practice chapter assigned to you by your instructor, you may wish to review the introductory comments on conversation practice in Chap. 2, 2-6 to 2-7.

A.   CARRYING /v/ INTO SPONTANEOUS DAILY CONVERSATION

This exercise requires you to use /v/ in daily conversation, starting with key words and expanding to all the /v/ words in your particular vocabulary. Complete instructions for this type of drill are given in Chap. 5, 5-5A, and there are some supplementary comments about the exercise in Chap. 2, 2-7A.

B.   GENERAL CLASSROOM EXERCISES IN SPEAKING

Your instructor will plan a series of classroom conversation activities, and each assignment will be discussed fully in class before you carry it out. When your instructor announces the first speaking activity, you may wish to review the introductory comments on classroom speaking in Chap. 2, 2-7B.

chapter nine

The Consonant Target
/s/ (sap)

COMMON SPELLINGS FOR /s/

The most frequent spellings are found in the words sap and cross; less frequent spellings include center, and the second sound of the letter x when it is equal to /ks/ as in box.

9–1. EAR TRAINING FOR THE /s/ TARGET

A.   A FEW REMINDERS ABOUT EAR TRAINING

The following test exercises will help you learn to recognize your /s/ target. If this is the first practice chapter assigned to you by your instructor, you may wish to review the discussion about listening practice in Chap. 2, 2-2B to 2-3C.

B.   RECOGNIZING /s/ IN WORDS

You will hear a list of words containing /s/. After listening to each word, write *B* if you heard /s/ at the beginning of the word, *M* if you heard /s/ in the middle, and *E* if you heard /s/ at the end of the word. The answers will be read to you at the end of the drill. This exercise is found in Appendix 1. If you have difficulty recognizing the target, you may find it worthwhile to review the test with somebody outside class.

C.   RECOGNIZING /s/ IN SENTENCES

You will listen to a series of sentences containing a number of /s/ words. Each sentence will be read several times. Try to locate the /s/ words in each sentence, and write them down. The /s/ words in each test sentence will be read to you at the end of the drill. The sentences appear later in the chapter in Section 9-4H. If you have difficulty recognizing the target, you may find it worthwhile to review the test with somebody outside class.

9–2.   DISCRIMINATING BETWEEN /s/ AND THE VARIOUS REPLACEMENTS

A.   PROBABLE TYPES OF REPLACEMENT

The following exercises will help you learn to compare /s/ with your replacement. You are probably using one of the following common replacements for /s/.

1.   You have a frontal lisp and substitute /θ/ as in **th**ought for /s/, or you may produce a distortion combining /θ/ and /s/.

2.   You have a lateral lisp and use a distortion that resembles a voiceless fricative /l/. This distortion is formed by touching your tongue tip or blade to some part of your upper front teeth, upper gum ridge, or front portion of your hard palate. One side of your tongue is lowered and the voiceless breath stream is forced over the side of your tongue with an unpleasant, slushy, friction-like quality. Your lips are parted slightly, and they are pulled toward the side through which your breath is escaping. Some lateral lispers lower both sides of the tongue.

3.   You use /z/ as in zip for /s/. Sometimes this problem is complicated by the spelling similarities between /s/ and /z/. If your replacement is /z/, look over the comments about spelling in Chapter 10.

4.   You distort /s/, because you pronounce the consonant with a sharp hissing or even a whistling quality.

5.   You distort /s/, because you pronounce the consonant with too little force and produce a weak, inaudible /s/.

Your instructor will tell you which replacement you are using. If, on the other hand, you are not employing one of the more common replacements, your teacher will tell you exactly how you are mispronouncing /s/ and provide you with some discrimination drills. Note that /s/ may be mispronounced in a wide manner of different ways, and your particular problem with /s/ may not fit the more common problems listed above. Regarding potential /s/ errors two noted authorities have stated: "Of all the sounds in English, not one has more error variety than does the /s/.[1]

B.   PAIRED LISTS OF WORDS

The words in the following paired lists are identical, except that the words in Column 1 contain the target and the words in Column 2 contain one of the replacements. Complete instructions for this type of exercise are given in Chap. 5, 5-2B.

1. Column 1 /s/	Column 2 /z/	2. Column 1 /s/	Column 2 /θ/[2]
sip	zip	sink	think
Sue	zoo	some	thumb
sink	zinc	sin	thin
racing	raising	sank	thank
ceasing	seizing	sought	thought
rice	rise	sick	thick
lace	lays	sing	thing
pace	pays	force	fourth
trace	trays	face	faith
race	rays	bass	bath
niece	knees	pass	path
piece	peas	mouse	mouth
loose	lose		
bus	buzz		
price	prize		
ice	eyes		

C.   PAIRED SENTENCES

The following paired sentences are identical except that the final word in the first sentence contains /s/, and the final word in the second sentence contains one of the replacements. Complete instructions for this type of exercise are given in Chap. 5, 5-2C.

/s/ – /θ/[3]	/s/ – /z/
1. Will he sink?	1. I like the juice.
Will he think?	I like the Jews.

---

[1]C. Van Riper and J. V. Irwin, *Voice and Articulation* (Englewood Cliffs, N.J.: Prentice-Hall, Inc., 1958), p. 83.

[2]If your replacement is a distortion combining /θ/ and /s/, your instructor will carry out this drill by imitating your distortion while pronouncing the /θ/ words.

[3]See footnote 2.

2. It doesn't look sick.
   It doesn't look thick.
3. I'd like a bass.
   I'd like a bath.
4. Can you find the pass?
   Can you find the path?
5. She lost face.
   She lost faith.
6. It's near his mouse.
   It's near his mouth.

2. What's the price?
   What's the prize?
3. Did you hear the bus?
   Did you hear the buzz?
4. He won the race.
   He won the raise.

D.   LISTENING FOR REPLACEMENTS IN FAMILIAR /s/ WORDS

You will hear a list of words containing /s/. Sometimes the words will be pronounced correctly with /s/; other times the words will be said incorrectly with your replacement. In the event that your replacement is some type of distortion, your instructor will imitate your distorted /s/. Complete instructions for this type of drill are found in Chap. 5, 5-2D.

9–3.   A FEW REMINDERS ABOUT ORAL PRACTICE PROCEDURES

If this is the first practice chapter assigned to you by your instructor, you may wish to review the comments about beginning oral practice in Chap. 2, 2-4. Before you actually begin practicing each individual pronunciation drill, you may also desire to review the supplementary explanations about the exercise in Chap. 2, 2-5.

9–4.   THE PRONUNCIATION OF /s/

A.   PRONOUNCING ISOLATED /s/

In the event that you cannot pronounce /s/ through imitation alone, your instructor will help you with the following suggestions about placement. Should placement be required, you should review the definition of a fricative in Chap. 4, 4-4H and the description of /s/ in Figure 5 in Chap. 4.

1.   *The Position of the Tongue, Teeth, and Lips*

Raise your tongue tip until it is close to the area in your mouth where your upper, middle front teeth join your upper gum ridge. The entire tongue tip and blade is characterized by a narrow, *v*-shaped groove or channel. Be careful not to touch either your gum ridge or your teeth with your tongue, because that will cause you to produce a frontal lisp rather than an acceptable /s/. Place the biting edges of your upper and lower, middle front teeth close together, and keep your lips spread as if in a slight smile. Press the edges of your tongue firmly against the bottoms of your upper back teeth. This will help prevent your breath from escaping over the sides of your tongue, causing a lateral lisp.

2.   The Escaping Breath

When you have placed your tongue, teeth, and lips in the basic position described above, begin blowing some breath out of your mouth in a smooth, steady stream. The breath passes through a narrow central passage between your grooved tongue and the upper gum ridge and is then driven between the biting edges of your upper and lower middle front teeth. The hissing friction-like quality of the escaping breath is the voiceless consonant /s/. If you have difficulty saying /s/ with your tongue tip raised, try pronouncing /s/ with your tongue tip pressed firmly against the bottoms of your lower, middle front teeth. The position of the rest of the mouth remains identical to the position described above.

B.   SPECIAL SUGGESTIONS FOR PRONOUNCING /s/ ACCEPTABLY

A few additional techniques are presented because of the complexity involved in pronouncing an acceptable /s/.

1.   The Lateral Lisp

The main problem in correcting a lateral lisp centers on a change in the direction of the breath stream. You must focus your attention on directing your breath out of your mouth through the narrow central passage formed between your grooved tongue and your upper gum ridge.

Pronounce /t/ and keep your tongue tip pressed firmly against your upper gum ridge. Observe how firmly the edges of your tongue are pressed against the bases of your upper back teeth. It is essential that you maintain this contact when you begin pronouncing /s/, because if you drop one or both sides of the tongue, your breath will escape laterally, and you will say a distorted /s/. Slowly lower your tongue tip and try to blow breath out of your mouth as you pronounce /s/. Keep your upper and lower front teeth positioned closely together, the biting edges of the teeth almost meeting. Do not move your lips or lower jaw while saying /s/. Watch your mouth in the mirror, and make certain that you are not pulling your lips or lower jaw to one side. Listen carefully, and determine whether you hear the hissing friction-like quality of an acceptable /s/, or whether you hear the slushy quality associated with a lateral lisp. Check your observations with your instructor. Another method of checking the escaping breath is by tapping the middle portion of your lips while pronouncing /s/. If you are pronouncing /s/ with central emission, the breath will have an interrupted quality; if you are saying /s/ with lateral emission, the escaping breath will have a steady quality.

2. *The Lateral or Frontal Lisp*

This technique is more useful for a lateral lisp, but it may also be helpful in correcting a frontal lisp. Use a mirror to help yourself visualize the procedure. Pronounce /θ/, and prolong the sound. Very gradually begin pulling your tongue back and up into your mouth until your tongue tip is close to your upper gum ridge. Although the tongue's position will not remain clearly visible, you can assume that a usable position has been reached when the quality of the escaping breath has altered from /θ/ to that of an acceptable /s/. Your instructor will help you determine when your achieve a good /s/. Actually, a reasonably acceptable /s/ should be heard as soon as you break the contact between the tongue tip and the teeth, provided you are directing the escaping breath out of a central opening in your mouth.

3. *The Sharp Hissing or Whistling* /s/

Two features of /s/ pronunciation may be modified if you are pronouncing a whistled or strongly hissed /s/. These are (1) the position of your tongue tip, and (2) the force or intensity of your outgoing breath. A whistled /s/ is often associated with a high tongue-tip position. Place your tongue tip very high and close to your upper gum ridge. Check that the biting edges of your upper and lower front teeth are positioned closely together, and do not alter this arrangement by moving your lower jaw when you say /s/. Pronounce /s/ a number of times. Each time you articulate the consonant, lower your tongue tip slightly. Continue doing this until your instructor indicates that your pronunciation of /s/ is acceptable. If this technique does not work, reverse the procedure. Use the lower tongue position, and press your tongue tip firmly against the bottoms of your lower, middle front teeth. Each time you articulate /s/, raise your tongue tip slightly. Continue doing this until you reach an acceptable position for the consonant. A strongly hissed and unpleasant sounding /s/ is frequently associated with too much force. Pronounce /s/ and vary your intensity until you achieve an acceptable /s/. If lessening the intensity of the outgoing breath is not sufficient, combine this procedure with different tongue-tip positions until your instructor is satisfied.

4. *The Weak* /s/

This pronunciation is the reverse of the strongly hissed /s/ mentioned above. To improve the quality of this /s/, simply increase your force while pronouncing /s/ until your instructor indicates that your pronunciation of /s/ is acceptable.

5. *The* /z/ *for* /s/ *Substitution*

The primary difference between /s/ and /z/ is voicing. Since your articulatory placement is correct, your objective is to pronounce your normal /z/ and then stop vocal-band vibration and begin pronouncing /s/. Check for the vibration of the bands by placing your fingers on your larynx as you pronounce /s/. Keep your fingers on your larynx until you can say /s/ without the bands vibrating.

C.   PRONOUNCING /s/ IN FAMILIAR WORDS

Pronounce each of the following words carefully. If you are either practicing with your instructor or listening to the exercise on tape, imitate your speech model as accurately as possible.

Beginning	Middle	End
1. said	1. also	1. case
2. same	2. answer	2. loss
3. sat	3. asleep	3. kiss
4. say	4. lesson	4. mass
5. sea	5. myself	5. face
6. side	6. upset	6. less
7. seem	7. racing	7. nice
8. seen	8. basket	8. ice
9. sand	9. useful	9. juice
10. so	10. asking	10. house
11. set	11. tossing	11. across
12. soft	12. disagree	12. advice
13. salt	13. chasing	13. dress
14. second	14. crossing	14. guess
15. celery	15. excited	15. grace
16. some	16. receive	16. notice
17. save	17. Pacific	17. brass
18. soon	18. hospital	18. grass
19. soap	19. eraser	19. bless
20. Sunday	20. excellent	20. loose
21. subject		
22. soup		
23. circle		
24. several		
25. suddenly		
26. sidewalk		

D.   PRONOUNCING WORD PAIRS CONTAINING /s/ AND A REPLACEMENT

Select some of the words from the paired lists in Section 9-2B containing /s/ and your replacement. Read one pair of words at a time, pronouncing the word with the target first (e.g., sing–thing). Make sure that you are saying /s/ first and /θ/ second. Reverse the procedure and pronounce the replacement word first and the target word second, making certain that you use /θ/ first and /s/ second. Try to develop speed and accuracy as you do the drill. If you are either practicing with your instructor or listening to the exercise on tape, imitate your speech model as accurately as possible. If you are listening to the taped exercise, listen *only* to the drill that compares the target with your particular replacement. You will find this drill more difficult than the word list in Section 9-4C because of the closeness of target and replacement.

E.   PRONOUNCING FAMILIAR WORDS
  CONTAINING FREQUENT /s/ CONSONANT CLUSTERS

You may find this exercise the most difficult of all the drills dealing with the pronunciation of /s/ in single words. It is often much more difficult to pronounce a consonant target when it is combined with another consonant in a cluster. Pronounce each of the words carefully. If you are either practicing with your instructor or listening to the drill on tape, imitate your speech model as accurately as possible.

/sk/	/sm/	/sp/	/st/	/sl/	/sn/
1. school	1. smile	1. speak	1. stand	1. sleep	1. snow
2. skin	2. small	2. space	2. stem	2. slide	2. snake
3. sky	3. smoke	3. special	3. state	3. slip	3. sneeze
4. skip	4. smell	4. spend	4. step	4. slow	4. snap
5. skate		5. spoke	5. still	5. sleeve	5. sniff
6. skirt		6. spoon	6. stamp		

/sw/	/skw/	/str/	/spr/	/skr/	/spl/
1. swamp	1. square	1. strange	1. spread	1. scratch	1. splash
2. swap	2. squeak	2. straight	2. spring	2. scream	2. splendid
3. swim	3. squeeze	3. strong	3. sprinkle	3. scrub	
4. swing		4. string		4. screen	
5. sweater		5. strike			
		6. street			

/st/	/ts/	/ns/	/sk/	/ps/	/ks/
1. against	1. peanuts	1. advance	1. desk	1. ropes	1. ax
2. almost	2. bits	2. fence	2. task	2. tops	2. box
3. best	3. its	3. chance	3. ask	3. mops	3. hooks
4. boast	4. let's	4. dance	4. mask	4. perhaps	4. speaks
5. cost	5. knots	5. distance		5. tips	5. mistakes

/sts/	/nst/	/nts/	/sks/	/kst/	/skt/
1. tastes	1. experienced	1. pants	1. desks	1. next	1. asked
2. nests	2. advanced	2. parents	2. tasks	2. mixed	2. masked
3. guests	3. danced	3. amounts	3. asks		3. risked
4. costs	4. bounced	4. accounts	4. masks		
5. dentists	5. fenced				
6. roasts					
7. pastes					

F. Pronouncing /s/ in Phrases

Pronounce each of the phrases carefully. If you mispronounce a word, say it over again several times and then repeat the entire phrase. If you are either practicing with your instructor or listening to the drill on tape, imitate your speech model as accurately as possible.

1. the **waitress sneezed** at **breakfast**
2. **six guests** at the **baseball** game
3. a **classroom** at **school**
4. **smell** of **gasoline** in the **bus**

5. **answer** the **question yourself**
6. **speak** on the **subject** of **chemistry**
7. **excellent advice** about drag **racing**

G. Pronouncing Short Phrases Containing /s/ and a Replacement

This drill is similar to the exercise in Section 9-4D, except that your replacement precedes the target in each phrase. Pronounce each of the phrases carefully. If you are either practicing with your instructor or listening to the exercise on tape, imitate your speech model as accurately as possible. If you are listening to the taped exercise, listen *only* to the drill that compares your target with your particular replacement. Although these phrases are shorter than those in the preceding drill, you may find this exercise more difficult, because your replacement directly precedes /s/ in each phrase.

$/\theta/ - /s/$

1. the north side
2. my math section
3. teeth seem clean
4. Beth sells candy
5. Ruth sat down
6. both salads are good
7. bath soap is needed

$/z/ - /s/$

1. those seem good
2. dries several now
3. prize soup
4. his soap
5. raise celery
6. pianos seen in the store

H. Pronouncing /s/ in Sentences

Pronounce each of the sentences carefully. If you use a replacement, say the word over again several times and then repeat the entire sentence. If you are either practicing with your instructor or listening to the exercise on tape, imitate your speech model as accurately as possible.

1. He **stopped smoking cigars** and **cigarettes yesterday** because of lung **cancer**.
2. The **excited nurse suddenly discovered** that the **medicine** was **harmless**.
3. The **Eskimo** girl had **six** or **seven sisters**.
4. **Susan served** baked **goose, sweet rice pancakes** with hot **sauce,** and **lettuce salad** for **supper last Saturday**.

5. The **customer asked** for a **frosty, ice-cold glass** of orange **juice** for **breakfast.**

6. She **lost** her **second fancy silver spoon this** morning.

7. He **expects** to take his **surfboard** and go **surfing** in the **race this** weekend.

I.   PRONOUNCING /s/ IN BEGINNING CONVERSATION

This exercise gives you an opportunity to begin using some of your previously learned /s/ words in beginning conversation. Complete instructions for this type of drill are given in Chap. 5, 5-4H. Read the instructions, and adapt them to practice with /s/.

1. "Did you **see** the **same** _____ ?"

2. "Can you **smell** the _____ ?"

3. "Did you **save some** of the **sweet** _____ ?"

4. "Did you **answer** his **question** about the _____ ?"

5. "Did you **receive** your _____ ?"

6. "Did you give the **customer** her _____ ?"

7. "Are you **interested** in the _____ ?"

8. "Did you **notice** the _____ ?"

9. "Is it **necessary** to **fix** the _____ ?"

10. "Do you **still** want **some** _____ ?"

11. "Did you **stop** buying the _____ ?"

12. "Did you **send** him the _____ ?"

13. "Was the _____ in the **box**?"

14. "Did he **speak** to you about the _____ ?"

15. "Did you get the _____ for **Christmas**?"

9–5.   CONVERSATION PRACTICE

So far you have learned how to pronounce your target by reading various kinds of exercises which contain /s/ words. Now you are ready to move into the final and most important part of your training program—learning to pronounce /s/ automatically while you are talking more or less spontaneously. If this is the first practice chapter assigned to you by your instructor, you may wish to review the introductory comments on conversation practice in Chap. 2, 2-6 to 2-7.

A.   CARRYING /s/ INTO SPONTANEOUS DAILY CONVERSATION

This exercise requires you to use /s/ in daily conversation, starting with key words and expanding to all the /s/ words in your particular vocabulary. Complete instructions for this type of drill are given in Chap. 5, 5-5A, and there are supplementary comments about the exercise in Chap. 2, 2-7A.

B. General Classroom Exercises in Speaking

Your instructor will plan a series of classroom conversation activities, and each assignment will be discussed fully in class before you carry it out. When your instructor announces the first speaking activity, you may wish to review the introductory comments on classroom speaking in Chap. 2, 2-7B.

chapter ten

The Consonant Target
/z/ (zip)

COMMON SPELLINGS FOR /z/

The most frequent spellings are found in the words dozen, puzzle, and cousin; less frequent spellings include nose and freeze.

An explanation is necessary and helpful at this point about words ending in the spellings **s** and **es**. The pronunciation of /z/ varies with /s/ in plural nouns, possessive nouns, and verbs in the present tense, third person singular, when these words end with the spellings **s** and **es**. Some simple rules determine the pronunciations of these English word types. The rules, which are given below, are based on the concept of voicing. You may wish to review the comments about voiced and voiceless consonants in Chap. 4, 4-3A. Pay particular attention to these rules if your instructor tells you that your replacement is the substitution of /s/ as in sip for /z/.

1. When the sound preceding the **s** or **es** ending is any one of the following voiceless sounds, the ending is pronounced /s/: /p/ (hops), (t) (hits), /k/ (picks), /f/ (puffs), and /θ/ (Ruth's).

2. When the sound preceding the **s** or **es** ending is any voiced sound, the ending is pronounced /z/. This´includes all vowels, diphthongs, and the following voiced consonants: /b/ (rubs), /d/ (reads), /g/ (bugs), /v/ (waves), /ð/ (bathes), /l/ (heels), /r/ (cars), /m/ (dimes), /n/ (hens), and /ŋ/ (rings).

3. When the sound preceding the **s** or **es** ending is any one of the following sounds, the ending is pronounced with a syllable. [The syllable may be pronounced as /əz) (/ə/ as in **a**bout) or /ɪz/ (/ɪ/ as in b**i**d).] Examples include /s/ (glasses), /z/ (sizes), /ʃ/ (ashes), /ʒ/ (rouges), /tʃ/ (peaches), and /dʒ/ (edges).[1]

10–1. EAR TRAINING FOR THE /z/ TARGET

A.   A FEW REMINDERS ABOUT EAR TRAINING

The following test exercises will help you learn to recognize your /z/ target. If this is the first practice chapter assigned to you by your instructor, you may wish to review the discussion about listening practice in Chap. 2, 2-2B to 2-3C.

B.   RECOGNIZING /z/ IN WORDS

You will hear a list of words containing /z/. After listening to each word, write *B* if you heard /z/ at the beginning of the word, *M* if you heard /z/ in the middle, and *E* if you heard /z/ at the end of the word. The answers will be read to you at the end of the drill. This exercise is found in Appendix 1. If you have difficulty recognizing the target, you may find it worthwhile to review the test with somebody outside of class.

C.   RECOGNIZING /z/ IN SENTENCES

You will listen to a series of sentences containing a number of /z/ words. Each sentence will be read several times. Try to locate the /z/ words in each sentence, and write them down. The /z/ words in each test sentence will be read to you at the end of the drill. The sentences appear later in the chapter in Section 10-4H. If you have difficulty recognizing the target, you may find it worthwhile to review the test with somebody outside class.

10–2. DISCRIMINATING BETWEEN /z/ AND THE VARIOUS REPLACEMENTS

A.   PROBABLE TYPES OF REPLACEMENT

The following exercises will help you learn to compare /z/ with your

---

[1]A further source of confusion because of s-spelled words which are pronounced /z/ comes from a list of identically spelled words. These words are pronounced with /z/ when they function as verbs and are pronounced with /s/ when they function as nouns. A few common nouns pronounced with /s/ include excuse, house, use, misuse, and abuse. The parallel verbs said with /z/ include excuse, house, use, misuse, and abuse. Whenever you are in doubt about whether to use /s/ or /z/, look the word up in a standard dictionary.

replacement. You are probably using one of the following common replacements for /z/.

1. You have a frontal lisp and substitute /ð/ as in (**th**em) for /z/, or you may produce a distortion combining /ð/ and /z/.

2. You have a lateral lisp and use a distortion that resembles a voiced fricative /l/. This distortion is formed by touching your tongue tip or blade to some part of your upper front teeth, upper gum ridge, or front portion of your hard palate. One side of your tongue is lowered, and the voiced breath stream is forced over the side of your tongue with an unpleasant, slushy, friction-like quality. Your lips are parted slightly and they are pulled toward the side through which your breath is escaping. Some lateral lispers lower both sides of the tongue.

3. You use /s/ as in sip for /z/. The potential mispronunciation problems associated with spelling have been mentioned earlier.

Your instructor will tell you which replacement you are using. If you are not employing one of the more common replacements, your teacher will tell you exactly how you are mispronouncing /z/ and provide you with some discrimination drills.

B. PAIRED LISTS OF WORDS

The words in the following paired lists are identical, except that the words in Column 1 contain the target, and the words in Column 2 contain one of the replacements. Complete instructions for this type of exercise are given in Chap. 5, 5-2B.

1. Column 1 /z/	Column 2 /ð/[2]	2. Column 1 /z/	Column 2 /s/
breeze	breathe	zip	sip
tease	teethe	zoo	Sue
close	clothe	zinc	sink
rise	writhe	raising	racing
		seizing	ceasing
		rise	rice
		lays	lace
		pays	pace

[2]If your replacement is a distortion combining /ð/ and /z/, your instructor will carry out this drill by imitating your distortion while pronouncing the /ð/ words.

2. Column 1 /z/   **Column 2** /s/

Column 1 /z/	Column 2 /s/
trays	trace
rays	race
knees	niece
peas	peace
lose	loose
buzz	bus
prize	price
eyes	ice

C.   PAIRED SENTENCES

The following paired sentences are identical, except that the final word in the first sentence contains /z/, and the final word in the second sentence contains /s/. Complete instructions for this type of exercise are given in Chap. 5, 5-2C.

/z/ – /s/

1. I like the Jews.
   I like the juice.
2. What's the prize?
   What's the price?

3. Did you hear the buzz?
   Did you hear the bus?
4. He won the raise.
   He won the race.

D.   LISTENING FOR REPLACEMENTS IN FAMILIAR /z/ WORDS

You will hear a list of words containing /z/. Sometimes the words will be pronounced correctly with /z/; other times the words will be said incorrectly with your replacement. In the event that your replacement is some type of distortion, your instructor will imitate your distorted /z/. Complete instructions for this type of drill are found in Chap. 5, 5-2D.

10–3.   A FEW REMINDERS ABOUT ORAL PRACTICE PROCEDURES

If this is the first practice chapter assigned to you by your instructor, you may wish to review the comments about beginning oral practice in Chap. 2, 2-4. Before you actually begin practicing each individual pronunciation drill, you may also desire to review the supplementary explanations about the exercise in Chap. 2, 2-5.

10–4.   THE PRONUNCIATION OF /z/

A.   PRONOUNCING ISOLATED /z/

In the event you cannot pronounce /z/ through imitation alone, your instructor will help you with the following suggestions about placement. Should placement be required, you should review the definition of a fricative in Chap. 4, 4-4H and the description of /z/ in Figure 5 in Chap. 4.

1.   The Position of the Tongue, Teeth, and Lips

Raise your tongue tip until it is close to the area in your mouth where your upper, middle front teeth join your upper gum ridge. The entire tongue tip and blade is characterized by a narrow, *v*-shaped groove or channel. Be careful not to touch either your gum ridge or your teeth with your tongue, because that will cause you to produce a frontal lisp rather than an acceptable /z/. Place the biting edges of your upper and lower, middle front teeth close together, and keep your lips spread as if in a slight smile. Press the edges of your tongue firmly against the bottoms of your upper back teeth. This will help prevent your breath from escaping over the sides of your tongue, causing a lateral lisp.

2.   The Escaping Breath

When you have placed your tongue, teeth, and lips in the basic position described above, begin blowing some breath out of your mouth in a smooth steady stream. The consonant is voiced, and the moderately friction-like vocalized breath passes through a narrow central passage between your grooved tongue and the upper gum ridge. It is then driven between the biting edges of the upper and lower front teeth. Check for the vibration of the bands by placing your fingers on your larynx as you pronounce /z/. If you are unable to feel the vibration from your own larynx, your instructor will place your fingers on his larynx and say /z/. Keep practicing until you can feel the vibration from your own larynx while saying /z/. When that happens you can double-check your pronunciation of /z/ by placing your hands over your ears while pronouncing the target. You should be able to hear the vibration. If your tongue is placed in the correct position, and you do not feel or hear the vibration, you are pronouncing /s/ rather than /z/. The primary difference between /s/ and /z/ is voicing. Finally, if you have difficulty saying /z/ with your tongue tip raised, try pronouncing /z/ with your tongue tip pressed firmly against the bottoms of your lower, middle front teeth. The position of the rest of the mouth remains identical to the position described above.

B.   Special Suggestions for Pronouncing /z/ Acceptably

A few additional techniques are presented because of the complexity involved in pronouncing an acceptable /z/.

1.   A Lateral Lisp

The main problem in correcting a lateral lisp centers on a change in the direction of the breath stream. You must focus your attention on directing your vocalized breath out of your mouth through the narrow central passage formed between your grooved tongue and your upper gum ridge.

Pronounce /d/ and keep your tongue tip pressed firmly against your upper gum ridge. Observe how firmly the edges of your tongue are pressed against the bases of your upper back teeth. It is essential that you maintain this contact when you begin pronuncing /z/, because if you drop one or both sides of the tongue, your breath will escape laterally and you will say a distorted /z/. Slowly lower your tongue tip and try to blow voiced breath out of your mouth as you pronounce /z/. Keep your upper and lower front teeth positioned closely together, the biting edges of the teeth almost meeting. Do not move your lips or lower jaw while saying /z/. Watch your mouth in a mirror, and make certain that you are not pulling your lips or lower jaw to one side. Listen carefully, and determine whether you hear the moderately friction-like quality of an acceptable /z/ or whether you hear the slushy voiced quality associated with a lateral lisp. Check your observations with your instructor. Another method of checking the escaping breath is by tapping the middle portion of your lips while pronouncing /z/. If you are pronouncing /z/ with central emission, the vocalized breath will have an interrupted quality; if you are saying /z/ with lateral emission, the escaping breath will have a steady quality.

2. A Lateral or Frontal Lisp

This technique is more useful for a lateral lisp, but it may also be helpful in correcting a frontal lisp. Use a mirror to help yourself visualize the procedure. Pronounce /ð/, and prolong the sound. Very gradually begin pulling your tongue back and up into your mouth until your tongue tip is close to your upper gum ridge. Although the tongue's position will not remain clearly visible, you can assume that a usable position has been reached when the quality of the escaping breath has altered from /ð/ to that of an acceptable /z/. Your instructor will help you determine when you achieve a good /z/. Actually, a reasonably acceptable /z/ should be heard as soon as you break the contact between the tongue tip and the teeth, provided you are directing the escaping breath out of a central opening in your mouth.

C. PRONOUNCING /z/ IN FAMILIAR WORDS

Pronounce each of the following words carefully. If you are either practicing with your instructor or listening to the exercise on tape, imitate your speech model as accurately as possible.

Beginning	Middle		End [3]	
1. zoo	1. present	4. desire	1. prize	4. those
2. zebra	2. pleasant	5. losing	2. cries	5. buys
3. zero	3. busy	6. puzzle	3. who's	6. teachers

[3]If you are having difficulty pronouncing final /z/, read footnote 3 in Chapter 8, and adapt the comments to the pronunciation of final voiced /z/.

Beginning	Middle		End	
4. zest	7. gazing	12. blizzard	7. checkers	14. mangoes
5. zipper	8. easy	13. blazing	8. cameras	15. pianos
6. zone	9. husband	14. thousand	9. barbers	16. washes
7. zip code	10. music	15. noisily	10. edges	17. charges
8. zinc	11. dozen		11. nose	18. bushes
			12. dries	19. was
			13. knees	20. goes

D.   PRONOUNCING WORD PAIRS CONTAINING /z/ AND A REPLACEMENT

Select some of the words from the paired lists in Section 10-2B containing /z/ and your replacement. Read one pair of words at a time, pronouncing the word with the target first (e.g., **rise–rice**). Make sure that you are saying /z/ first and /s/ second. Reverse the procedure, and pronounce the replacement word first and the target word second, making certain that you are using /s/ first and /z/ second. Try to develop speed and accuracy as you do the drill. If you are either practicing with your instructor or listening to the drill on tape, imitate your speech model as accurately as possible. If you are listening to the taped exercise, listen *only* to the drill that compares the target with your particular replacement. You will find this drill more difficult than the word list in Section 10-4C because of the closeness of target and replacement.

E.   PRONOUNCING FAMILIAR WORDS CONTAINING /z/ AND /s/

This drill is similar to the preceding exercise, except that the /s/ replacement precedes /z/ in each word. Pronounce each of the words carefully. If you are either practicing or listening to the exercise on tape, imitate your speech model as accurately as possible. You will find this drill more difficult than the preceding one, because your replacement precedes the target in each practice word.

/s/ – /z/

1. says	6. skies	11. sailors	16. dresses	21. masses
2. saws	7. snows	12. Sundays	17. erasers	22. dances
3. size	8. studies	13. Saturdays	18. glasses	23. straws
4. season	9. stays	14. seesaws	19. passes	24. screws
5. sees	10. slows	15. September's	20. misses	25. busses

F.   PRONOUNCING FAMILIAR WORDS
CONTAINING FREQUENT /z/ CONSONANT CLUSTERS

You may find this exercise the most difficult of all the drills dealing with the pronunciation of /z/ in single words. It is often much more difficult to pronounce a consonant target when it is combined with another consonant in a cluster. Pronounce each of the words carefully. If you are either practicing with your instructor or listening to the drill on tape, imitate your speech model as accurately as possible.

/bz/	/gz/	/lz/	/mz/	/nz/
1. clubs	1. bags	1. bells	1. drums	1. begins
2. cubs	2. bugs	2. peels	2. exclaims	2. grins
3. grabs	3. eggs	3. heels	3. limbs	3. cleans
4. rubs	4. hugs	4. wheels	4. dimes	4. chins
5. scrubs	5. begs	5. pulls	5. tames	5. napkins
	6. drugs	6. nails	6. palms	6. guns

/ŋz/	/vz/	/dz/	/ndz/	/rz/
1. rings	1. receives	1. reads	1. seconds	1. jars
2. hangs	2. hives	2. leads	2. hands	2. pears
3. bangs	3. drives	3. beads	3. winds	3. where's
4. wings	4. waves	4. beds	4. extends	4. fears
5. wrongs	5. knives	5. feeds	5. ends	5. tears
		6. seeds	6. bands	6. here's
				7. years
				8. cars

G.   PRONOUNCING /z/ IN PHRASES

Pronounce each of the phrases carefully. If you mispronounce a word, say it over again several times, and then repeat the entire phrase. If you are either practicing with your instructor or listening to the drill on tape, imitate your speech model as accurately as possible.

1.   **uses pillows** for the **babies**
2.   the **branches** of the **trees** fell **easily**
3.   **allows music** on **radios** at the **zoo**
4.   **buys matches** for **his cousin**
5.   **boxes** of **raisins** for the **busy president**

H.   PRONOUNCING /z/ IN SENTENCES

Pronounce each of the sentences carefully. If you use a replacement, say the word over again several times, and then repeat the entire sentence. If you are either practicing with your instructor or listening to the exercise on tape, imitate your speech model as accurately as possible.

1.   She **appears pleased** by her **lazy husband's pleasant present.**
2.   He didn't **realize** that **his fingers** and **his nose** were almost **frozen** by the **freezing** weather.

3. We **always** found **ourselves** buying **pies** and **cookies** for **dessert** at **Susan's parties.**

4. He bought several **pounds** of **peaches, oranges, apples,** and **cherries** for **Thursday's** picnic.

5. **George's puzzle** contained a garden of **tomatoes, cucumbers, potatoes,** and **radishes.**

I.   PRONOUNCING /z/ IN BEGINNING CONVERSATION

This exercise gives you an opportunity to begin using some of your previously learned /z/ words in beginning conversation. Complete instructions for this type of drill are given in Chap. 5, 5-4H. Read the instructions and adapt them to practice with /z/.

1. "**Does** he **use these** _____?"

2. "**Is** he too **busy** to take the _____ home?"

3. "**Is** he **raising** _____ in **his** yard?"

4. "**Are those** _____ **yours** or **ours**?"

5. "**Did his mother's** friend like the _____?"

6. "**Who's** _____ did you find?"

7. "**Has** he **frozen** the _____ yet?"

8. "**Was** she **surprised** by the _____?"

9. "I often drive to _____ on **weekends**."

10. "**Where's** your _____?"

11. "Give me five **pounds** of _____."

10-5.   CONVERSATION PRACTICE

So far you have learned how to pronounce your target by reading various kinds of exercises which contain /z/ words. Now you are ready to move into the final and most important part of your training program—learning to pronounce /z/ automatically while you are talking more or less spontaneously. If this is the first practice chapter assigned to you by your instructor, you may wish to review the introductory comments on conversation practice in Chap. 2, 2-6 to 2-7.

A.   CARRYING /z/ INTO SPONTANEOUS DAILY CONVERSATION

This exercise requires you to use /z/ in daily conversation, starting with key words and expanding to all the /z/ words in your particular vocabulary. Complete instructions for this type of drill are given in Chap. 5, 5-A, and there are supplementary comments about the exercise in Chap. 2, 2-7A.

B. GENERAL CLASSROOM EXERCISES IN SPEAKING

Your instructor will plan a series of classroom conversation activities, and each assignment will be discussed fully in class before you carry it out. When your instructor announces the first speaking activity, you may wish to review the introductory comments on classroom speaking in Chap. 2, 2-7B.

chapter eleven

The Consonant Target
/ʃ/ (**ship**)

COMMON SPELLINGS FOR /ʃ/

The most frequent spelling is found in the word **ship**; less frequent spellings include **s**ugar, ma**ch**ine, na**ti**on, o**c**ean, and is**s**ue.

11-1. EAR TRAINING FOR THE /ʃ/ TARGET

A. A FEW REMINDERS ABOUT EAR TRAINING

The following test exercises will help you learn to recognize your /ʃ/ target. If this is the first practice chapter assigned to you by your instructor, you may wish to review the discussion about listening practice in Chap. 2, 2-2B to 2-3C.

B. RECOGNIZING /ʃ/ IN WORDS

You will hear a list of words containing /ʃ/. After listening to each word, write *B* if you heard /ʃ/ at the beginning of the word, *M* if you heard /ʃ/ in the middle, and *E* if you heard /ʃ/ at the end of the word. The answers will be read to you at the end of the drill. This exercise is found in Appendix 1. If you have difficulty recognizing the target, you may find it worthwhile to review the test with somebody outside class.

C.   Recognizing /ʃ/ in Sentences

You will listen to a series of sentences containing a number of /ʃ/ words. Each sentence will be read several times. Try to locate the /ʃ/ words in each sentence, and write them down. The /ʃ/ words in each test sentence will be read to you at the end of the drill. The sentences appear later in the chapter in Section 11-4H. If you have difficulty recognizing the target, you may find it worthwhile to review the test with somebody outside class.

11–2.   DISCRIMINATING BETWEEN /ʃ/ AND THE VARIOUS REPLACEMENTS

A.   Probable Types of Replacement

The following exercises will help you learn to compare /ʃ/ with your replacement. You are probably substituting one of the following common replacements for /ʃ/: (1) /s/ as in **s**ap, or (2) /tʃ/ as in **ch**ip, or (3) you may have a lateral lisp and use a distortion that resembles a voiceless fricative /l/.[1] Your instructor will tell you which replacement you are using. If you are not employing one of the more common replacements, your teacher will tell you exactly how you are mispronouncing /ʃ/ and provide you with some discrimination drills.

B.   Paired Lists of Words

The words in the following paired lists are identical, except that the words in Column 1 contain the target, and the words in Column 2 contain one of the replacements. Complete instructions for this type of exercise are given in Chap. 5, 5-2B.

1. Column 1 /ʃ/	Column 2 /s/	2. Column 1 /ʃ/	Column 2 /tʃ/
shame	same	shoes	choose
ship	sip	she's	cheese
short	sort	sheet	cheat
shoe	Sue	shop	chop
shore	sore	ship	chip
she	see	washing	watching
shine	sign	dishing	ditching
sheet	seat	wash	watch
shelf	self	cash	catch
shell	sell	wish	witch
shed	said	dish	ditch
shower	sour	mash	match
swish	Swiss	mush	much
clash	class		

[1] A description of this lateral lisp is found in Chapter 9, Section 9-2A.

C. PAIRED SENTENCES

The following paired sentences are identical, except that the final word in the first sentence contains /ʃ/, and the final word in the second sentence contains one of the replacements. Complete instructions for this type of exercise are given in Chap. 5, 5-2C.

/ʃ/ – /s/	/ʃ/ – /tʃ/
1. He likes my shoe.	1. I see the shop.
He likes my Sue.	I see the chop.
2. It has a shine.	2. I found the ship.
It has a sign.	I found the chip.
3. It began to shower	3. What's he washing?
It began to sour.	What's he watching?
4. Is it a white sheet?	4. He fell over the dish.
Is it a white seat?	He fell over the ditch.

D. LISTENING FOR REPLACEMENTS IN FAMILIAR /ʃ/ WORDS

You will hear a list of words containing /ʃ/. Sometimes the words will be pronounced correctly with /ʃ/; other times the words will be said incorrectly with your replacement. In the event that your replacement is a lateral lisp, your instructor will imitate your distorted /ʃ/. Complete instructions for this type of drill are found in Chap. 5, 5-2D.

11–3. A FEW REMINDERS ABOUT ORAL PRACTICE PROCEDURES

If this is the first practice chapter assigned to you by your instructor, you may wish to review the comments about beginning oral practice in Chap. 2, 2-4. Before you actually begin practicing each individual pronunciation drill, you may also desire to review the supplementary explanations about the exercise in Chap. 2, 2-5.

11–4. THE PRONUNCIATION OF /ʃ/

A. PRONOUNCING ISOLATED /ʃ/

In the event that you cannot pronounce /ʃ/ through imitation alone, your instructor will help you with the following suggestions about placement. Should placement be required, you should review the definition of a fricative in Chap. 4, 4-4H and the description of /ʃ/ in Figure 5 in Chap. 4.

1. The Position of the Tongue, Teeth, and Lips

Raise the blade of your tongue until it is just behind the area where your hard palate joins the upper gum ridge. Point your tongue tip toward your upper gum ridge. The blade is characterized by a broad, shallow groove or channel. Be careful not to touch your hard palate, upper gum ridge, or teeth with your tongue, because that will cause you to produce /tʃ/ or a distortion similar to /tʃ/. Place the biting edges of your upper and lower, middle front teeth close together, and press the edges of your tongue firmly against the bottoms of your upper back teeth. This will help prevent your breath from escaping over the sides of your tongue, causing a lateral lisp. Push your lips forward and round them slightly.

2. The Escaping Breath

When you have placed your tongue, teeth, and lips in the basic position described above, begin blowing some breath out of your mouth in a smooth steady stream. The breath passes through a wide shallow passage between your grooved tongue and the front of the hard palate, and is then driven between the biting edges of the upper and lower, middle front teeth. The definitely noisy or friction-like quality of the escaping breath is the voiceless consonant /ʃ/. If you have difficulty saying /ʃ/ with the tip of your tongue raised, try pronouncing /ʃ/ with the blade of the tongue lowered slightly and the tongue tip pointed close to the gum area below the lower, middle front teeth. The position of the rest of the mouth remains identical to the position described above.

B. SPECIAL SUGGESTIONS FOR PRONOUNCING /ʃ/ ACCEPTABLY

A few additional suggestions are offered because of the complexity involved in pronouncing an acceptable /ʃ/.

1. Avoiding /s/

The fundamental tongue position for /ʃ/ is further back in the mouth than the tongue position for /s/. Slowly pull your tongue back from your /s/ position, simultaneously trying to raise the tongue blade toward your hard palate. You should detect a change from /s/ to /ʃ/ as your tongue moves up and back. If necessary, experiment with your tongue tip, trying the raised and lowered positions described earlier. Remember that your lips are pushed forward and somewhat rounded. Use a mirror to check your lips while pronouncing /ʃ/. Listen carefully for the friction-like quality of an acceptable /ʃ/, and check your observations with your instructor.

2. Avoiding a Lateral Lisp

The main problem in correcting a lateral lisp centers on a change in the direction of the breath stream. You must focus your attention on directing your breath out of your mouth through the broad central passage formed between your grooved tongue blade and the hard palate. Watch your mouth in a mirror, and make certain that you are not pulling your lips or lower jaw to one side. Listen carefully, and determine whether you hear the friction-like quality of an acceptable /ʃ/ or whether you hear the slushy quality associated with a lateral lisp. Check your observations with your instructor. Another method of checking the escaping breath is by tapping the middle portion of your lips while pronouncing /ʃ/. If you are pronouncing /ʃ/ with central emission, the breath will have an interrupted quality; if you are saying /ʃ/ with lateral emission, the escaping breath will have a steady quality.

3. Additional Comments

If you continue having difficulty achieving an acceptable /ʃ/, experiment in the following ways: (1) make small backward and forward adjustments in your basic tongue position, (2) vary the amount of lip rounding and protrusion, and (3) vary the force or intensity of your escaping breath. Keep practicing until your instructor agrees that you are producing an acceptable /ʃ/.

C. PRONOUNCING /ʃ/ IN FAMILIAR WORDS

Pronounce each of the following words carefully. If you are either practicing with your instructor or listening to the exercise on tape, imitate your speech model as accurately as possible.

Beginning	Middle	End
1. ship	1. ashamed	1. brush
2. should	2. ashes	2. bush
3. show	3. delicious	3. wash
4. sure	4. direction	4. crash
5. shape	5. issue	5. dash
6. shop	6. machine	6. dish
7. shore	7. vacation	7. finish
8. she	8. wishing	8. flash
9. shady	9. bushel	9. foolish
10. shine	10. national	10. fresh
11. shelf	11. washing	11. wish
12. shell	12. fishing	12. push
13. shook	13. brushing	13. rush
14. shower	14. Washington	14. English
15. shall	15. smashing	15. radish
16. shoes	16. ocean	
17. Chicago	17. Russia	
18. chef	18. mushroom	
19. sugar		
20. shoulder		

D.   PRONOUNCING WORD PAIRS
     CONTAINING /ʃ/ AND A REPLACEMENT

Select some of the words from the paired lists in Section 11-2B containing /ʃ/ and your replacement. Read one pair of words at a time, pronouncing the word with the target first (e.g., **shame–same**). Make sure that you are saying /ʃ/ first and /s/ second. Reverse the procedure, and pronounce the replacement word first and the target word second, making certain that you are using /s/ first and /ʃ/ second. Try to develop speed and accuracy as you do the drill. If you are either practicing with your instructor or listening to the drill on tape, imitate your speech model as accurately as possible. If you are listening to the taped exercise, listen *only* to the drill that compares the target with your particular replacement. You will find this drill more difficult than the word list in Section 11-4C because ·of the closeness of target and replacement.

E.   PRONOUNCING FAMILIAR WORDS
     CONTAINING FREQUENT /ʃ/ CONSONANT CLUSTERS

You may find this exercise the most difficult of all the drills that deal with the pronunciation of /ʃ/ in single words. It is often much more difficult to pronounce a consonant target when it is combined with another consonant in a cluster. Pronounce each of the words carefully. If you are either practicing with your instructor or listening to the drill on tape, imitate your speech model as accurately as possible.

/ʃt/

1. dashed
2. crashed
3. finished
4. flashed
5. washed
6. brushed
7. fished
8. wished
9. rushed
10. pushed

F.   PRONOUNCING /ʃ/ IN PHRASES

Pronounce each of the phrases carefully. If you mispronounce a word, say it over again several times, and then repeat the entire phrase. If you are either practicing with your instructor or listening to the drill on tape, imitate your speech model as accurately as possible.

1.   **wishing** to **wash** in the **ocean**
2.   **shaving** the **Spanish dishwasher**
3.   **rushed** to **finish** the **dictionary**
4.   **anxious** to **show** us **Sharon's** barber **shop**
5.   an **especially selfish fisherman**

G. Pronouncing Short Phrases Containing /ʃ/ and a Replacement

This drill is similar to the exercise in Section 11-4D, except that your replacement precedes the target in each phrase. Pronounce each of the phrases carefully. If you are either practicing with your instructor or listening to the exercise on tape, imitate your speech model as accurately as possible. If you are listening to the taped exercise, listen *only* to the drill that compares your target with your particular replacement. Although these phrases are shorter than those in the preceding drill, you may find this exercise more difficult because your replacement directly precedes /ʃ/ in each phrase.

/s/ – /ʃ/	/tʃ/ – /ʃ/
1. dress shop	1. to teach shoppers
2. nice shower	2. which shadow
3. loose shelf	3. rich shoppers
4. across Chicago	4. much sugar
5. the grass shore	5. each shoulder
6. a house shaking	6. church should be
7. a brass ship	7. beach shoes
8. less sugar	8. lunch show
9. notice should come	

H. Pronouncing /ʃ/ in Sentences

Pronounce each of the sentences carefully. If you use a replacement, say the word over again several times, and then repeat the entire sentence. If you are either practicing with your instructor or listening to the exercise on tape, imitate your speech model as accurately as possible.

1. The **shower** had passed and the sun was **shining** at the **seashore.**
2. The **shoemaker** had a **bushel** of **delicious mushrooms** and **radishes.**
3. The **shoppers** were looking at **English shirts, Irish shawls,** and **Polish sheets** in the **showcase.**
4. "Are you **sure she's finished washing** the **dishes?" Shirley** asked.
5. The children were **shivering** and **shaking** from the **sharp** cold.

I. Pronouncing /ʃ/ in Beginning Conversation

This exercise gives you an opportunity to begin using some of your previously learned /ʃ/ words in beginning conversation. Complete instructions for this type of drill are given in Chap. 5, 5-4H. Read the instructions and adapt them to practice with /ʃ/.

1. "Did the **shower** get the _____ wet?"
2. "Is the _____ in the **shade**?"
3. "Did you **rush** to buy the _____ in the **shop**?"
4. "Can **she wash** the _____?"
5. "Will **she polish** the _____?"
6. "Is the _____ **fresh**?"
7. "Can **Charlotte brush** off the _____?"
8. "I want a _____ milk **shake**."
9. "The _____ that **she** made was **delicious**."
10. "What **direction** is _____ from here?"

11–5. CONVERSATION PRACTICE

So far you have learned how to pronounce your target by reading various kinds of exercises which contain /ʃ/ words. Now you are ready to move into the final and most important part of your training program—learning to pronounce /ʃ/ automatically while you are talking more or less spontaneously. If this is the first practice chapter assigned to you by your instructor, you may wish to review the introductory comments on conversation practice in Chap. 2, 2-6, to 2-7.

A. CARRYING /ʃ/ INTO SPONTANEOUS DAILY CONVERSATION

This exercise requires you to/use /ʃ/ in daily conversation, starting with key words and expanding to all the /ʃ/ words in your particular vocabulary. Complete instructions for this type of drill are given in Chap. 5, 5-5A, and there are supplementary comments about the exercise in Chap. 2, 2-7A.

B. GENERAL CLASSROOM EXERCISES IN SPEAKING

Your instructor will plan a series of classroom conversation activities, and each assignment will be discussed fully in class before you carry it out. When your instructor announces the first speaking activity, you may wish to review the introductory comments on classroom speaking in Chap. 2, 2-7B.

chapter twelve

The Consonant Target
/ʒ/ (measure)

COMMON SPELLINGS FOR /ʒ/

The most frequent spelling is found in the word measure; less frequent spellings include massage and division.

12–1. EAR TRAINING FOR THE /ʒ/ TARGET

A. A Few Reminders About Ear Training

The following test exercises will help you learn to recognize your /ʒ/ target. If this is the first practice chapter assigned to you by your instructor, you may wish to review the discussion about listening practice in Chap. 2, 2-2B to 2-3C.

B. Recognizing /ʒ/ in Words

You will hear a list of words containing /ʒ/. After listening to each word, write *M* if you heard /ʒ/ in the middle of the word and *E* if you heard /ʒ/ at the end of the word. The answers will be read to you at the end of the drill. This

exercise is found in Appendix 1. If you have difficulty recognizing the target, you may find it worthwhile to review the test with somebody outside class.

C.   Recognizing /ʒ/ in Sentences

You will listen to a series of sentences containing a number of /ʒ/ words. Each sentence will be read to you several times. Try to locate the /ʒ/ words in each sentence, and write them down. The /ʒ/ words in each test sentence will be read to you at the end of the drill. The sentences appear later in the chapter in Section 12-4D. If you have difficulty recognizing the target, you may find it worthwhile to review the test with somebody outside class.

12–2.   DISCRIMINATING BETWEEN /ʒ/ AND THE VARIOUS REPLACEMENTS

A.   Probable Types of Replacement

The following exercises will help you learn to compare /ʒ/ with your replacement. You are probably substituting one of the following common replacements for /ʒ/: (1) /dʒ/ as in **juice**, (2) /z/ as in **zip**, (3) /ʃ/ as in **ship**, or (4) you may have a lateral lisp and use a distortion that resembles a voiced fricative /l/.[1] Your instructor will tell you which replacement you are using. If you are not employing one of the more common replacements, your teacher will tell you exactly how you are mispronouncing /ʒ/ and provide you with some discrimination drills.

B.   Listening for Replacements in Familiar /ʒ/ Words

You will hear a list of words containing /ʒ/. Sometimes the words will be pronounced correctly with /ʒ/; other times the words will be said incorrectly with your replacement. In the event that your replacement is a lateral lisp, your instructor will imitate your distorted /ʒ/. Complete instructions for this type of drill are found in Chap. 5, 5-2D.

12–3.   A FEW REMINDERS ABOUT ORAL PRACTICE PROCEDURES

If this is the first practice chapter assigned to you by your instructor, you may wish to review the comments about beginning oral practice in Chap. 2, 2-4. Before you actually begin practicing each individual pronunciation drill, you

---

[1] A description of this lateral lisp is found in Chapter 10, Section 10-2A.

may also desire to review the supplementary explanations about the exercise in Chap. 2, 2-5.

12–4.   THE PRONUNCIATION OF /ʒ/

A.   PRONOUNCING ISOLATED /ʒ/

In the event that you cannot pronounce /ʒ/ through imitation alone, your instructor will help you with the following suggestions about placement. Should placement be required, you should review the definition of a fricative in Chap. 4, 4-4H and the description of /ʒ/ in Figure 5 in Chap. 4.

1.   *The Position of the Tongue, Teeth, and Lips*

Raise the blade of your tongue until it is just behind the area where your hard palate joins the upper gum ridge. Point your tongue tip toward your upper gum ridge. The blade is characterized by a broad, shallow groove or channel. Be careful not to touch your hard palate, upper gum ridge, or teeth with your tongue, because that will cause you to produce /dʒ/ or a distortion similar to /dʒ/. Place the biting edges of your upper and lower, middle front teeth close together, and press the edges of your tongue firmly against the bottoms of your upper back teeth. This will help prevent your breath from escaping over the sides of your tongue, causing a lateral lisp. Push your lips forward and round them slightly.

2.   *The Escaping Breath*

When you have placed your tongue, teeth, and lips in the basic position described above, begin blowing some breath out of your mouth in a smooth steady stream. The consonant is voiced, and the moderately friction-like vocalized breath passes through a wide shallow passage between your grooved tongue and the front of the hard palate, and is then driven between the biting edges of the upper and lower, middle front teeth. Check for the vibration of the bands by placing your fingers on your larynx as you pronounce /ʒ/. If you are unable to feel the vibration from your own larynx, your instructor will place your fingers on his larynx and say /ʒ/. Keep practicing until you can feel the vibration from your own larynx while saying /ʒ/. When that happens, you can double-check your pronunciation of /ʒ/ by placing your hands over your ears while pronouncing the target. You should be able to hear the vibration. If your tongue is placed in the correct position and you do not feel or hear the vibration, you are pronouncing /ʃ/ rather than /ʒ/. The primary difference between /ʃ/ and /ʒ/ is voicing. Finally, if you have difficulty saying /ʒ/ with the tip of your tongue raised, try pronouncing /ʒ/ with the blade slightly lower and the tongue tip pointed close to the gum area below the lower, middle front teeth. The position of the rest of the mouth remains identical to the position described above.

B.   Special Suggestions for Pronouncing /ʒ/ Acceptably

A few additional suggestions are offered because of the complexity involved in pronouncing an acceptable /ʒ/.

1.   Avoiding /z/

The fundamental tongue position for /ʒ/ is further back in the mouth than the tongue position for /z/. Slowly pull your tongue back from your /z/ position, simultaneously trying to raise the tongue blade toward your hard palate. You should detect a change from /z/ to /ʒ/ as your tongue moves up and back. If necessary, experiment with your tongue tip, trying the raised and lowered positions described earlier. Remember that your lips are pushed forward and somewhat rounded. Use a mirror to check your lips while pronouncing /ʒ/. Listen carefully for the moderately friction-like quality of an acceptable /ʒ/, and check your observations with your instructor.

2.   Avoiding a Lateral Lisp

The main problem in correcting a lateral lisp centers on a change in the direction of the breath stream. You must focus your attention on directing your vocalized breath out of your mouth through the broad central passage formed between your grooved tongue blade and the hard palate. Watch your mouth in a mirror to make certain that you are not pulling your lips or lower jaw to one side. Listen carefully and determine whether you hear the moderately friction-like quality of an acceptable /ʒ/, or whether you hear the slushy quality associated with a lateral lisp. Check your observations with your instructor. Another method of checking the escaping breath is by tapping the middle portion of your lips while pronouncing /ʒ/. If you are pronouncing /ʒ/ with central emission, the breath will have an interrupted quality; if you are saying /ʒ/ with lateral emission, the escaping breath will have a steady quality.

3.   Additional Comments

If you continue having difficulty achieving an acceptable /ʒ/, experiment in the following ways: (1) make small backward and forward adjustments in your basic tongue position, (2) vary the amount of lip rounding and protrusion, and (3) vary the force or intensity of your escaping breath. Keep practicing until your instructor agrees that you are producing an acceptable /ʒ/.

C.   Pronouncing /ʒ/ in Familiar Words

Pronounce each of the following words carefully. If you are either practicing with your instructor or listening to the exercise on tape, imitate your speech model as accurately as possible.

	Middle		**End**[2]
1. leisure	7. television	1. rouge
2. measure	8. collision	2. garage
3. treasure	9. division	3. massage
4. usual	10. measuring	4. beige
5. unusual	11. invasion	5. barrage
6. unusually	12. Asia	

D.   PRONOUNCING /ʒ/ IN SENTENCES

Pronounce each of the sentences carefully. If you use a replacement, say the word over again several times, and then repeat the entire sentence. If you are either practicing with your instructor or listening to the exercise on tape, imitate your speech model as accurately as possible.

1.   She dropped the **measuring** cup by the **television** set.
2.   As **usual** he had a **collision** with the **garage** door.
3.   He **usually** found **division** problems a **pleasure**.
4.   The **Asian** student tried different kinds of **rouge** during her **leisure** time.
5.   After the **invasion** was over, they found the **treasure** in a **beige** trunk.

E.   PRONOUNCING /ʒ/ IN BEGINNING CONVERSATION

This exercise gives you an opportunity to begin using some of your previously learned /ʒ/ words in beginning conversation. Complete instructions for this type of drill are given in Chap. 5, 5-4H. Read the instructions and adapt them to practice with /ʒ/.

1.   "Do you **usually** buy _____?"
2.   "Can you **measure** the _____?"
3.   "Did you watch _____ on **television**?"
4.   "Is the _____ in the **garage**?"
5.   "_____ is a country in **Asia**."

12–5.   CONVERSATION PRACTICE

So far you have learned how to pronounce your target by reading various kinds of exercises which contain /ʒ/ words. Now you are ready to move into the

---

[2]If you are having difficulty pronouncing final /ʒ/, read footnote 3 in Chapter 8, and adapt the comments to the pronunciation of final voiced /ʒ/.

final and most important part of your training program—learning to pronounce /ʒ/ automatically while you are talking more or less spontaneously. If this is the first practice chapter assigned to you by your instructor, you may wish to review the introductory comments on conversation practice in Chap. 2, 2-6 to 2-7.

A.   CARRYING /ʒ/ INTO SPONTANEOUS DAILY CONVERSATION

This exercise requires you to use /ʒ/ in daily conversation, starting with key words and expanding to all the /ʒ/ words in your particular vocabulary. Complete instructions for this type of drill are given in Chap. 5, 5-5A, and there are supplementary comments about the exercise in Chap. 2, 2-7A.

B.   GENERAL CLASSROOM EXERCISES IN SPEAKING

Your instructor will plan a series of classroom conversation activities, and each assignment will be discussed fully in class before you carry it out. When your instructor announces the first speaking activity, you may wish to review the introductory comments on classroom speaking in Chap. 2, 2-7B.

chapter thirteen

The Consonant Target
/h/ (**how**)

COMMON SPELLINGS FOR /h/

The most frequent spellings are found in the words **h**ow, and **wh**o.

13–1. EAR TRAINING FOR /h/

A. A FEW REMINDERS ABOUT EAR TRAINING

The following test exercises will help you learn to recognize your /h/ target. If this is the first practice chapter assigned to you by your instructor, you may wish to review the discussion about listening practice in Chap. 2, 2-B to 2-3C.

B. RECOGNIZING /h/ IN WORDS

You will hear a list of words containing /h/. After listening to each word, write *B* if you heard /h/ at the beginning of the word and *M* if you heard /h/ in the middle of the word. The answers will be read to you at the end of the drill.

This exercise is found in Appendix 1. If you have difficulty recognizing the target, you may find it worthwhile to review the test with somebody outside class.

C.   RECOGNIZING /h/ IN SENTENCES

You will listen to a series of sentences containing a number of /h/ words. Each sentence will be read to you several times. Try to locate the /h/ words in each sentence, and write them down. The /h/ words in each test sentence will be read to you at the end of the drill. The sentences appear later in the chapter in Section 13-4D. If you have difficulty recognizing the target, you may find it worthwhile to review the test with somebody outside class.

13–2.   DISCRIMINATING BETWEEN /h/ AND THE VARIOUS REPLACEMENTS

A.   PROBABLE TYPES OF REPLACEMENT

The following exercises will help you learn to compare /h/ with your replacement. You are probably substituting one of the following common replacements for /h/: (1) you omit initial /h/,[1] or (2) you pronounce a more tense and forceful fricative /h/ by raising the back of your tongue up toward the soft palate and sharply constricting the escaping breath. Your instructor will tell you which replacement you are using. If you are not using one of the more common replacements, your teacher will tell you exactly how you are mispronouncing /h/ and provide you with some discrimination drills.

B.   PAIRED LISTS OF WORDS

The words in the following paired list are identical, except that the words in Column 1 contain the target, and the words in Column 2 contain the replacement. Complete instructions for this type of exercise are given in Chap. 5, 5-2B.

Column 1 /h/	Column 2 (omitted /h/)
ham	am
hand	and
hat	at
hair	air
harm	arm

[1]This type of error should not be confused with the normal tendency in American English to alter the weak-stressed pronunciation of words like **him, her,** and **his** by dropping /h/. A full discussion of weak or unstressed forms is found in Chapter 48.

Column 1 /h/	Column 2 (omitted /h/)
hear	ear
heat	eat
hold	old
hill	ill
hit	it
high	I
hate	ate

C.   LISTENING FOR REPLACEMENTS IN FAMILIAR /h/ WORDS

You will hear a list of words containing /h/. Sometimes the words will be pronounced correctly with /h/; other times the words will be said incorrectly with your replacement. Complete instructions for this type of drill are found in Chap. 5, 5-2D.

13–3.   A FEW REMINDERS
ABOUT ORAL PRACTICE PROCEDURES

If this is the first practice chapter assigned to you by your instructor, you may wish to review the comments about beginning oral practice in Chap. 2, 2-4. Before you actually begin practicing each individual pronunciation drill, you may also desire to review the supplementary explanations about the exercise in Chap. 2, 2-5.

13–4.   THE PRONUNCIATION OF /h/

A.   PRONOUNCING ISOLATED /h/

In the event that you cannot pronounce /h/ through imitation alone, your instructor will help you with the following suggestions about placement. Should placement be required, you should review the definition of a fricative in Chap. 4, 4-4H and the description of /h/ in Figure 5 in Chap. 4.

1.   *The Escaping Breath*

The consonant /h/ is formed in the glottis rather than in your mouth. Your vocal bands are brought closely enough together to create a definitely noisy or friction-like quality as you blow your breath between the bands. The escaping breath passes steadily over the tongue and out of the mouth; the tongue and lips tend to adopt the position of the following vowel or diphthong. If your replacement is the tense /h/ that is produced in the back of your mouth, concentrate on keeping your tongue flat in your mouth while blowing breath gently out of your mouth.

B.   PRONOUNCING /h/ IN FAMILIAR WORDS

Pronounce each of the following words carefully. If you are either practicing with your instructor or listening to the exercise on tape, imitate your speech model as accurately as possible.

Beginning		Middle
1. hail	11. hurry	1. behind
2. halfway	12. whole	2. perhaps
3. handsome	13. who	3. unhappy
4. halt	14. whom	4. behave
5. happen	15. whose	5. ahead
6. happy	16. hello	6. overhead
7. hardly	17. help	7. anyhow
8. hear	18. home	8. schoolhouse
9. hungry	19. hold	9. sawhorse
10. hurt	20. herself	10. downhill

C.   PRONOUNCING /h/ IN PHRASES

Pronounce each of the phrases carefully. If you mispronounce a word, say it over again several times, and then repeat the entire phrase. If you are either practicing with your instructor or listening to the drill on tape, imitate your speech model as accurately as possible.

1.   a **hamburger** and a **hotdog** at **Halloween**
2.   no **honey** in the **beehive**
3.   a **hot hard-boiled** egg in the **hospital**
4.   a **heavy hammer** for the **handle** bars
5.   a **hair** cut for a **half** dollar

D.   PRONOUNCING /h/ IN SENTENCES

Pronounce each of the sentences carefully. If you use a replacement, say the word over again several times and then repeat the entire sentence. If you are either practicing with your instructor or listening to the exercise on tape, imitate your speech model as accurately as possible.

1.   The **hungry** cat was **hunting** mice near the **mousehole**.
2.   My **husband** accidently **happened** to bump his **head** in the **hallway** and went to the **hospital**.
3.   She **hopped halfway** down the **hill** to the **highway**.
4.   She **hoped** to move the **heavy sawhorse herself**.
5.   They **hurried home** to **help** cook the **wholesome ham**.

E.   Pronouncing /h/ in Beginning Conversation

This exercise gives you an opportunity to begin using some of your previously learned /h/ words in beginning conversation. Complete instructions for this type of drill are given in Chap. 5, 5-4H. Read the instructions and adapt them to practice with /h/.

1.   "My **husband** brought some _____ **home**."
2.   "Did you **help Henry** with the _____?"
3.   "**Hurry** over to my **house** and I'll give you the _____."
4.   "Did the baby **hide** the _____ **behind** the chair?"
5.   "The **hotel** is on _____ street."
6.   "She was **unhappy** about the new _____ that she bought."
7.   "**How** many _____ did you see?"

13–5.   CONVERSATION PRACTICE

So far you have learned how to pronounce your target by reading various kinds of exercises which contain /h/ words. Now you are ready to move into the final and most important part of your training program—learning to pronounce /h/ automatically while you are talking more or less spontaneously. If this is the first practice chapter assigned to you by your instructor, you may wish to review the introductory comments on conversation practice in Chap. 2, 2-6 to 2-7.

A.   Carrying /h/ into Spontaneous Daily Conversation

This exercise requires you to use /h/ in daily conversation, starting with key words and expanding to all the /h/ words in your particular vocabulary. Complete instructions for this type of drill are given in Chap. 5, 5-5A, and there are supplementary comments about the exercise in Chap. 2, 2-7A.

B.   General Classroom Exercises in Speaking

Your instructor will plan a series of classroom conversation activities, and each assignment will be discussed fully in class before you carry it out. When your instructor announces the first speaking activity, you may wish to review the introductory comments on classroom speaking in Chap. 2, 2-7B.

chapter fourteen

The Consonant Target
/tʃ/ (chip)

COMMON SPELLINGS FOR /tʃ/

The most frequent spelling is found in the word **ch**ip; less frequent spellings include ma**tch**, ques**ti**on, and na**tu**re.

14–1. EAR TRAINING FOR THE /tʃ/ TARGET

A. A FEW REMINDERS ABOUT EAR TRAINING

The following test exercises will help you learn to recognize your /tʃ/ target. If this is the first practice chapter assigned to you by your instructor, you may wish to review the discussion about listening practice in Chap. 2, 2-2B to 2-3C.

B. RECOGNIZING /tʃ/ IN WORDS

You will hear a list of words containing /tʃ/. After listening to each word, write *B* if you heard /tʃ/ at the beginning of the word, *M* if you heard /tʃ/ in the middle, and *E* if you heard /tʃ/ at the end of the word. The answers will be read to you at the end of the drill. This exercise is found in Appendix 1. If you have difficulty recognizing the target, you may find it worthwhile to review the test with somebody outside class.

C. RECOGNIZING /tʃ/ IN SENTENCES

You will listen to a series of sentences containing a number of /tʃ/ words. Each sentence will be read several times. Try to locate the /tʃ/ words in each sentence and write them down. The /tʃ/ words in each test sentence will be read to you at the end of the drill. The sentences appear later in the chapter in Section 14-4H. If you have difficulty recognizing the target, you may find it worthwhile to review the test with somebody outside class.

14–2. DISCRIMINATING BETWEEN /tʃ/ AND THE VARIOUS REPLACEMENTS

A. PROBABLE TYPES OF REPLACEMENT

The following exercises will help you learn to compare /tʃ/ with your replacement. You are probably substituting one of the following common replacements for /tʃ/: (1) /ʃ/ as in (*ship*), (2) the consonant cluster /ts/ as in beets, or (3) you may have a lateral lisp on the /ʃ/ portion of the target and use a distortion that resembles a voiceless fricative /l/.[1] Your instructor will tell you which replacement you are using. If you are not employing one of the more common replacements, your teacher will tell you exactly how you are mispronouncing /tʃ/ and provide you with some discrimination drills.

B. PAIRED LISTS OF WORDS

The words in the following paired lists are identical, except that the words in Column 1 contain the target and the words in Column 2 contain one of the replacements. Complete instructions for this type of exercise are given in Chap. 5, 5-2B.

1. Column 1 /tʃ/	Column 2 /ʃ/	2. Column 1 /tʃ/	Column 2 /ts/
cheat	sheet	match	mats
cheese	she's	which	wits
choose	shoes	watch	watts
chip	ship	patch	pats
chew	shoe	hitch	hits
chop	shop	each	eats
watching	washing	coach	coats

[1]A description of this lateral lisp is found in Chapter 9, Section 9-2A.

1. Column 1 /tʃ/	Column 2 /ʃ/	2. Column 1 /tʃ/	Column 2 /ts/
ditching	dishing	peach	Pete's
watch	wash	hatch	hats
catch	cash	batch	bats
much	mush	pitch	pits
ditch	dish		
match	mash		

C.   PAIRED SENTENCES

The following paired sentences are identical, except that the final word in the first sentence contains /tʃ/, and the final word in the second sentence contains one of the replacements. Complete instructions for this type of exercise are given in Chap. 5, 5-2C.

/tʃ/ – /ʃ/	/tʃ/ – /ts/
1. It's a small chip.	1. I see the match.
It's a small ship.	I see the mats.
2. I see the chop.	2. He needs the batch.
I see the shop.	He needs the bats.
3. What's he watching?	3. I found the coach.
What's he washing?	I found the coats.
4. He fell over the ditch.	4. He threw the pitch.
He fell over the dish.	He threw the pits.
5. Do you have my watch?	
Do you have my wash?	

D.   LISTENING FOR REPLACEMENTS IN FAMILIAR /tʃ/ WORDS

You will hear a list of words containing /tʃ/. Sometimes the words will be pronounced correctly with /tʃ/; other times the words will be said incorrectly with your replacement. In the event that you have a lateral lisp, your instructor will imitate your distorted /tʃ/. Complete instructions for this type of drill are found in Chap. 5, 5-2D.

14–3.   A FEW REMINDERS
ABOUT ORAL PRACTICE PROCEDURES

If this is the first practice chapter assigned to you by your instructor, you may wish to review the comments about beginning oral practice in Chap. 2, 2-4. Before you actually begin practicing each individual pronunciation drill, you may also desire to review the supplementary explanations about the exercise in Chap. 2, 2-5.

14–4.   THE PRONUNCIATION OF /tʃ/

A.   Pronouncing Isolated /tʃ/

In the event you cannot pronounce /tʃ/ through imitation alone, your instructor will help you with the following suggestions about placement. Should placement be required, you should review the definition of an affricate in Chap. 4, 4-4H and the description of /tʃ/ in Figure 5 in Chapter 4.

1.   The Position of the Tongue, Teeth, and Lips

The initial position for /tʃ/ is similar to the placement of the stop sound /t/. Place the front of your tongue in broad firm contact with the back of your upper gum ridge. Press the edges of your tongue firmly against the bottoms of your upper back teeth, helping to compress the breath trapped behind your tongue. This contact will also prevent your breath from escaping over the sides of your tongue, causing a lateral lisp. Push your lips forward and round them slightly.

2.   The Escaping Breath

The second position for /tʃ/ resembles an explosively pronounced /ʃ/. Slowly begin lowering the front of your tongue. As your tongue pulls away from your upper gum ridge, blow the breath out of your mouth with an explosive friction-like quality. The combination of the initial stop and the final slow, explosive frictionlike movement into /ʃ/ creates the affricate /tʃ/.

B.   Special Suggestions for Pronouncing /tʃ/ Acceptably

A few additional suggestions are offered because of the complexity involved in pronouncing an acceptable /tʃ/.

1.   The Lateral Lisp

Review the comments about avoiding a lateral lisp when pronouncing /ʃ/ in Chap. 11, 11-4B.

2.   The Substitution of /ʃ/ for /tʃ/

Concentrate on feeling your tongue in contact with the upper gum ridge as you begin pronuncing the target. Without gum ridge contact you will produce /ʃ/.

3.   The Substitution of /ts/ for /tʃ/

Concentrate on pulling your tongue back in the mouth for /ʃ/. /s/ is formed in the area of the mouth where the front teeth join the upper gum ridge, while

/ʃ/ is formed just behind the area where the hard palate joins the upper gum ridge. If you do not move your tongue back as you pull it away from your upper gum ridge, you will pronounce /s/.

C.   Pronouncing /tʃ/ in Familiar Words

Pronounce each of the following words carefully. If you are either practicing with your instructor or listening to the exercise on tape, imitate your speech model as accurately as possible.

Beginning	Middle	End
1. cheerful	1. adventure	1. rich
2. chance	2. butcher	2. which
3. change	3. benches	3. match
4. charge	4. perching	4. perch
5. chase	5. hitching	5. pouch
6. cheer	6. reaching	6. patch
7. chew	7. matching	7. reach
8. chief	8. watching	8. hitch
9. children	9. branching	9. ditch
10. chilly	10. bunching	10. each
11. chopping	11. pitcher	11. church
12. chair	12. patching	12. beach
13. chin	13. beaches	
14. choose	14. peaches	
15. cherry	15. furniture	
16. chain	16. lunchroom	
17. chess		

D.   Pronouncing Word Pairs Containing /tʃ/ and a Replacement

Select some of the words from the paired lists in Section 14-2B containing /tʃ/ and your replacement. Read one pair of words at a time, pronouncing the word with the target first (e.g., **match–mats**). Make sure that you are saying /tʃ/ first and /ts/ second. Reverse the procedure, and pronounce the replacement word first and the target word second, making certain that you use /ts/ first and /tʃ/ second. Try to develop speed and accuracy as you do the drill. If you are either practicing with your instructor or listening to the exercise on tape, imitate your speech model as accurately as possible. If you are listening to the taped exercise, listen *only* to the drill that compares the target with your particular replacement. You will find this drill more difficult than the word list in Section 14-4C because of the closeness of target and replacement.

E. PRONOUNCING FAMILIAR WORDS
CONTAINING FREQUENT /tʃ/ CONSONANT CLUSTERS

You may find this exercise the most difficult of all the drills dealing with the pronunciation of /tʃ/ in single words. It is often much more difficult to pronounce a consonant target when it is combined with another consonant in a cluster. Pronounce each of the words carefully. If you are either practicing with your instructor or listening to the drill on tape, imitate your speech model as accurately as possible.

/ntʃ/	/tʃt/
1. lunch	1. hitched
2. bunch	2. patched
3. branch	3. reached
4. French	4. searched
5. bench	5. watched
6. pinch	6. marched
7. ranch	
8. inch	

F. PRONOUNCING /tʃ/ IN PHRASES

Pronounce each of the phrases carefully. If you mispronounce a word, say it over again several times, and then repeat the entire phrase. If you are either practicing with your instructor or listening to the drill on tape, imitate your speech model as accurately as possible.

1. eight **Dutch children**
2. **pinch** the pork **chops**
3. **charge** the bill **cheerfully**
4. **reached** to **touch** the **chip** of wood
5. **watched** too **much hitchhiking**

G. PRONOUNCING SHORT PHRASES
CONTAINING /tʃ/ AND A REPLACEMENT

This drill is similar to the exercise in Section 14-4D, except that your replacement precedes the target in each phrase. Pronounce each of the phrases carefully. If you are either practicing with your instructor or listening to the exercise on tape, imitate your speech model as accurately as possible. If you are listening to the taped exercise, listen *only* to the drill that compares your target with your particular replacement. Although these phrase are shorter than those in the preceding drill, you may find this exercise more difficult because your replacement directly precedes /tʃ/ in each phrase.

/ʃ/ – /tʃ/		/ts/ – /tʃ/
1. English cheese	6. fish chowder	1. eats cheerfully
2. fresh chicken	7. crash charge	2. Pete's chair
3. foolish child	8. fish chips	3. hits children
4. finish chewing	9. selfish choosing	4. cuts cherries
5. fresh cherries		5. coats charged

H. PRONOUNCING /tʃ/ IN SENTENCES

Pronounce each of the sentences carefully. If you use a replacement, say the word over again several times and then repeat the entire sentence. If you are either practicing with your instructor or listening to the exercise on tape, imitate your speech model as accurately as possible.

1. They **chose** some **benches** and **chairs** to bring to the **church.**
2. They gave **each** of the **rich children** a **chocolate chicken** egg for Easter.
3. The **teacher** gave the **child** another **chance** to answer the **question.**
4. The **butcher chased** us along the **chilly beach** but he couldn't **catch** us.
5. He wanted a **cheese sandwich** and a slice of **peach** or **cherry** pie for **lunch.**
6. From **Charlie's porch** the **ranch stretched** for miles across the **pasture** land.

I. PRONOUNCING /tʃ/ IN BEGINNING CONVERSATION

This exercise gives you an opportunity to begin using some of your previously learned /tʃ/ words in beginning conversation. Complete instructions for this type of drill are given in Chap. 5, 5-4H. Read the instructions, and adapt them to practice with /tʃ/.

1. "Did you **watch** _____ on television?"
2. "Did you **choose** the _____ ?"
3. "Are you **searching** for a _____ ?"
4. "Did you **exchange** the _____ ?"
5. "Is the _____ in the **kitchen**?"
6. "Will you have a **chance** to buy the _____ ?"
7. "Can you **reach** the _____ ?"
8. "Do the **children** want some _____ for dinner?"
9. "Is the _____ on the **porch**?"
10. "Please buy me a **bunch** of _____ at the florists."

14–5.   CONVERSATION PRACTICE

So far you have learned how to pronounce your target by reading various kinds of exercises which contain /tʃ/ words. Now you are ready to move into the final and most important part of your training program—learning to pronounce /tʃ/ automatically while you are talking more or less spontaneously. If this is the first practice chapter assigned to you by your instructor, you may wish to review the introductory comments on conversation practice in Chap. 2, 2-6 to 2-7.

A.   CARRYING /tʃ/ INTO SPONTANEOUS DAILY CONVERSATION

This exercise requires you to use /tʃ/ in daily conversation, starting with key words and expanding to all the /tʃ/ words in your particular vocabulary. Complete instructions for this type of drill are given in Chap. 5, 5-5A, and there are supplementary comments about the exercise in Chap. 2, 2-7A.

B.   GENERAL CLASSROOM EXERCISES IN SPEAKING

Your instructor will plan a series of classroom conversation activities, and each assignment will be discussed fully in class before you carry it out. When your instructor announces the first speaking activity, you may wish to review the introductory comments on classroom speaking in Chap. 2, 2-7B.

chapter fifteen

The Consonant Target
/dʒ/ (juice)

COMMON SPELLINGS FOR /dʒ/

The most frequent spellings are found in the following words: **j**uice and he**dge**; less frequent spellings include sol**di**er, ma**g**ic, and e**du**cation.

15–1. EAR TRAINING FOR THE /dʒ/ TARGET

A. A Few Reminders About Ear Training

The following test exercises will help you learn to recognize your /dʒ/ target. If this is the first practice chapter assigned to you by your instructor, you may wish to review the discussion about listening practice in Chap. 2, 2-2B to 2-3C.

134

B.   RECOGNIZING /dʒ/ IN WORDS

You will hear a list of words containing /dʒ/. After listening to each word, write *B* if you heard /dʒ/ at the beginning of the word, *M* if you heard /dʒ/ in the middle, and *E* if you heard /dʒ/ at the end of the word. The answers will be read to you at the end of the drill. This exercise is found in Appendix 1. If you have difficulty recognizing the target, you may find it worthwhile to review the test with somebody outside of class.

C.   RECOGNIZING /dʒ/ IN SENTENCES

You will listen to a series of sentences containing a number of /dʒ/ words. Each sentence will be read several times. Try to locate the /dʒ/ words in each sentence and write them down. The /dʒ/ words in each test sentence will be read to you at the end of the drill. The sentences appear later in the chapter in Section 15-4H. If you have difficulty recognizing the target, you may find it worthwhile to review the test with somebody outside class.

15–2.   DISCRIMINATING BETWEEN /dʒ/ AND
         THE VARIOUS REPLACEMENTS

A.   PROBABLE TYPES OF REPLACEMENT

The following exercises will help you learn to compare /dʒ/ with your replacement. You are probably substituting one of the following common replacements for /dʒ/: (1) /ʒ/ as in measure, (2) /tʃ/ as in **ch**ip, (3) /j/ as in **y**ellow, (4) the consonant cluster /dz/ as in lea**ds**, or (5) you may have a lateral lisp on the /ʒ/ portion of the target and use a distortion that resembles a voiced fricative /l/.[1] Your instructor will tell you which replacement you are using. If you are not employing one of the more common replacements, your teacher will tell you exactly how you are mispronouncing /dʒ/ and provide you with some discrimination drills.

B.   PAIRED LISTS OF WORDS

The words in the following paired lists are identical, except that the words in Column 1 contain the target and the words in Column 2 contain one of the replacements. Complete instructions for this type of exercise are given in Chap. 5, 5-2B.

---

[1]A description of this lateral lisp is found in Chapter 10, 10-2A.

1.	Column 1	Column 2	2.	Column 1	Column 2	3.	Column 1	Column 2
	/dʒ/	/dz/		/dʒ/	/j/		/dʒ/	/tʃ/
	age	aids		jam	yam		Jew	chew
	rage	raids		jail	Yale		gin	chin
	edge	Ed's		jello	yellow		Jerry	cherry
	hedge	heads		jet	yet		Jill	chill
	ridge	rids		Jew	you		joke	choke
	budge	buds		joke	yoke		Joe's	chose
	wage	wades					jump	chump
							Jane	chain
							jar	char
							edging	etching
							lunging	lunching
							edge	etch
							lunge	lunch
							Madge	match
							ridge	rich

C.   PAIRED SENTENCES

The following paired sentences are identical except that the key word in the first sentence contains /dʒ/, and the key word in the second sentence contains one of the replacements. Complete instructions for this type of exercise are given in Chap. 5, 5-2C.

/dʒ/ – /j/

1. I ate the jam.
   I ate the yam.
2. He went to jail.
   He went to Yale.
3. He likes jello.
   He likes yellow.
4. I like the joke.
   I like the yoke.

/dʒ/ – /tʃ/

1. It's near his gin.
   It's near his chin.
2. The joke was old.
   The choke was old.
3. He was edging the grass.
   He was etching the grass.

D.   LISTENING FOR REPLACEMENTS IN FAMILAR /dʒ/ WORDS

You will hear a list of words containing /dʒ/. Sometimes the words will be pronounced correctly with /dʒ/; other times the words will be said incorrectly with your replacement. In the event that you have a lateral lisp, your instructor will imitate your distorted /dʒ/. Complete instructions for this type of drill are found in Chap. 5, 5-2D.

15–3.   A FEW REMINDERS ABOUT ORAL PRACTICE PROCEDURES

If this is the first practice chapter assigned to you by your instructor, you may wish to review the comments about beginning oral practice in Chap. 2,

2-4. Before you actually begin practicing each individual pronunciation drill, you may also desire to review the supplementary explanations about the exercise in Chap. 2, 2-5.

15–4.   THE PRONUNCIATION OF /dʒ/

A.   PRONOUNCING ISOLATED /dʒ/

In the event that you cannot pronounce /dʒ/ through imitation alone, your instructor will help you with the following suggestions about placement. Should placement be required, you should review the definition of an affricate in Chap. 4, 4-4H and the description of /dʒ/ in Figure 5 in Chapter 4.

1.   The Position of the Tongue, Teeth, and Lips

The initial position for /dʒ/ is similar to the placement of the stop sound /d/. Place the front of your tongue in broad firm contact with the back of your upper gum ridge. Press the edges of your tongue firmly against the bottoms of your upper back teeth, helping to compress the breath trapped behind your tongue. This contact will also prevent your breath from escaping over the sides of your tongue, causing a lateral lisp. Push your lips forward and round them slightly.

2.   The Escaping Breath

The second position for /dʒ/ resembles an explosively pronounced /ʒ/. Slowly begin lowering the front of your tongue. As your tongue pulls away from your upper gum ridge, blow the voiced breath out of your mouth with an explosive friction-like quality. The combination of the initial stop and the final slow, explosive, vocalized friction-like movement into /ʒ/ creates the affricate /dʒ/. Make sure that you are producing vocal-band vibration by placing your fingers on your larynx as you pronounce /dʒ/. If you are unable to feel the vibration from your own larynx, your instructor will place your fingers on his larynx and say /dʒ/. Keep practicing until you can feel the vibration from your own larynx while saying /dʒ/. When that happens, you can double-check your pronunciation of /dʒ/ by placing your hands over your ears while pronouncing the target. You should be able to hear the vibration. If your tongue is placed in the correct position, and you do not feel or hear the vibration, you are pronouncing /tʃ/ rather than /dʒ/. The primary difference between /tʃ/ and /dʒ/ is voicing.

B.   SPECIAL SUGGESTIONS FOR PRONOUNCING /dʒ/ ACCEPTABLY

A few additional suggestions are offered because of the complexity involved in pronouncing an acceptable /dʒ/.

1. The Lateral Lisp

Review the comments about avoiding a lateral lisp when pronouncing /ʒ/ in Chap. 12, 12-4B.

2. The Substitution of /j/ for /dʒ/

Concentrate on feeling your tongue in contact with the upper gum ridge as you begin pronouncing the target. Without gum-ridge contact you will produce /j/.

3. The Substitution of /dz/ for /dʒ/

Concentrate on pulling your tongue back in the mouth for /ʒ/. /z/ is formed in the area of the mouth where the front teeth join the upper gum ridge, while /ʒ/ is formed just behind the area where the hard palate joins the upper gum ridge. If you do not move your tongue back as you pull it away from your upper gum ridge, you will pronounce /z/.

C. Pronouncing /dʒ/ in Familiar Words

Pronounce each of the following words carefully. If you are either practicing with your instructor or listening to the exercise on tape, imitate your speech model as accurately as possible.

Beginning		Middle		End[2]	
1. jam	11. joke	1. engine	1. George	11. hedge
2. jacket	12. joy	2. enjoy	2. judge	12. language
3. June	13. Joe	3. imagine	3. bridge	13. manage
4. July	14. juicy	4. magic	4. cage	14. package
5. January	15. just	5. vegetable	5. cabbage	15. rage
6. jelly	16. job	6. magician	6. stage	
7. jail	17. John	7. pigeon	7. page	
8. gym	18. Japan	8. soldier	8. badge	
9. Jim	19. jaw	9. angel	9. college	
10. jungle	20. general	10. major	10. age	

D. Pronouncing Word Pairs Containing /dʒ/ and a Replacement

Select some of the words from the paired lists in Section 15-2B containing /dʒ/ and your replacement. Read one pair of words at a time, pronouncing the word with the target first (e.g., **age**–**aids**.) Make sure that you are saying /dʒ/ first and /dz/ second. Reverse the procedure and pronounce the replacement

[2]If you have difficulty pronouncing final /dʒ/, read footnote 3 in Chapter 8, and adapt the comments to the pronunciation of final voiced /dʒ/.

word first and the target word second, making certain that you use /dz/ first and /dʒ/ second. Try to develop speed and accuracy as you do the drill. If you are either practicing with your instructor or listening to the exercise on tape, imitate your speech model as accurately as possible. If you are listening to the taped exercise, listen *only* to the drill that compares the target with your particular replacement. You will find this drill more difficult than the word list in Section 15-4C because of the closeness of target and replacement.

E.   PRONOUNCING FAMILIAR WORDS CONTAINING FREQUENT /dʒ/ CONSONANT CLUSTERS

You may find this exercise the most difficult of all the drills dealing with the pronunciation of /dʒ/ in single words. It is often much more difficult to pronounce a consonant target when it is combined with another consonant in a cluster. Pronounce each of the words carefully. If you are either practicing with your instructor or listening to the drill on tape, imitate your speech model as accurately as possible.

/dʒd/	/ndʒ/	/ndʒd/
1. caged	1. strange	1. changed
2. judged	2. change	2. sponged
3. edged	3. orange	3. arranged
4. raged	4. arrange	
5. managed		

F.   PRONOUNCING /dʒ/ IN PHRASES

Pronounce each of the phrases carefully. If you mispronounce a word, say it over again several times and then repeat the entire phrase. If you are either practicing with your instructor or listening to the drill on tape, imitate your speech model as accurately as possible.

1.   a **package** of **orange juice**
2.   a **jet engine changed**
3.   a **junior** in **college**
4.   **just** some **ginger** ale for the **soldier**
5.   **enjoying Jim's** blue **jeans**

G.   PRONOUNCING SHORT PHRASES CONTAINING /dʒ/ AND A REPLACEMENT

This drill is similar to the exercise in Section 15-4D, except that your replacement precedes the target in each phrase. Pronounce each of the phrases carefully.

If you are either practicing with your instructor or listening to the exercise on tape, imitate your speech model as accurately as possible. If you are listening to the taped exercise, listen *only* to the drill that compares your target with your particular replacement. Although these phrases are shorter than those in the preceding drill, you may find this exercise more difficult, because your replacement directly precedes /dʒ/ in each phrase.

/tʃ/ – /dʒ/		/dz/ – /dʒ/
1. catch judy	7. reach John	1. aids John
2. match George	8. peach juice	2. needs joy
3. watch Jack	9. peach jam	3. adds just fine
4. touch Jim	10. French general	4. feeds Joe
5. teach Jill	11. rich judge	5. bird's jaw
6. scratch Joe	12. lunch jars	6. weds Jane

H. PRONOUNCING /dʒ/ IN SENTENCES

Pronounce each of the sentences carefully. If you use a replacement, say the word over again several times, and then repeat the entire sentence. If you are either practicing with your instructor or listening to the exercise on tape, imitate your speech model as accurately as possible.

1. **George, Judy,** and **Roger enjoy** eating boiled **cabbage.**
2. The **bluejay** saw the **dangerous** cat and **jumped** out of the **hedge** near the **garbage** truck.
3. The **strange**-looking **passenger** took his **large package** and walked across the **bridge.**
4. **Jill** put some **juicy oranges,** some **gingerbread,** and a **jar** of **jam** into the **refrigerator.**
5. **Jean** couldn't understand the **jolly German gentleman's language.**

I. PRONOUNCING /dʒ/ IN BEGINNING CONVERSATION

This exercise gives you an opportunity to begin using some of your previously learned /dʒ/ words in beginning conversation. Complete instructions for this type of drill are given in Chap. 5, 5-4H. Read the instructions and adapt them to practice with /dʒ/.

1. "Will you **graduate** in _____?"
2. "Were you **jaywalking** on _____?"
3. "Is the color of your new **Dodge** _____?"
4. "Did he **exchange** the _____?"

5. "Can the **magician** make the _____ disappear?"

6. "Did you lose your _____ in the **gym**?"

7. "**Joe** is the **manager** of the _____."

8. "Did you leave your _____ on the **stage**?"

9. "The **major** went to _____."

15–5.   CONVERSATION PRACTICE

So far you have learned how to pronounce your target by reading various kinds of exercises which contain /dʒ/ words. Now you are ready to move into the final and most important part of your training program—learning to pronounce /dʒ/ automatically while you are talking more or less spontaneously. If this is the first practice chapter assigned to you by your instructor, you may wish to review the introductory comments on conversation in Chap. 2, 2-6 to 2-7.

A.   CARRYING /dʒ/ INTO SPONTANEOUS DAILY CONVERSATION

This exercise requires you to use /dʒ/ in daily conversation, starting with key words and expanding to all the /dʒ/ words in your particular vocabulary. Complete instructions for this type of drill are given in Chap. 5, 5-5A, and there are supplementary comments about the exercise in Chap. 2, 2-7A.

B.   GENERAL CLASSROOM EXERCISES IN SPEAKING

Your instructor will plan a series of classroom conversation activities, and each assignment will be discussed fully in class before you carry it out. When your instructor announces the first speaking activity, you may wish to review the introductory comments on classroom speaking in Chap. 2, 2-7B.

chapter sixteen

The Consonant Target
/l/ (lap)[1]

COMMON SPELLINGS FOR /l/

The most frequent spelling is found in the word lap; a less frequent spelling is found in the word till.

[1] There are two basic types or variants of /l/: (1) the "light" or "clear" /l/, and (2) the "dark" /l/. The light /l/ is generally found initially before front vowels (e.g., leave, live, and laugh). The dark /l/ is generally found initially before back vowels and in other positions (e.g., lose, telephone, gulf, and full). Wise indicates that in General American speech all /l/ sounds are dark. In Eastern American and Southern American English the consonant /l/ is clear when it occurs before a front vowel and is dark elsewhere. See C. M. Wise, *Applied Phonetics* (Englewood Cliffs, N.J.: Prentice-Hall, Inc., 1957), pp. 131–132. For this reason all /l/ sounds are considered dark in this chapter. If you live in an area where clear /l/ is used, retain this pronunciation. If you have any questions about the use of clear /l/ in your dialect, ask your instructor. The difference between light and dark /l/ depends upon variations in tongue position. The description of these differences is found in Sections 16-1 to 16-4, and it is essential that you read this discussion carefully in order to clarify the preceding comments about the two types of English /l/.

16–1. EAR TRAINING FOR THE /l/ TARGET

A. A FEW REMINDERS ABOUT EAR TRAINING

The following test exercises will help you learn to recognize your /l/ target. If this is the first practice chapter assigned to you by your instructor, you may wish to review the discussion about listening practice in Chap. 2, 2-B to 2-3C.

The ear training exercises for /l/ require a few additional special remarks, because the replacements differ so decisively. Note the following types of replacements.

1. You substitute /r/ as in rap for /l/.
2. You substitute /n/ as in not for /l/.
3. You substitute clear /l/ for dark /l/ in all /l/ words.
4. You substitute a vowel for /l/. The vowel is usually /ə/ as in about, /ʊ/ as in pull, or /o/ as in post. This type of replacement is typically found before stop sounds and in place of final /l/, as in build, milk, and mill.
5. You omit /l/ after vowels in words like self, help, and twelve.
6. You substitute a vowel—usually /ə/—for syllabic /l̩/ in words like battle and saddle, which forms /əl/ rather than /l̩/.[2]

Because of these various types of replacement pronunciations, several kinds of ear training drills are used in this chapter. Your instructor will tell you which exercise he wants you to carry out.

B. RECOGNIZING /l/ IN WORDS
WHEN THE REPLACEMENT IS /r/, /n/, A VOWEL, OR AN OMISSION

You will hear a list of words containing /l/. After listening to each word, write *B* if you heard /l/ at the beginning of the word, *M* if you heard /l/ in the middle, and *E* if you heard /l/ at the end of the word. The answers will be read to you at the end of the drill. This exercise is found in Appendix 1. If you have difficulty recognizing the target, you may find it worthwhile to review the test with somebody outside class.

C. RECOGNIZING /l/ IN SENTENCES
WHEN THE REPLACEMENT IS /r/, /n/, A VOWEL, OR AN OMISSION

You will listen to a series of sentences containing a number of /l/ words. Each sentence will be read several times. Try to locate the /l/ words in each sen-

---

[2]/l/ may become syllabic and replace a vowel when it has a common point of articulation with the preceding consonant. Thus /t/ as in tie, /d/ as in die, and /l/ are all formed on the upper gum ridge, and /l/ becomes syllabic after them in words like battle and saddle. A description of syllabic /l̩/ is found in Section 16-4.

tence and write them down. The /l/ words in each test sentence will be read to you at the end of the drill. The sentences appear later in the chapter in Section 16-4I. If you have difficulty recognizing the target, you may find it worthwhile to review the test with somebody outside class.

D. RECOGNIZING DARK /l/

In the following exercise your instructor will help you learn to recognize the quality of dark /l/. You will hear a list of words containing /l/ in various positions. Listen carefully to your instructor's pronunciation, and familiarize yourself with the quality of dark /l/. This exercise is found in Appendix 1. If you have difficulty recognizing dark /l/, you may find it worthwhile to review the test with somebody outside class.

E. RECOGNIZING SYLLABIC /l̩/

In the following exercise your instructor will help you learn to recognize the pronunciation of syllabic /l̩/. You will hear a list of words containing syllabic /l̩/. Listen carefully to your instructor's pronunciation and familiarize yourself with the pronunciation of syllabic /l̩/. This exercise is found in Appendix 1. If you have difficulty recognizing syllabic /l̩/, you may find it worthwhile to review the test with somebody outside class.

16–2. DISCRIMINATING BETWEEN /l/ AND THE VARIOUS REPLACEMENTS

A. PROBABLE TYPES OF REPLACEMENT

The following exercises will help you learn to compare /l/ with your replacement. Your instructor has already told you which of the more common replacements you are using. If you are not employing one of these more common replacements, your instructor will tell you exactly how you are mispronouncing /l/ and provide you with some discrimination drills.

B. PAIRED LISTS OF WORDS

The words in the following paired lists are identical, except that the words in Column 1 contain the target, and the words in Column 2 contain one of the replacements. Complete instructions for this type of exercise are given in Chap. 5, 5-2B.

1.	**Column 1** /l/	**Column 2** /r/	2.	**Column 1** /l/	**Column 2** /n/
	load	road		lock	knock
	low	row		lice	nice
	lock	rock		lead	need
	leaf	reef		life	knife
	lamp	ramp		lap	nap
	liver	river		let	net
	lice	rice		loose	noose
	long	wrong		lot	knot
	lap	rap		lip	nip
	lungs	rungs		mile	mine
	lead	reed		meal	mean
	led	red		seal	seen
	lake	rake		pail	pain
	laid	raid		fill	fin
	alive	arrive			

C. Paired Sentences

The following paired sentences are identical except that the final word in the first sentence contains /l/, and the final word in the second sentence contains one of the replacements. Complete instructions for this type of drill are given in Chap. 5, 5-2C.

/l/ – /r/	/l/ – /n/
1. Where's the load?	1. He has a lead.
Where's the road?	He has a need.
2. He has the lock.	2. It's my life.
He has the rock.	It's my knife.
3. I see the leaf.	3. He has a lot.
I see the reef.	He has a knot.
4. Put it on the lamp.	4. He has a pail.
Put it on the ramp.	He has a pain.
5. I think it's long.	
I think it's wrong.	
6. Did you see the liver?	
Did you see the river?	

D. Listening for Replacements in Familiar /l/ Words

You will hear a list of words containing /l/. Sometimes the words will be pronounced correctly with /l/; other times the words will be said incorrectly with your replacement. Complete instructions for this drill are found in Chap. 5, 5-2D.

16–3. A FEW REMINDERS ABOUT ORAL PRACTICE PROCEDURES

If this is the first practice chapter assigned to you by your instructor, you may wish to review the comments about beginning oral practice in Chap. 2, 2-4. Before you actually begin practicing each individual pronunciation drill, you may also desire to review the supplementary explanations about the exercise in Chap. 2, 2-5.

16–4. THE PRONUNCIATION OF /l/

A. PRONOUNCING ISOLATED /l/

In the event that you cannot pronounce /l/ through imitation alone, your instructor will help you with the following suggestions about placement. Should placement be required, you should review the definition of a lateral in Chap. 4, 4-4H and the description of /l/ in Figure 5 in Chapter 4.

1. The Position of the Tongue for Dark /l/

The tongue tip is pressed firmly against the upper gum ridge, and the back of the tongue is raised high in the mouth toward the soft palate. The high tongue tip and the high back create a depression in the middle of the tongue. Your contact against the upper gum ridge is particularly important, because if you fail to make this contact you are likely to substitute /r/, a vowel, or simply omit the target. Concentrate on feeling your tongue tip in contact with the upper gum ridge as you pronounce /l/. The contact is clearly visible, and a small mirror should help you see what you are doing.

2. The Position of the Tongue for Clear /l/

The contact between the tongue tip and the upper gum ridge is identical to the contact for dark /l/. There are two differences, however: (1) the back of the tongue is low in the mouth for clear /l/, and (2) a larger portion of the front of the tongue is raised in the front of the mouth for clear /l/. These positional tongue differences are particularly important if you substitute clear /l/ for/dark /l/. In this event, be certain to concentrate on keeping the back of your tongue high in your mouth and avoid raising the front of your tongue too much.

3. The Escaping Breath

The escape of the breath is identical for both /l/ variants. The consonant /l/ is voiced. When your tongue is properly positioned, force the voiced breath stream steadily out of your mouth around one or both sides of your tongue. This part of pronouncing /l/ is especially important if your replacement is /n/. When you produce /n/ your tongue is also pressed against your upper gum ridge, but you are sending your voiced breath stream out of your nose. Check this aspect of your pronunciation by saying the target and lightly placing your fingers on your nostrils. If you pronounce /n/ you should feel some vibration as the breath escapes through your nose; if you pronounce /l/ you will not feel this vibration.

B. PRONOUNCING SYLLABIC /l̩/

We noted earlier that the target may become syllabic when it has a common point of articulation with a preceding consonant such as /t/ or /d/. Syllabic /l̩/ always occurs in a weak-stressed syllable. It is formed by keeping the tongue tip on the upper gum ridge after the preceding /t/ or /d/, and then laterally exploding the /t/ or /d/ by quickly lowering the sides of the tongue. Try saying the word **battle** slowly. If you are successful in keeping your tongue tip pressed against your gum ridge for /t/ and /l/, you will pronounce syllabic /l̩/. If, however, you remove your tongue tip from the gum ridge after having pronounced /t/ and then bring it back up for /l/, you will produce /əl/. If this occurs, say **battle** several times, and concentrate on keeping your tongue tip pressed against your gum ridge until you can keep it there while exploding /t/ over the sides of your tongue. You should be able to feel a puff of air striking your cheeks as you drop the sides of your tongue and complete the syllabic /l̩/.

C. PRONOUNCING /l/ IN FAMILIAR WORDS

Pronounce each of the following words carefully. If you are either practicing with your instructor or listening to the exercise on tape, imitate your speech model as accurately as possible.

Beginning	Middle	End
1. lad	1. alike	1. coal
2. law	2. allow	2. heel
3. lazy	3. almost	3. hole
4. less	4. along	4. hail
5. life	5. aloud	5. fill
6. luck	6. also	6. fall
7. lying	7. asleep	7. awful
8. lose	8. collect	8. cool
9. lost	9. fellow	9. hall
10. ladder	10. hello	10. hill
11. lettuce	11. believe	11. mail
12. lips	12. ceiling	12. fool
13. large	13. smelling	13. bill
14. laugh	14. swallowing	14. call
15. loud	15. mailbox	15. spoil
16. lesson	16. million	16. steal
	17. William	17. mill
	18. college	18. will
		19. chill
		20. feel
		21. pill

D.   PRONOUNCING WORD PAIRS CONTAINING /l/ AND A REPLACEMENT

Select some of the words from the paired lists in Section 16-2B containing /l/ and your replacement. Read one pair of words at a time, pronouncing the word with the target first (e.g., **low–row**.) Make sure that you are saying /l/ first and /r/ second. Reverse the procedure, and pronounce the replacement word first and the target word second, making certain that you use /r/ first and /l/ second. Try to develop speed and accuracy as you do the drill. If you are either practicing with your instructor or listening to the exercise on tape, imitate your speech model as accurately as possible. If you are listening to the taped exercise, listen *only* to the drill that compares the target with your replacement. You will find this drill more difficult than the word list in Section 16-4C because of the closeness of target and replacement.

E.   PRONOUNCING FAMILIAR WORDS CONTAINING FREQUENT /l/ CONSONANT CLUSTERS

You may find this exercise the most difficult of all the drills dealing with the pronunciation of /l/ in single words. It is often much more difficult to pronounce a consonant target when it is combined with another consonant in a cluster. Pronounce each of the words carefully. If you are either practicing with your instructor or listening to the drill on tape, imitate your speech model as accurately as possible.

/bl/	/kl/	/fl/	/gl/	/pl/	/sl/
1. blaze	1. close	1. flame	1. glue	1. plain	1. slide
2. bless	2. class	2. float	2. glance	2. plan	2. slow
3. blew	3. clean	3. flow	3. glare	3. plenty	3. slap
4. block	4. club	4. flies	4. glow	4. pleasant	4. slip
5. bloom	5. clear	5. flour	5. glass	5. place	5. sloppy

/spl/	/ld/	/lf/	/lt/	/ld/	/lz/
1. splash	1. field	1. myself	1. halt	1. failed	1. feels
2. splendid	2. hold	2. itself	2. melt	2. build	2. shells
	3. old	3. himself	3. salt	3. mold	3. miles
		4. shelf	4. built	4. told	
		5. gulf	5. felt	5. cold	

/lk/	/lp/	/lv/	/lm/	/lvz/
1. silk	1. help	1. twelve	1. film	1. ourselves
2. milk				2. themselves
				3. yourselves

F.   PRONOUNCING SYLLABIC /l̩/ IN FAMILIAR WORDS

Pronounce each of the following words carefully. If you are either practicing with your instructor or listening to the exercise on tape, imitate your speech model as accurately as possible.

1. battle	9. model
2. cradle	10. cattle
3. gentle	11. needle
4. handle	12. petal
5. kettle	13. rattle
6. little	14. medal
7. middle	15. saddle
8. riddle	16. paddle

G.   PRONOUNCING /l/ IN PHRASES

Pronounce each of the phrases carefully. If you mispronounce a word, say it over again several times and then repeat the entire phrase. If you are either practicing with your instructor or listening to the drill on tape, imitate your speech model as accurately as possible.

1.   a pleasant smile in the library
2.   calling to leave the bill early
3.   seal the letter in the envelope
4.   lying by the lovely full blue pool
5.   the loud alarm bell rang at eleven

H.   PRONOUNCING SHORT PHRASES CONTAINING /l/ AND A REPLACEMENT

This drill is similar to the exercise in Section 16-4D, except that your replacement precedes the target in each phrase. Pronounce each of the phrases carefully. If you are either practicing with your instructor or listening to the exercise on tape, imitate your speech model as accurately as possible. If you are listening to the taped exercise, listen *only* to the drill that compares your target with your particular replacement. Although these phrases are shorter than those in the preceding drill, you may find this exercise more difficult, because your replacement directly precedes /l/ in each phrase.

/r/ – /l/	/n/ – /l/
1. far light	1. run loose
2. star lost	2. tin lid
3. jar loose	3. train load
4. more lettuce	4. find ladder
5. door lock	5. seen life
6. car lamp	6. tan liver
7. four lakes	7. none left

I.   PRONOUNCING /l/ IN SENTENCES

Pronounce each of the sentences carefully. If you use a replacement, say the word over again several times and then repeat the entire sentence. If you are

either practicing with your instructor or listening to the exercise on tape, imitate your speech model as accurately as possible.

1. **Billy always slept** in a **black** and **yellow sleeping** bag **while** camping at **Long Lake.**
2. The **gentle lady slipped** and **fell while** running across the **middle** of the **lawn.**
3. **Lee** was **allowed** a **late** snack of **cold milk** and a **little slice** of **lime** pie.
4. **Ellen** didn't **believe** that **English** was an easy **language** to **learn.**
5. The **laughing children** were **leaping** and **yelling** among the **petals** on the **cool hillside.**

J.   PRONOUNCING /l/ IN BEGINNING CONVERSATION

This exercise gives you an opportunity to begin using some of your previously learned /l/ words in beginning conversation. Complete instructions for this type of drill are given in Chap. 5, 5-4H. Read the instructions and adapt them to practice with /l/.

1. "Do you **like** the _____?"
2. "**Will** you **load** the _____ on the truck?"
3. "Did you see the **little** _____?"
4. "I need the **needle** to sew the _____."
5. "Did you **place** the _____ on the **shelf**?"
6. "**Will** you **help** me find the _____?"
7. "Did you **look** for the _____?"
8. "Did you **lose** your _____?"
9. "Do you have **plenty** of _____?"
10. "Was the **telephone call** about the _____?"
11. "**Please** send a **telegram** about the _____."
12. "Did you take the _____ to **school last** week?"
13. "Was the _____ painted **yellow** or **black**?"

16–5.   CONVERSATION PRACTICE

So far you have learned how to pronounce your target by reading various kinds of exercises which contain /l/ words. Now you are ready to move into the final and most important part of your training program—learning how to pronounce /l/ automatically while you are talking more or less spontaneously. If this is the first practice chapter assigned to you by your instructor, you may wish to review the introductory comments on conversation in Chap. 2, 2-6 to 2-7.

A.   CARRYING /l/ INTO SPONTANEOUS DAILY CONVERSATION

This exercise requires you to use /l/ in daily conversation, starting with key words and expanding to all the /l/ words in your particular vocabulary. Complete instructions for this type of drill are given in Chap. 5, 5-5A, and there are supplementary comments about the exercise in Chap. 2, 2-7A.

B.   GENERAL CLASSROOM EXERCISES IN SPEAKING

Your instructor will plan a series of classroom conversation activities, and each assignment will be discussed fully in class before you carry it out. When your instructor announces the first speaking activity, you may wish to review the introductory comments on classroom speaking in Chap. 2, 2-7B.

chapter seventeen

The Consonant Target
/r/ (rap)[1]

COMMON SPELLINGS FOR /r/

The most frequent spelling is found in the word **r**ap; a less frequent spelling is found in the word ma**rr**y.

[1]Certain regional variations among standard American English dialects need to be mentioned in connection with the improvement of the /r/ target. If you speak General American, you normally always pronounce /r/, and you will practice pronouncing /r/ in all of the practice items in this chapter. However, if you speak Eastern or Southern American English your standard pronunciation of /r/ is different. Your dialect is considered to be an "r"-less dialect, because you normally eliminate the consonant /r/ in certain instances. When /r/ follows the vowel /ɑ/ as in **j**ar and **f**ar the final /r/ is typically replaced by a prolonged /ɑ/ (e.g., /fɑ/ and /dʒɑ/). When /r/ is final in other words such as near and sure, the final /r/ is replaced by the vowel /ə/ as in about (e.g., /nɪə/ and /ʃʊə/. When /r/ follows a vowel but precedes another consonant as in **far**m and **four**th, /r/ is either omitted or replaced by /ə/ (e.g., /fɑm/, /fɑəm/, and /fɔəθ/. Thus when you study the target /r/, you will not practice words containing final /r/ or words containing /r/ before a final consonant. Practice only beginning /r/ as in red, middle /r/ between two vowels as in around, and /r/ in beginning consonant clusters as in drew. If you have any questions about the pronunciation of /r/ in your dialect, ask your instructor. If you speak Eastern or Southern American, note the discussion of your regional pronunciation of /ə/ in place of General American "r"-colored /ɚ/ as in (paper) in footnote 1 in Chapter 43. Your Eastern or Southern pronunciation of /ɜ/ as in **b**ird in place of General American "r"-colored

17–1. EAR TRAINING FOR THE /r/ TARGET

A. A Few Reminders About Ear Training

The following test exercises will help you learn to recognize your /r/ target. If this is the first practice chapter assigned to you by your instructor, you may wish to review the discussion about listening practice in Chap. 2, 2-B to 2-3C.

B. Recognizing /r/ in Words

You will hear a list of words containing /r/. After listening to each word, write *B* if you heard /r/ at the beginning of the word, *M* if you heard /r/ in the middle, and *E* if you heard /r/ at the end of the word. The answers will be read to you at the end of the drill. This exercise is found in Appendix 1. If you have difficulty recognizing the target, you may find it worthwhile to review the test with somebody outside class.

C. Recognizing /r/ in Sentences

You will listen to a series of sentences containing a number of /r/ words. Each sentence will be read several times. Try to locate the /r/ words in each sentence, and write them down. The /r/ words in each test sentence will be read to you at the end of the drill. The sentences appear later in the chapter in Section 17-4H. If you have difficulty recognizing the target, you may find it worthwhile to review the test with somebody outside class.

17–2. DISCRIMINATING BETWEEN /r/ AND THE VARIOUS REPLACEMENTS

A. Probable Types of Replacement

The following exercises will help you learn to compare /r/ with your replacement. You are probably substituting one of the following common replacements for /r/: (1) /l/ as in lap, (2) /w/ as in we, (3) a /r/ that is pronounced with a gum-ridge trill—that is, the /r/ is made with one or more strokes or taps of the tongue tip against the upper gum ridge, or (4) a /r/ that is made with a uvula trill—that is, the back of the tongue is raised and placed in contact with the uvula; the uvula then vibrates from the force of the escaping breath. Your instructor will tell you which replacement you are using. If you are not employing

---

/ɝ/ as in bird is discussed in footnote 1 in Chapter 42. Keep in mind that the speaker who does not always pronounce /r/ in his dialect generally uses /ə/ and /ɜ/ in his speech. Conversely, the speaker who always uses /r/ also employs /ɚ/ and /ɝ/ in his speech.

one of the more common replacements, your teacher will tell you exactly how you are mispronouncing /r/ and provide you with some discrimination drills.

B.   Paired Lists of Words

The words in the following paired lists are identical, except that the words in Column 1 contain the target and the words in Column 2 contain one of the replacements. Complete instructions for this type of exercise are given in Chap. 5, 5-2B.

1.	Column 1 /r/	Column 2 /l/	2.	Column 1 /r/	Column 2 /w/
	road	load		reads	weeds
	row	low		rent	went
	rock	lock		ride	wide
	reef	leaf		ring	wing
	ramp	lamp		rise	wise
	river	liver		rest	west
	rice	lice		rake	wake
	wrong	long		rag	wag
	rap	lap		run	one
	rungs	lungs		roar	wore
	reed	lead		ripe	wipe
	red	led		reap	weep

C.   Paired Sentences

The following paired sentences are identical, except that the final word in the first sentence contains /r/, and the final word in the second sentence contains one of the replacements. Complete instructions for this type of drill are found in Chap. 5, 5-2C.

/r/ – /l/	/r/ – /w/
1. Where's the road? Where's the load?	1. He's trying to read. He's trying to weed.
2. He has the rock. He has the lock.	2. I see the ring. I see the wing.
3. I see the reef. I see the leaf.	3. I like the rest. I like the west.
4. Put it on the ramp. Put it on the lamp.	4. Was he reaping? Was he weeping?
5. I think it's wrong. I think it's long.	
6. Did you see the river? Did you see the liver?	

D.   Listening for Replacements in Familiar /r/ Words

You will hear a list of words containing /r/. Sometimes the words will be pronounced correctly with /r/; other times the words will be said incorrectly with your replacement. Complete instructions for this drill are found in Chap. 5, 5-2D.

17–3.   A FEW REMINDERS ABOUT ORAL PRACTICE PROCEDURES

If this is the first practice chapter assigned to you by your instructor, you may wish to review the comments about beginning oral practice in Chap. 2, 2-4. Before you actually begin practicing each individual pronunciation drill, you may also desire to review the supplementary explanations about the exercise in Chap. 2, 2-5.

17–4.   THE PRONUNCIATION OF /r/

A.   Pronouncing /r/ in a Simple Syllable

In the event that you cannot pronounce /r/ through imitation alone, your instructor will help you with the following suggestions about placement. Should placement be required, you should review the definition of a glide in Chap. 4, 4-4H, and the description of /r/ in Figure 5 in Chapter 4. Note that because of the glide characteristics of the consonant, the target cannot be pronounced in isolation.

1.   The Position of the Tongue

The basic position for your tongue is very close to the /ɝ/ or /ɚ/ vowel positions. Press the edges of your tongue against the bottoms of your upper back teeth. Now try to curl and raise your tongue tip back toward the area just behind your upper gum ridge. Be careful not to touch your gum ridge with your tongue tip. If you do this, you are liable to pronounce the trilled gum ridge replacement or the /l/ replacement. If you find that you cannot avoid touching your gum ridge, you might try an alternative position. Arch the blade of your tongue toward the front of your hard palate, and keep your tongue tip low and pointed toward the bottoms of your lower front teeth. Always keep the back of your tongue low in order to avoid the uvula trill. When you place your tongue properly either way, you are basically in the position for /ɝ/ or /ɚ/.

2.   The Movement of the Tongue

/r/ is a voiced glide which is heard as your tongue moves from one position to another; it is literally an in-motion sound. The quality of /r/ becomes clear *only* as the tongue moves or glides from position to position. When /r/ precedes a vowel, the second position occurs as your tongue quickly glides from /ɝ/ or /ɚ/ to the position of the following vowel (e.g., **rea**d). The lips adopt the position of the following vowel. When /r/ follows a vowel the glide is from that vowel in the direction of either /ɝ/ or /ɚ/ (e.g., **far**).

B.   SPECIAL SUGGESTIONS FOR PRONOUNCING /r/ ACCEPTABLY

Many students, regardless of the nature of their /r/ problem, have difficulty pronouncing this target. The following steps are suggested to help you begin producing an acceptable /r/. Essentially the procedure is to learn to pronounce an acceptable /ɝ/, and then learn to develop the required gliding movement.

1.   Begin pronouncing /ɑ/.
2.   As you say /ɑ/, gradually raise your tongue and lower jaw until the edges of your tongue contact the bottoms of your upper back teeth.
3.   Continue raising your tongue tip, and begin curling it behind your upper gum ridge. Tense your tongue slightly. As your tongue comes into position, you should begin hearing the sound of /ɝ/. The amount of curl varies from speaker to speaker. Experiment until your instructor tells you that you are producing an acceptable /ɝ/. Continue practicing until you can glide your tongue easily and rapidly from /ɑ/ to /ɝ/. When you develop a quick gliding movement away from /ɑ/ you will begin hearing final /r/ as in /ɑr/. Now you are read for the next step, pronouncing initial /r/.[2]
4.   Plan to say a syllable beginning with initial /r/ such as /rɑ/. Pronounce /ɝ/, prolong it for a second, and then glide your tongue to the vowel /ɑ/. If you handle the glide correctly, you will hear /ɝrɑ/ as you pass through /r/ on the way to /ɑ/. If you fail to develop the glide, you will pronounce only the vowels /ɝ/ and /ɑ/. Keep working for a smooth gliding movement away from /ɝ/. Remember that without the gliding movement you will not produce the /r/ target. Continue practicing until you can pronounce /rɑ/ without starting with a prolonged /ɝ/. Begin attempting other syllables, and then proceed into words containing initial /r/. Then attempt medial and final /r/ words.

C.   PRONOUNCING /r/ IN FAMILIAR WORDS

Pronounce each of the following words carefully. If you are either practicing with your instructor or listening to the exercise on tape, imitate your speech model as accurately as possible.

---

[2]Note that there is little acoustical difference between /ɑɝ/ or /ɑɚ/ and /ɑr/. Some instructors consider final spelled *r* as in *far* or *pear* to be /ɚ/.

Beginning		**Middle**		**End**	
1. remember	11. writing	1. around	11. married	1. pear	10. care
2. reach	12. reaching	2. vary	12. material	2. far	11. dear
3. ribbon	13. rich	3. berry	13. parade	3. jar	12. tear
4. radio	14. round	4. carried	14. appearing	4. sure	13. door
5. rope	15. refuse	5. direct	15. caring	5. appear	14. fair
6. raincoat	16. result	6. orange	16. nearing	6. more	15. bear
7. rice	17. receive	7. forest	17. fearing	7. there	16. car
8. rainbow	18. remain	8. tomorrow	18. staring	8. cigar	17. bar
9. raisin	19. roast	9. cherry	19. cigarette	9. hair	18. poor
10. running	20. reason	10. hurry	20. typewriter		

D.   PRONOUNCING WORD PAIRS CONTAINING /r/ AND A REPLACEMENT

Select some of the words from the paired lists in Section 17-2B containing /r/ and your replacement. Read one pair of words at a time, pronouncing the word with the target first (e.g., **road**–**load**). Make sure that you are saying /r/ first and /l/ second. Reverse the procedure, and pronounce the replacement word first and the target word second, making certain that you use /l/ first and /r/ second. Try to develop speed and accuracy as you do the drill. If you are either practicing with your instructor or listening to the exercise on tape, imitate your speech model as accurately as possible. If you are listening to the taped exercise, listen *only* to the drill that compares the target with your replacement. You will find this drill more difficult than the word list in Section 17-4C because of the closeness of target and replacement.

E.   PRONOUNCING FAMILIAR WORDS CONTAINING FREQUENT /r/ CONSONANT CLUSTERS

You may find this exercise the most difficult of all the drills dealing with the pronunciation of /r/ in single words. It is often much more difficult to pronounce a consonant target when it is combined with another consonant in a cluster. Pronounce each of the words carefully. If you are either practicing with your instructor or listening to the drill on tape, imitate your speech model as accurately as possible.

/tr/[3]	/dr/[3]	/br/	/pr/	/kr/	/gr/
1. track	1. drew	1. bright	1. priest	1. crack	1. great
2. trade	2. driver	2. bring	2. president	2. crash	2. grant
3. travel	3. drown	3. broom	3. prison	3. crawl	3. grew
4. treat	4. dry	4. broken	4. present	4. crowd	4. grade
5. trick	5. drop	5. brother	5. pretty	5. creep	5. ground
6. trunk	6. drugs	6. bread	6. pray	6. cracker	6. green
7. train	7. dress	7. breakfast	7. proper	7. ice cream	7. grapes
8. truck	8. drink	8. brown	8. protect	8. crayon	8. grass

[3]Note that the /r/ takes on a slightly friction-like quality after /t/ and /d/. This fricative quality is the correct pronunciation for /r/ in these clusters.

/fr/	/θr/	/skr/	/str/	/rm/	/rn/
1. friend	1. through	1. scramble	1. stretch	1. arm	1. barn
2. from	2. throw	2. scrap	2. stroke	2. charm	2. horn
3. fresh	3. three	3. scream	3. struck	3. harm	3. warn
4. frighten	4. thrilling	4. scrub	4. strange	4. farm	
5. frost	5. thread	5. scratch	5. strength	5. warm	
	6. throat	6. screen	6. straw		
		7. screwdriver	7. strike		
			8. string		

/rt/	/rd/	/rk/	/rs/	/rz/
1. heart	1. hard	1. fork	1. force	1. jars
2. court	2. cord	2. cork	2. course	2. pears
3. smart	3. card	3. dark	3. divorce	3. fears
4. short	4. guard	4. mark		4. tears
				5. years
				6. cars

F. Pronouncing /r/ in Phrases

Pronounce each of the phrases carefully. If you mispronounce a word, say it over again several times, and then repeat the entire phrase. If you are either practicing with your instructor or listening to the drill on tape, imitate your speech model as accurately as possible.

1. **care** to **read** a book **tomorrow**
2. **writing there** without **erasing**
3. **here** to **drive** to the **railroad** station
4. **before** the **parade** in the **rain**

G. Pronouncing Short Phrases Containing /r/ and /l/

This drill is similar to the exercise in Section 17-4D, except that your replacement precedes the target in each phrase. Pronounce each of the phrases carefully. If you are either practicing with your instructor or listening to the exercise on tape, imitate your speech model as accurately as possible. Although these phrases are shorter than those in the preceding drill, you may find this exercise more difficult, because your replacement directly precedes /r/ in each phrase.

/l/ – /r/

1. an awful ribbon
2. a cool roast
3. feel rich
4. smell rice
5. call right now
6. a mile race
7. a small room
8. the hole remained
9. a full river
10. all right
11. fall rain
12. steal radios
13. real reason
14. sail ready

H.   PRONOUNCING /r/ IN SENTENCES

Pronounce each of the sentences carefully. If you use a replacement, say the word over again several times and then repeat the entire sentence. If you are either practicing with your instructor or listening to the exercise on tape, imitate your speech model as accurately as possible.

1. They stopped in the **drugstore** and bought **more cigarettes** and ice **cream.**
2. He **tried** not to **drop** the bags of **red cherries, green grapes,** and **ripe oranges.**
3. He ate a **pear** and **rice cereal** with **raisins** and sweet **cream** at **breakfast.**
4. Wild **roses** and **raspberries grow near** the **river.**
5. The **carefully** made **scarecrow remained dressed** in **red** and **gray rags.**
6. His **friend promised** the **grocer** that he would **hurry** and clean the back **room right** away.
7. **Everybody** wanted to **appear** in the **great spring parade.**
8. **Robert refused** to **bring** some **fresh crackers** to us.

I.   PRONOUNCING /r/ IN BEGINNING CONVERSATION

This exercise gives you an opportunity to begin using some of your previously learned /r/ words in beginning conversation. Complete instructions for this type of drill are given in Chap. 5, 5-4H. Read the instructions, and adapt them to practice with /r/.

1. "Did you **wrap** up the _____?"
2. "Is the _____ **very** small?"
3. "Did you put the **ripe** _____ in the **freezer**?"
4. "I **drew** a picture of a _____."
5. "Can he **carry** the _____ to my **brother**?"
6. "Did she **crack** the _____?"
7. "Did you **drop** the _____?"
8. "Did my **parents promise** you a _____?"
9. "Will you **hurry** and **bring** me the _____?"
10. "Can **Richard drive** out to see the _____?"
11. "Will **Mary try** to **repair** the _____?"
12. "Do you know the **price** of that _____?"
13. "Does **Roger** want **more** _____?"
14. "How **far** is _____ from **here**?"

17–5.   CONVERSATION PRACTICE

So far you have learned how to pronounce your target by reading various kinds of exercises which contain /r/ words. Now you are ready to move into the final and most important part of your training program—learning how to pronounce /r/ automatically while you are talking more or less spontaneously. If this is the first practice chapter assigned to you by your instructor, you may wish to review the introductory comments on conversation in Chap. 2, 2-6 to 2-7.

A.   CARRYING /r/ INTO SPONTANEOUS DAILY CONVERSATION

This exercise requires you to use /r/ in daily conversation, starting with key words and expanding to all the /r/ words in your particular vocabulary. Complete instructions for this type of drill are given in Chap. 5, 5-5A, and there are supplementary comments about the exercise in Chap. 2, 2-7A.

B.   GENERAL CLASSROOM EXERCISES IN SPEAKING

Your instructor will plan a series of classroom conversation activities, and each assignment will be discussed fully in class before you carry it out. When your instructor announces the first speaking activity, you may wish to review the introductory comments on classroom speaking in Chap. 2, 2-7B.

chapter eighteen

The Consonant Target
/j/ (**yellow**)

COMMON SPELLINGS FOR /j/

The most frequent spelling is found in the word yellow; a less frequent spelling is found in the word onion.

18–1.   EAR TRAINING FOR THE /j/ TARGET

A.   A Few Reminders About Ear Training

The following test exercises will help you learn to recognize your /j/ target. If this is the first practice chapter assigned to you by your instructor, you may wish to review the discussion about listening practice in Chap. 2, 2-2B to 2-3C.

B.   Recognizing /j/ in Words

You will hear a list of words containing /j/. After listening to each word, write *B* if you heard /j/ at the beginning of the word and *M* if you heard /j/ in the middle of the word. The answers will be read to you at the end of the drill. This

exercise is found in Appendix 1. If you have difficulty recognizing the target, you may find it worthwhile to review the test with somebody outside class.

C.   RECOGNIZING /j/ IN SENTENCES

You will listen to a series of sentences containing a number of /j/ words. Each sentence will be read to you several times. Try to locate the /j/ words in each sentence, and write them down. The /j/ words in each test sentence will be read to you at the end of the drill. The sentences appear later in the chapter in Section 18-4H. If you have difficulty recognizing the target, you may find it worthwhile to review the test with somebody outside class.

18–2.   DISCRIMINATING BETWEEN /j/ AND THE VARIOUS REPLACEMENTS

A.   PROBABLE TYPES OF REPLACEMENT

The following exercises will help you learn to compare /j/ with your replacement. You are probably substituting one of the following common replacements for /j/: (1) /dʒ/ as in (juice), (2) /ʒ/ as in (measure), or (3) the omission of /j/. Your instructor will tell you which replacement you are using. If you are not employing one of the more common replacements, your teacher will tell you exactly how you are mispronouncing /j/ and provide you with some discrimination drills.

B.   PAIRED LISTS OF WORDS

The words in the following paired list are identical, except that the words in Column 1 contain the target, and the words in Column 2 contain the /dʒ/ replacement. Complete instructions for this type of exercise are given in Chap. 5, 5-2B.

Column 1 /j/	Column 2 /dʒ/
yard	jarred
year	jeer
yellow	jello
yes	Jess
yet	jet
Yale	jail
yam	jam
yolk	joke
use (n.)	juice
mayor	major

C.   PAIRED SENTENCES

The following paired sentences are identical, except that the final word in the first sentence contains /j/, and the final word in the second sentence contains the /dʒ/ replacement. Complete instructions for this type of drill are found in Chap. 5, 5-2C.

$$/j/ - /dʒ/$$

1. I think it's yellow.
   I think its jello.
2. He went to Yale.
   He went to jail.
3. He wants the yam.
   He wants the jam.

4. It's an old yolk.
   It's an old joke.
5. He's a mayor.
   He's a major.

D. LISTENING FOR REPLACEMENTS IN FAMILIAR /j/ WORDS

You will hear a list of words containing /j/. Sometimes the words will be pronounced correctly with /j/; other times the words will be said incorrectly with your replacement. Complete instructions for this drill are found in Chap. 5, 5-2D.

18–3. A FEW REMINDERS ABOUT ORAL PRACTICE PROCEDURES

If this is the first practice chapter assigned to you by your instructor, you may wish to review the comments about beginning oral practice in Chap. 2, 2-4. Before you actually begin practicing each individual pronunciation drill, you may also desire to review the supplementary explanations about the exercise in Chap. 2, 2-5.

18–4. THE PRONUNCIATION OF /j/

A. PRONOUNCING /j/ IN A SIMPLE SYLLABLE

In the event that you cannot pronounce /j/ through imitation alone, your instructor will help you with the following suggestions about placement. Should placement be required, you should review the definition of a glide in Chap. 4, 4-4H, and the description of /j/ in Figure 5 in Chapter 4. Note that because of the glide characteristics of the consonant, the target cannot be pronounced in isolation.

1. The Position of the Tongue

The basic position for your tongue is very close to the /i/ or /ɪ/ vowel positions, as in bead and bid. Press the edges of your tongue against the bottoms of your upper back teeth. Arch the blade of your tongue close to the front of the hard palate, and keep your tongue tip low and pointed toward the biting edges of your lower, middle front teeth. You may or may not touch your teeth with your tongue tip. Avoid contact between your tongue tip and the upper gum ridge, because that may cause you to use the /dӡ/ replacement.

2. The Movement of the Tongue

/j/ is a voiced glide which is heard as your tongue moves from position to position; it is literally an in-motion sound. The quality of /j/ becomes clear *only* as the tongue moves or glides from one position to another position. The second position of /j/ occurs as your tongue quickly glides from /i/ or /ɪ/ to the position of the following vowel. The lips adopt the position of the following vowel.

B. A GENERAL TECHNIQUE FOR PRONOUNCING /j/

This suggestion is particularly suited for students who omit /j/, and the procedures are based on the close similarity in position between /i/ and /j/.

1. Pronounce /i/ several times so that you can establish an awareness of your arched tongue blade, the low tongue tip, and the unrounded lip position. Observe the unrounded lips in a mirror.

2. When you are familiar with /i/, say /i/, and then slowly glide your tongue to the vowel /ae/ as in b**a**d. If you handle the glide correctly, you will pass through /j/ on the way to /ae/ and pronounce /ijae/. If you fail to develop the glide, you will pronounce only the vowels /i/ and /ae/. As you begin to feel the movement of your tongue—and to hear the quality of /j/—start increasing the speed of your tongue glide. As you increase your tempo, your gliding movement from /i/ to /ae/ will become assimilated into the equivalent of /jae/.

3. Continue practicing until you can pronounce /jae/ without going through the intermediate steps. Begin attempting other syllables, and then proceed into words containing initial /j/.

C. PRONOUNCING /j/ IN FAMILIAR WORDS

Pronounce each of the following words carefully. If you are either practicing with your instructor or listening to the exercise on tape, imitate your speech model as accurately as possible.

Beginning		Middle
1. your	11. year	1. barnyard
2. yours	12. using	2. unusual
3. yawn	13. useful	3. onion
4. you	14. you'd	4. opinion
5. use	15. yesterday	5. companion
6. yet	16. you'll	6. beyond
7. young	17. yelling	7. million
8. university	18. usually	8. senior
9. United States	19. yellow	9. lawyer
10. you've	20. yard	10. communion

D. PRONOUNCING WORD PAIRS CONTAINING /j/ AND THE /dʒ/ REPLACEMENT

Select some of the words from the paired list in Section 18-2B containing /j/ and your /dʒ/ replacement. Read one pair of words at a time, pronouncing the word with the target first (e.g., **year–jeer**). Make sure that you are saying /j/ first and /dʒ/ second. Reverse the procedure, and pronounce the replacement word first and the target word second, making certain that you use /dʒ/ first and /j/ second. Try to develop speed and accuracy as you do the drill. If you are either practicing with your instructor or listening to the exercise on tape, imitate your speech model as accurately as possible. You will find this drill more difficult than the word list in Section 18-4C because of the closeness of target and replacement.

E. PRONOUNCING FAMILIAR WORDS CONTAINING FREQUENT /j/ CONSONANT CLUSTERS

You may find this exercise the most difficult of all the drills dealing with the pronunciation of /j/ in single words. It is often much more difficult to pronounce a consonant target when it is combined with another consonant in a cluster. Pronounce each of the words carefully. If you are either practicing with your instructor or listening to the drill on tape, imitate your speech model as accurately as possible.

/mj/	/fj/	/vj/	/pj/	/bj/	/kj/
1. museum	1. few	1. view	1. pure	1. beauty	1. cube
2. music	2. fuse		2. pupil	2. beautiful	2. Cuba
3. musician				3. bugle	3. cute
4. mule					

/nj/[1]	/tj/[1]	/dj/[1]	/sj/[1]	/stj/[1]
1. newspaper	1. Tuesday	1. due	1. suit	1. student
2. new	2. tube	2. duty	2. suit case	2. stupid
3. New England	3. tune			
4. New York				

F. PRONOUNCING /j/ IN PHRASES

Pronounce each of the phrases carefully. If you mispronounce a word, say it over again several times, and then repeat the entire phrase. If you are either practicing with your instructor or listening to the drill on tape, imitate your speech model as accurately as possible.

---

[1] Not all speakers pronounce these words with /j/. In addition to using /ju/, some speakers pronounce these words with either /u/ or /ɪu/. Although there seems to be a preference in words of this type for /u/, the words have been included in this chapter for those of you who prefer to employ the /ju/ pronunciation. If you have any questions about which pronunciation—if any—is the preferred one in your area, ask your instructor.

1. **using** the **yams** at breakfast
2. a **companion** for **yourself**
3. **beyond** the **farmyard**
4. an **Italian lawyer** at **Yale**
5. a **young banyan** tree in the **yard**

G. PRONOUNCING SHORT PHRASES CONTAINING /j/ AND /dʒ/

This drill is similar to the exercise in Section 18-4D except that your /dʒ/ replacement precedes the target in each phrase. Pronounce each of the phrases carefully. If you are either practicing with your instructor or listening to the exercise on tape, imitate your speech model as accurately as possible. Although these phrases are shorter than those in the preceding drill, you may find this exercise more difficult, because your replacement directly precedes /j/ in each phrase.

$$/dʒ/ - /j/$$

1. charge yours	4. bridge used
2. manage usually	5. package yesterday
3. college year	6. George yawned

H. PRONOUNCING /j/ IN SENTENCES

Pronounce each of the sentences carefully. If you use a replacement, say the word over again several times, and then repeat the entire sentence. If you are either practicing with your instructor or listening to the exercise on tape, imitate your speech model as accurately as possible.

1. **Yes,** his **uniform** was stained **yellow** by the egg **yolk.**
2. Did **you** eat a **few onions yesterday**?
3. **William** saw his **younger** brother **yawning** in class.
4. **Daniel** thought that the **music** was **unusually beautiful.**
5. The **youth usually yelled** at every game.
6. What is **your opinion** about the **United** Nations?
7. In **your senior year you** will visit the Grand **Canyon.**

I. PRONOUNCING /j/ IN BEGINNING CONVERSATION

This exercise gives you an opportunity to begin using some of your previously learned /j/ words in beginning conversation. Complete instructions for this type of drill are given in Chap. 5, 5-4H. Read the instructions and adapt them to practice with /j/.

1. "Are **you** going to the **University** of _____ ?"

2. "Do **you use your** _____ ?"

3. "He **usually** flies to _____ every **year**."

4. "Did he **yell** about the _____ ?"

5. "What is **your opinion** about the _____ ?"

6. "Did **you** see a **few** _____ ?"

18–5.   CONVERSATION PRACTICE

So far you have learned how to pronounce your target by reading various kinds of exercises which contain /j/ words. Now you are ready to move into the final and most important part of your training program—learning how to pronounce /j/ automatically while you are talking more or less spontaneously. If this is the first practice chapter assigned to you by your instructor, you may wish to review the introductory comments on conversation in Chap. 2, 2-6 to 2-7.

A.   CARRYING /j/ INTO SPONTANEOUS DAILY CONVERSATION

This exercise requires you to use /j/ in daily conversation, starting with key words and expanding to all the /j/ words in your particular vocabulary. Complete instructions for this type of drill are given in Chap. 5, 5-5A, and there are supplementary comments about the exercise in Chap. 2, 2-7A.

B.   GENERAL CLASSROOM EXERCISES IN SPEAKING

Your instructor will plan a series of classroom conversation activities, and each assignment will be discussed fully in class before you carry it out. When your instructor announces the first speaking activity, you may wish to review the introductory comments on classroom speaking in Chap. 2, 2-7B.

chapter nineteen

The Consonant Target
/w/ (we)

COMMON SPELLINGS FOR /w/

The most frequent spelling is found in the word **wet**; two less frequent spellings are **qu**een and the first sound of the letter **o** in **o**ne—/wʌn/.

19–1. EAR TRAINING FOR THE /w/ TARGET

A. A FEW REMINDERS ABOUT EAR TRAINING

The following test exercises will help you learn to recognize your /w/ target. If this is the first practice chapter assigned to you by your instructor, you may wish to review the discussion about listening practice in Chap. 2, 2-2B to 2-3C.

B. RECOGNIZING /w/ IN WORDS

You will hear a list of words containing /w/. After listening to each word, write *B* if you heard /w/ at the beginning of the word and *M* if you heard /w/ in the middle of the word. The answers will be read to you at the end of the drill. This exercise is found in Appendix 1. If you have difficulty recognizing the target, you may find it worthwhile to review the test with somebody outside class.

C.   RECOGNIZING /w/ IN SENTENCES

You will listen to a series of sentences containing a number of /w/ words. Each sentence will be read to you several times. Try to locate the /w/ words in each sentence, and write them down. The /w/ words in each test sentence will be read to you at the end of the drill. The sentences appear later in the chapter in Section 4H. If you have difficulty recognizing the target, you may find it worthwhile to review the test with somebody outside class.

19–2.   DISCRIMINATING BETWEEN /w/ AND THE VARIOUS REPLACEMENTS

A.   PROBABLE TYPES OF REPLACEMENT

The following exercises will help you learn to compare /w/ with your replacement. You are probably using one of the following common replacements for /w/: (1) (v) as in vine, or (2) the omission of /w/. Your instructor will tell you which replacement you are using. If you are not employing one of the more common replacements, your teacher will tell you exactly how you are mispronouncing /w/ and provide you with some discrimination drills.

B.   PAIRED LISTS OF WORDS

The words in the following paired list are identical, except that the words in Column 1 contain the target, and the words in Column 2 contain the /v/ replacement. Complete instructions for this type of exercise are given in Chap. 5, 5-2B.

Column 1 /w/	**Column 2** /v/
wine	vine
went	vent
west	vest
worse	verse
wail	veil
wary	vary
wend	vend

C.   PAIRED SENTENCES

The following paired sentences are identical, except that the final word in the first sentence contains /w/, and the final word in the second sentence contains the /v/ replacement. Complete instructions for this type of drill are found in Chap. 5, 5-2C.

$$/w/ - /v/$$

1. Give me the wine.
   Give me the vine.
2. Is it worse?
   Is it verse?
3. It's in the west.
   It's in the vest.

D.   LISTENING FOR REPLACEMENTS IN FAMILIAR /w/ WORDS

You will hear a list of words containing /w/. Sometimes the words will be pronounced correctly with /w/; other times the words will be said incorrectly with your replacement. Complete instructions for this drill are found in Chap. 5, 5-2D.

19–3.   A FEW REMINDERS ABOUT ORAL PRACTICE PROCEDURES

If this is the first practice chapter assigned to you by your instructor, you may wish to review the comments about beginning oral practice in Chap. 2, 2-4. Before you actually begin practicing each individual pronunciation drill, you may also desire to review the supplementary explanations about the exercise in Chap. 2, 2-5.

19–4.   THE PRONUNCIATION OF /w/

A.   PRONOUNCING /w/ IN A SIMPLE SYLLABLE

In the event that you cannot pronounce /w/ through imitation alone, your instructor will help you with the following suggestions about placement. Should placement be required, you should review the definition of a glide in Chap. 4, 4-4H, and the description of /w/ in Figure 5 in Chapter 4. Note that because of the glide characteristics of the consonant, the target cannot be pronounced in isolation.

1.   The Position of the Tongue

The basic position for your tongue is very close to the /u/ or /ʊ/ vowel positions, as in pool and pull. Press the edges of your tongue against the bottoms of your upper back teeth. Arch the back of your tongue high and close to your soft palate, and keep your tongue tip low and pointed toward the biting edges of your lower front teeth. You may or may not touch your teeth with your tongue tip.

2. The Movement of the Tongue

/w/ is a voiced glide which is heard as your tongue moves from position to position; it is literally an in-motion sound. The quality of /w/ becomes clear *only* as the tongue moves or glides from one position to another position. The second position of /w/ occurs as your tongue quickly glides from /u/ or /ʊ/ to the position of the following vowel. The lips are round but tend to be more rounded before round vowels, as in **wool** than before unround vowels, as in **we**.

B. A GENERAL TECHNIQUE FOR PRONOUNCING /w/

This suggestion is particularly suited for students who omit /w/, and the procedures are based on the close similarity in position between /u/ and /w/.

1. Pronounce /u/ several times so that you can establish an awareness of your high back tongue position and rounded lips. Observe the rounded lips in a mirror.

2. When you are familiar with /u/, say /u/, and then slowly glide your tongue to the vowel /ɑ/, as in father. If you handle the glide correctly, you will pass through /w/ on the way to /ɑ/ and pronounce /uwɑ/. If you fail to develop the glide, you will pronounce only the vowels /u/ and /ɑ/. As you begin to feel the movement of your tongue—and to hear the quality of /w/, start increasing the speed of your tongue glide. As you increase your tempo, your gliding movement from /u/ to /ɑ/ will become assimilated into the equivalent of /wɑ/.

3. Continue practicing until you can pronounce /wɑ/ without going through the intermediate steps. Begin attempting other syllables, and then proceed into words containing initial /w/.

C. PRONOUNCING /w/ IN FAMILAR WORDS

Pronounce each of the following words carefully. If you are either practicing with your instructor or listening to the exercise on tape, imitate your speech model as accurately as possible.

Beginning		Middle	
1. want	11. welcome	1. away	9. sidewalk
2. warning	12. went	2. awake	10. highway
3. was	13. were	3. always	11. seaweed
4. waste	14. women	4. between	12. doorway
5. water	15. woolen	5. awoke	13. driveway
6. wave	16. wouldn't	6. otherwise	14. Halloween
7. we	17. wound	7. backward	15. sandwich
8. wearing	18. wall	8. anyone	
9. weather	19. wasp		
10. week	20. wagon		

D. PRONOUNCING WORD PAIRS CONTAINING /w/ AND THE /v/ REPLACEMENT

Select some of the words from the paired list in Section 19-2B containing /w/ and your /v/ replacement. Read one pair of words at a time, pronouncing the word with the target first (e.g., **wine–vine**). Make sure that you are saying /w/ first and /v/ second. Reverse the procedure, and pronounce the replacement word first and the target word second, making certain that you use /v/ first and /w/ second. Try to develop speed and accuracy as you do the drill. If you are either practicing with your instructor or listening to the exercise on tape, imitate your speech model as accurately as possible. You will find this drill more difficult than the word list in Section 19-4C because of the closeness of target and replacement.

E. PRONOUNCING FAMILIAR WORDS CONTAINING FREQUENT /w/ CONSONANT CLUSTERS

You may find this exercise the most difficult of all the drills dealing with the pronunciation of /w/ in single words. It is often much more difficult to pronounce a consonant target when it is combined with another consonant in a cluster. Pronounce each of the words carefully. If you are either practicing with your instructor or listening to the drill on tape, imitate your speech model as accurately as possible.

/sw/	/kw/	/tw/	/skw/
1. sweet	1. quarter	1. twelve	1. square
2. swift	2. queen	2. twenty	2. squirrel
3. sweep	3. quiet	3. twist	3. squeal
4. swing	4. question	4. twin	4. squawk
5. swam	5. queer	5. twice	5. squeeze
6. swamp	6. quick		6. squeak
	7. quit		
	8. quite		

F. PRONOUNCING /w/ IN PHRASES

Pronounce each of the phrases carefully. If you mispronounce a word, say it over again several times, and then repeat the entire phrase. If you are either practicing with your instructor or listening to the drill on tape, imitate your speech model as accurately as possible.

1. the **quiet wife's woolen wig**
2. a **wagon** of **wood** in **winter**
3. **always** some **way** to **win quickly**
4. **someone's wallet** last **week**
5. no **water** in the **swimming** pool

G.   Pronouncing Short Phrases Containing /w/ and /v/

This drill is similar to the exercise in Section 19-4D, except that your /v/ replacement precedes the target in each phrase. Pronounce each of the phrases carefully. If you are either practicing with your instructor or listening to the exercise on tape, imitate your speech model as accurately as possible. Although these phrases are shorter than those in the preceding drill, you may find this exercise more difficult, because your replacement directly precedes /w/ in each phrase.

/v/ – /w/

1. leave wood
2. drive west
3. save wallpaper
4. give wool
5. have wallets
6. love work
7. serve water
8. expensive wife
9. love walking

H.   Pronouncing /w/ in Sentences

Pronounce each of the sentences carefully. If you use a replacement, say the word over again several times, and then repeat the entire sentence. If you are either practicing with your instructor or listening to the exercise on tape, imitate your speech model as accurately as possible.

1. The **waiter** and the **waitress wouldn't work** on **Halloween.**
2. They ordered some **waffles** and **sweet squash sandwiches** last **Wednesday.**
3. **We** lost a **wristwatch** on the **sidewalk** in **Washington** last **winter.**
4. The **wild wind was always** chasing the **swamp weeds** through the open **doorway.**
5. The **workers will** be **washing windows** and **sweeping** floors next **week.**

I.   Pronouncing /w/ in Beginning Conversation

This exercise gives you an opportunity to begin using some of your previously learned /w/ words in beginning conversation. Complete instructions for this type of drill are given in Chap. 5, 5-4H. Read the instructions and adapt them to practice with /w/.

1. "I need a **quarter** for some _____."
2. "Did you **waste** any _____?"
3. "**Will** you **wash** the _____ next **week**?"
4. "Is the _____ **wet**?"
5. "**Would** you like the _____ **Wednesday**?"
6. "**Was** the _____ in the **driveway**?"
7. "Do you **always** use the _____?"
8. "**Were** you going to _____ this summer?"

9. "**Will** they take the _____ **away**?"

10. "Do you have a choice **between** the two _____ ?"

11. "Does **anyone** need the _____ ?"

12. "Is your new _____ made of **wool**?"

19–5. CONVERSATION PRACTICE

So far you have learned how to pronounce your target by reading various kinds of exercises which contain /w/ words. Now you are ready to move into the final and most important part of your training program—learning how to pronounce /w/ automatically while you are talking more or less spontaneously. If this is the first practice chapter assigned to you by your instructor, you may wish to review the introductory comments on conversation in Chap. 2, 2-6 to 2-7.

A. CARRYING /w/ INTO SPONTANEOUS DAILY CONVERSATION

This exercise requires you to use /w/ in daily conversation, starting with key words and expanding to all the /w/ words in your particular vocabulary. Complete instructions for this type of drill are given in Chap. 5, 5-5H, and there are supplementary comments about the exercise in Chap. 2, 2-7A.

B. GENERAL CLASSROOM EXERCISES IN SPEAKING

Your instructor will plan a series of classroom conversation activities, and each assignment will be discussed fully in class before you carry it out. When your instructor announces the first speaking activity, you may wish to review the introductory comments on classroom speaking in Chap. 2, 2-7B.

chapter twenty

The Consonant Target
/ʍ/ (**wheat**)[1]

COMMON SPELLINGS FOR /ʍ/

The only spelling for /ʍ/ is **wh** as in **wh**eat. Note that spelled **wh** is pronounced /h/ in certain common words, e.g., **wh**o, **wh**ose, and **wh**ole.

20–1. EAR TRAINING FOR THE /ʍ/ TARGET

A. A FEW REMINDERS ABOUT EAR TRAINING

The following test exercises will help you learn to recognize your /ʍ/ target. If this is the first practice chapter assigned to you by your instructor, you

---

[1]Although most speakers of American English distinguish between /w/ as in **we** and /ʍ/—words spelled **w** and **wh** respectively—there are many other individuals who do not make this distinction. These speakers use the /w/ pronunciation in all **w** and **wh** words. If you live in an area where /ʍ/ is the preferred pronunciation, learn this target. If /w/ is the preferred pronunciation in your area, omit studying /ʍ/. If you have any questions about the pronunciation of /ʍ/ in your dialect, ask your instructor. In the event that you are a nonnative speaker of English, the use of /w/ should be sufficient in your oral English.

may wish to review the discussion about listening practice in Chap. 2, 2-2B to 2-3C.

B.   RECOGNIZING /ʍ/ IN WORDS

You will hear a list of words containing /ʍ/. After listening to each word, write *B* if you heard /ʍ/ at the beginning of the word and *M* if you heard /ʍ/ in the middle of the word. The answers will be read to you at the end of the drill. This exercise is found in Appendix 1. If you have difficulty recognizing the target, you may find it worthwhile to review the test with somebody outside class.

C.   RECOGNIZING /ʍ/ IN SENTENCES

You will listen to a series of sentences containing a number of /ʍ/ words. Each sentence will be read to you several times. Try to locate the /ʍ/ words in each sentence and write them down. The /ʍ/ words in each sentence will be read to you at the end of the drill. The sentences appear later in the chapter in Section 20-4G. If you have difficulty recognizing the target, you may find it worthwhile to review the test with somebody outside class.

20–2.   DISCRIMINATING BETWEEN /ʍ/ AND THE VARIOUS REPLACEMENTS

A.   PROBABLE TYPES OF REPLACEMENT

The following exercises will help you learn to compare /ʍ/ with your replacement. You are probably substituting one of the following common replacements for /ʍ/: (1) you use the previously mentioned /w/ in an area where /ʍ/ is the preferred pronounciation, or (2) you use /f/ as in fun.[2] Your instructor will tell you which replacement you are using. If you are not employing one of the more common replacements, your teacher will tell you exactly how you are mispronouncing /ʍ/ and provide you with some discrimination drills.

B.   PAIRED LISTS OF WORDS

The words in the following paired lists are identical, except that the words in Column 1 contain the target, and the words in Column 2 contain one of the replacements. Complete instructions for this type of exercise are given in Chap. 5, 5-2B.

---

[2]If this is your substitution and you live in an area where speakers do not distinguish between /w/ and /ʍ/, you may wish to consider learning only /w/.

1.	**Column 1** /ʍ/	**Column 2** /w/	2.	**Column 1** /ʍ/	**Column 2** /f/
	where	wear		wheat	feet
	whether	weather		wheel	feel
	whale	wail		where	fair
	whine	wine		while	file
	which	witch		white	fight
				whale	fail
				whine	fine

C.   PAIRED SENTENCES

The following paired sentences are identical, except that the key word in the first sentence contains /ʍ/, and the key word in the second sentence contains one of the replacements. Complete instructions for this type of exercise are given in Chap. 5, 5-2C.

/ʍ/ – /w/
1. Did you hear the whale?
   Did you hear the wail?
2. His whine is good.
   His wine is good.

/ʍ/ – /f/
1. I see the wheat.
   I see the feet.
2. It will be a while.
   It will be a file.
3. He wants to make it white.
   He wants to make it fight.

D.   LISTENING FOR REPLACEMENTS IN FAMILIAR /ʍ/ WORDS

You will hear a list of words containing /ʍ/. Sometimes the words will be pronounced correctly with /ʍ/; other times the words will be said incorrectly with your replacement. Complete instructions for this drill are found in Chap. 5, 5-2D.

20–3.   A FEW REMINDERS ABOUT ORAL PRACTICE PROCEDURES

If this is the first practice chapter assigned to you by your instructor, you may wish to review the comments about beginning oral practice in Chap. 2, 2-4. Before you actually begin practicing each individual pronunciation drill, you may also desire to review the supplementary explanations about the exercise in Chap. 2, 2-5.

20–4. THE PRONUNCIATION OF /ʍ/

A. PRONOUNCING /ʍ/ IN A SIMPLE SYLLABLE

In the event that you cannot pronounce /ʍ/ through imitation alone, your instructor will help you with the following suggestions about placement. Should placement by required, you should review the definition of a glide in Chap. 4, 4-4H, and the description of /ʍ/ in Figure 5 in Chapter 4. Note that because of the glide characteristics of the consonant, the target cannot be pronounced in isolation.

1. The Position of the Tongue

The basic position for your tongue is very close to the /u/ or /ʊ/ vowel positions, as in **pool** and **pull**. Press the edges of your tongue against the bottoms of your upper back teeth. Arch the back of your tongue high and close to your soft palate, and keep your tongue tip low and pointed toward the biting edges of your lower front teeth. You may or may not touch your teeth with your tongue tip.

2. The Movement of the Tongue

/ʍ/ is a voiceless glide which is heard as your tongue moves from position to position; it is literally an in-motion sound. The quality of /ʍ/ becomes clear *only* as the tongue moves or glides from one position to another position. The second position of /ʍ/ occurs as your tongue quickly glides from /u/ or /ʊ/ to the position of the following vowel. A friction-like quality accompanies this movement as you blow breath noisily out of your mouth through your rounded lips.

B. SPECIAL SUGGESTIONS FOR PRONOUNCING /ʍ/ ACCEPTABLY

Remember that /ʍ/ is essentially an unvoiced /w/ with an added friction-like quality. Review the suggestions in Chap. 19, 19-4B for producing /w/, and try pronouncing /w/ by unvoicing it and blowing voiceless breath out of your mouth. Some textbooks use an /hw/ symbol for /ʍ/, and it may help you to think of the target as beginning with a voiceless fricative /h/ which glides into /w/. If your replacement is /f/, be sure to keep your lips rounded and your upper teeth from touching your lower lip.

C. PRONOUNCING /ʍ/ IN FAMILIAR WORDS

Pronounce each of the following words carefully. If you are either practicing with your instructor or listening to the exercise on tape, imitate your speech model as accurately as possible.

Beginning		**Middle**
1. what	10. whisper	1. bobwhite
2. wheat	11. whistle	2. anywhere
3. wheel	12. whizzed	3. everywhere
4. white	13. why	4. somewhere
5. when	14. wherever	5. nowhere
6. where	15. whirl	
7. whether	16. whine	
8. which	17. whiskey	
9. while	18. whip	

D.   Pronouncing Word Pairs Containing /ʍ/ and a Replacement

Select some of the words from the paired lists in Section 20-2B containing /ʍ/ and your replacement. Read one pair of words at a time, pronouncing the word with the target first (e.g., **whine–wine**). Make sure that you are saying /ʍ/ first and /w/ second. Reverse the procedure, and pronounce the replacement word first and the target word second, making certain that you use /w/ first and /ʍ/ second. Try to develop speed and accuracy as you do the drill. If you are either practicing with your instructor or listening to the exercise on tape, imitate your speech model as accurately as possible. If you are listening to the taped exercise, listen *only* to the drill that compares the target with your replacement. You will find this drill more difficult than the word list in Section 20-4C because of the closeness of target and replacement.

E.   Pronouncing /ʍ/ in Phrases

Pronounce each of the phrases carefully. If you mispronounce a word, say it over again several times, and then repeat the entire phrase. If you are either practicing with your instructor or listening to the drill on tape, imitate your speech model as accurately as possible.

1. **whirlybird whizzed** overhead
2. **whales wherever** you go
3. **somewhere** in the **White House**
4. **what white wheelchair**
5. **whiskers whenever** he shaved

F.   Pronouncing Short Phrases Containing /ʍ/ and /f/

This drill is similar to the exercise in Section 20-4D, except that your /f/ replacement precedes the target in each phrase. Pronounce each of the phrases carefully. If you are either practicing with your instructor or listening to the exercise on tape, imitate your speech model as accurately as possible. Although these phrases are shorter than those in the preceding drill, you may find this exercise more difficult, because your replacement directly precedes /ʍ/ in each phrase.

/f/ – /ʍ/

1. rough whiskers   1. off what
2. chief whispered   5. if when
3. calf whined   6. roof where

G.   PRONOUNCING /ʍ/ IN SENTENCES

Pronounce each of the sentences carefully. If you use a replacement, say the word over again several times, and then repeat the entire sentence. If you are either practicing with your instructor or listening to the exercise on tape, imitate your speech model as accurately as possible.

1.   **When** did he lose the **wheel**?
2.   **What** kind of car **whizzed** past?
3.   **Where** did you see the **bobwhite**?
4.   **Everywhere** they saw fields of **wheat**.
5.   The happy boy was **whistling while** pushing his **wheelbarrow**.
6.   Do you know **why** the **white** dog is **whining**?

H.   PRONOUNCING /ʍ/ IN BEGINNING CONVERSATION

This exercise gives you an opportunity to begin using some of your previously learned /ʍ/ words in beginning conversation. Complete instructions for this type of drill are given in Chap. 5, 5-4H. Read the instructions, and adapt them to practice with /ʍ/.

1.   "Do you know **whether** or not he wants the _____?"
2.   "Do you know **when** he saw the _____?"
3.   "Do you know **where** he found the _____?"
4.   "Did you see the _____ **while** waiting for me?"
5.   "Was the _____ **white**?"
6.   "Can you tell me **which** _____ you want?"

20–5.   CONVERSATION PRACTICE

So far you have learned how to pronounce your target by reading various kinds of exercises which contain /ʍ/ words. Now you are ready to move into the final and most important part of your training program—learning how to pronounce /ʍ/ automatically while you are talking more or less spontaneously. If this is the first practice chapter assigned to you by your instructor, you may wish to review the introductory comments on conversation in Chap. 2, 2-6 to 2-7.

A.   CARRYING /ʍ/ INTO SPONTANEOUS DAILY CONVERSATION

This exercise requires you to use /ʍ/ in daily conversation, starting with key words and expanding to all the /ʍ/ words in your particular vocabulary. Complete instructions for this type of drill are given in Chap. 5, 5-5A, and there are supplementary comments about the exercise in Chap. 2, 2-7A.

B.   GENERAL CLASSROOM EXERCISES IN SPEAKING

Your instructor will plan a series of classroom conversation activities, and each assignment will be discussed fully in class before you carry it out. When your instructor announces the first speaking activity, you may wish to review the introductory comments on classroom speaking in Chap. 2, 2-7B.

chapter twenty-one

The Consonant Target
/m/ (**me**)[1]

COMMON SPELLINGS FOR /m/

The most frequent spelling is found in the word **me**; less frequent spellings include au**tum**n and cli**mb**.

21–1. EAR TRAINING FOR THE /m/ TARGET

A. A FEW REMINDERS ABOUT EAR TRAINING

The following test exercises will help you learn to recognize your /m/ target. If this is the first practice chapter assigned to you by your instructor, you may wish to review the discussion about listening practice in Chap. 2, 2-2B to 2-3C.

B. RECOGNIZING /m/ IN WORDS

You will hear a list of words containing /m/. After listening to each word, write *B* if you heard /m/ at the beginning of the word, *M* if you heard /m/ in the

[1]This chapter presents only final /m/ as a single consonant and /m/ in final consonant clusters. These appear to be the only major problem areas with this target.

middle, and *E* if you heard /m/ at the end of the word. Concentrate on being able to locate the target at the end of words. The answers will be read to you at the end of the drill. This exercise is found in Appendix 1. If you have difficulty recognizing the target, you may find it worthwhile to review the test with somebody outside class.

C.   RECOGNIZING /m/ IN SENTENCES

You will listen to a series of sentences containing a number of final /m/ words. Each sentence will be read to you several times. Try to locate the final /m/ words in each sentence, and write them down. The final /m/ words in each sentence will be read to you at the end of the drill. The sentences appear later in the chapter in Section 21-4F. If you have difficulty recognizing the target, you may find it worthwhile to review the test with somebody outside class.

21–2.   DISCRIMINATING BETWEEN /m/ AND THE VARIOUS REPLACEMENTS

A.   PROBABLE TYPES OF REPLACEMENT

The following exercises will help you learn to compare /m/ with your replacement. You are probably substituting one of the following common replacements for /m/: (1) /n/ as in **n**ot for final /m/, or (2) /ŋ/ as in goi**ng** for final /m/. Your instructor will tell you which replacement you are using. If you are not employing one of the more common replacements, your teacher will tell you exactly how you are mispronouncing /m/ and provide you with some discrimination drills.

B.   PAIRED LISTS OF WORDS

The words in the following paired lists are identical, except that the words in Column 1 contain the target, and the words in Column 2 contain one of the replacements. Complete instructions for this type of exercise are given in Chap. 5, 5-2B.

1. Column 1 /m/	Column 2 /n/	2. Column 1 /m/	Column 2 /ŋ/
Tim	tin	hum	hung
seem	seen	ram	rang
same	sane	swim	swing
Jim	gin	clam	clang
comb	cone	Sam	sang
dime	dine	ham	hang
lime	line	slam	slang
game	gain		
ram	ran		
clam	clan		

C. Paired Sentences

The following paired sentences are identical, except that the final word in the first sentence contains /m/, and the final word in the second sentence contains one of the replacements. Complete instructions for this type of exercise are given in Chap. 5, 5-2C.

/m/ – /n/	/m/ – /ŋ/
1. Is it Tim?	1. Can you swim?
Is it tin?	Can you swing?
2. I like Jim.	2. I think it's slam.
I like gin.	I think it's slang.
3. I need a comb.	
I need a cone.	
4. Give me the lime.	
Give me the line.	
5. Is it a game?	
Is it a gain?	

D. Listening for Replacements in Familiar /m/ Words

You will hear a list of words containing /m/. Sometimes the words will be pronounced correctly with /m/; other times the words will be said incorrectly with your replacement. Complete instructions for this drill are found in Chap. 5, 5-2D.

21–3. A FEW REMINDERS ABOUT ORAL PRACTICE PROCEDURES

If this is the first practice chapter assigned to you by your instructor, you may wish to review the comments about beginning oral practice in Chap. 2, 2-4. Before you actually begin practicing each individual pronunciation drill, you may also desire to review the supplementary explanations about the exercise in Chap. 2, 2-5.

21–4. THE PRONUNCIATION OF /m/

A. Pronouncing Isolated /m/

In the event that you cannot pronounce /m/ through imitation alone, your instructor will help you with the following suggestions about placement. Should placement be required, you should review the definition of a nasal in Chap. 4, 4-4H, and the description of /m/ in Figure 5 in Chapter 4.

1. The Position of the Lips

The position of the articulators is clearly visible when you pronounce /m/, and if you use a mirror, you should easily see what you are doing. Look at your mouth, and simply press your lips firmly together. This position is important, If you are substituting /n/, you are pressing your tongue tip against your upper gum ridge; if you are substituting /ŋ/, you are pressing the back of your tongue against your soft palate. The lips are *open* for the pronunciation of /n/ and /ŋ/.

2. The Escaping Breath

The consonant /m/ is voiced, and the soft palate is lowered. When your lips are firmly pressed together, force the voiced breath out through your nose in a smooth steady stream.

B.   Pronouncing /m/ in Familiar Words

Pronounce each of the following words carefully. If you are either practicing with your instructor or listening to the exercise on tape, imitate your speech model as accurately as possible.

End

1. aim	5. clam	9. seem	13. bottom	17. arm	21. steam
2. became	6. Jim	10. Tim	14. come	18. dime	22. drum
3. him	7. limb	11. Tom	15. some	19. jam	23. room
4. home	8. Sam	12. them	16. swim	20. crumb	24. gum

C.   Pronouncing Word Pairs Containing /m/ and a Replacement

Select some of the words from the paired lists in Section 21-2B containing /m/ and your replacement. Read one pair of words at a time, pronouncing the word with the target first (e.g., **seem–seen**). Make sure that you are saying /m/ first and /n/ second. Reverse the procedure, and pronounce the replacement word first and the target word second, making certain that you use /n/ first and /m/ second. Try to develop speed and accuracy as you do the drill. If you are either practicing with your instructor or listening to the exercise on tape, imitate your speech model as accurately as possible. If you are listening to the taped exercise, listen *only* to the drill that compares the target with your replacement. You will find this drill more difficult than the word list in Section 21-4B because of the closeness of target and replacement.

D. PRONOUNCING FAMILIAR WORDS CONTAINING FREQUENT /m/ CONSONANT CLUSTERS

You may find this exercise the most difficult of all the drills dealing with the pronunciation of /m/ in single words. It is often much more difficult to pronounce a consonant target when it is combined with another consonant in a cluster. Pronounce each of the words carefully. If you are either practicing with your instructor or listening to the drill on tape, imitate your speech model as accurately as possible.

/mp/	/md/	/mz/	/lm/	/mpt/
1. pump	1. steamed	1. swims	1. film	1. pumped
2. stamp	2. climbed	2. clams		2. jumped
3. jump	3. aimed	3. dimes		3. stamped
4. camp	4. ashamed	4. drums		4. camped
5. lamp	5. seemed	5. exclaims		5. bumped
6. damp	6. exclaimed	6. seems		

E. PRONOUNCING /m/ IN PHRASES

Pronounce each of the phrases carefully. If you mispronounce a word, say it over again several times, and then repeat the entire phrase. If you are either practicing with your instructor or listening to the drill on tape, imitate your speech model as accurately as possible.

1. sour **cream** and **lamb** for dinner
2. **lime** pie for **Tim** and **Tom**
3. **scream** at the **same game**
4. **trim** the **palm stem** at **camp**
5. **rum** or **plum** ice **cream**

F. PRONOUNCING /m/ IN SENTENCES

Pronounce each of the sentences carefully. If you use a replacement, say the word over again several times, and then repeat the entire sentence. If you are either practicing with your instructor or listening to the exercise on tape, imitate your speech model as accurately as possible.

1. **Sam seemed** to like eating the **same rum** candy and ice **cream**.
2. He **came home from** the office at **suppertime** for a **ham** dinner.
3. **Jim jumped** at the chance to cook **steamed clams**.
4. He bought a **comb** for a **dime** last **autumn**.
5. **Tom** didn't **seem** able to **come** to the **workroom** on **time**.

G. Pronouncing /m/ in Beginning Conversation

This exercise gives you an opportunity to begin using some of your previously learned /m/ words in beginning conversation. Complete instructions for this type of drill are given in Chap. 5, 5-4H. Read the instructions, and adapt them to practice with /m/.

1. "That **stamp** is **from** _____."
2. "I'm going to **camp** at _____."
3. "He **became** class president in _____."
4. "Did **Jim** give **him** the _____?"
5. "Did **Tom** tell **them** about the _____?"
6. "Will he **come** for the _____?"
7. "Is the _____ at **home** in **Jim's room**?"
8. "Does **Sam** have **some time** to see the _____?"
9. "Does he **seem** to like his new _____?"

21–5. CONVERSATION PRACTICE

So far you have learned how to pronounce your target by reading various kinds of exercises which contain /m/ words. Now you are ready to move into the final and most important part of your training program—learning how to pronounce /m/ automatically while you are talking more or less spontaneously. If this is the first practice chapter assigned to you by your instructor, you may wish to review the introductory comments on conversation in Chap. 2, 2-6 to 2-7.

A. Carrying /m/ into Spontaneous Daily Conversation

This exercise requires you to use /m/ in daily conversation, starting with key words and expanding to all the /m/ words in your particular vocabulary. Complete instructions for this type of drill are given in Chap. 5, 5-5A, and there are supplementary comments about the exercise in Chap. 2, 2-7A.

B. General Classroom Exercises in Speaking

Your instructor will plan a series of classroom conversation activities, and each assignment will be discussed fully in class before you carry it out. When your instructor announces the first speaking activity, you may wish to review the introductory comments on classroom speaking in Chap. 2, 2-7B.

chapter twenty-two

The Consonant Target
/n/ (**not**)

COMMON SPELLINGS FOR /n/

The most frequent spellings are found in the words ru**n** and ru**nn**ing; a less frequent spelling is found in the word **kn**ife.

22–1.   EAR TRAINING FOR THE /n/ TARGET

A.   A Few Reminders About Ear Training

The following test exercises will help you learn to recognize your /n/ target. If this is the first practice chapter assigned to you by your instructor, you may wish to review the discussion about listening practice in Chap. 2, 2-B to 2-3C.

The ear training exercises for /n/ require a few additional special remarks, because the replacements differ so widely. Note the following types of replacements.

1. You substitute /m/ as in **me** for /n/, particularly when /n/ is at the end of the word.
2. You substitute /ŋ/ as in **going** for /n/, particularly when /n/ is at the end of the word.
3. You substitute /l/ as in **lap** for /n/, particularly when /n/ is at the beginning or in the middle of the word.
4. You substitute a vowel—usually /ə/ as in **about**—for syllabic /n̩/ in words like **cotton, hidden,** and **didn't.** This forms /ən/ rather than /n̩/.[1]

Because of these various types of replacement pronunciations, several kinds of ear training drills are used in this chapter. Your instructor will tell you which exercise he wants you to carry out.

B.   Recognizing /n/ in Words

You will hear a list of words containing /n/. After listening to each word, write *B* if you heard /n/ at the beginning of the word, *M* if you heard /n/ in the middle, and *E* if you heard /n/ at the end of the word. The answers will be read to you at the end of the drill. This exercise is found in Appendix 1. If you have difficulty recognizing the target, you may find it worthwhile to review the test with somebody outside class.

C.   Recognizing /n/ in Phrases

You will listen to a series of phrases containing a number of /n/ words. Each phrase will be read to you several times. Try to locate the /n/ words in each phrase and write them down. The /n/ words in each phrase will be read to you at the end of the drill. The phrases appear later in the chapter in Section 22-4G. If you have difficulty recognizing the target, you may find it worthwhile to review the test with somebody outside class.

D.   Recognizing Syllabic /n̩/

In the following exercise your instructor will help you learn to recognize the pronunciation of syllabic /n̩/. You will hear a list of words containing syllabic /n̩/. Listen carefully to your instructor's pronunciation and familiarize yourself with the pronunciation of syllabic /n̩/. This exercise is found in Appendix 1. If you have difficulty recognizing syllabic /n̩/, you may find it worthwhile to review the test with somebody outside class.

---

[1] /n/ may become syllabic and replace a vowel when it has a common point of articulation with the preceding consonant. Thus /t/ as in **tie**, /d/ as in **die** and /n/ are all formed on the upper gum ridge, and /n/ becomes syllabic after them in words like **cotton, hidden** and **didn't.** A description of syllabic /n̩/ is found in Section 22-4.

22–2. DISCRIMINATING BETWEEN /n/ AND THE VARIOUS REPLACEMENTS

A. PROBABLE TYPES OF REPLACEMENT

The following exercises will help you learn to compare /n/ with your replacement. Your instructor has already told you which of the more common replacements you are using. If you are not employing one of these more common replacements, your instructor will tell you exactly how you are mispronouncing /n/ and provide you with some discrimination drills.

B. PAIRED LISTS OF WORDS

The words in the following paired lists are identical, except that the words in Column 1 contain the target, and the words in Column 2 contain one of the replacements. Complete instructions for this type of exercise are given in Chap. 5, 5-2B.

1.	Column 1 /n/	Column 2 /m/	2.	Column 1 /n/	Column 2 /ŋ/	3.	Column 1 /n/	Column 2 /l/
	tin	Tim		ran	rang		knock	lock
	seen	seem		sin	sing		nice	lice
	sane	same		win	wing		need	lead
	gin	Jim		been	Bing		knife	life
	cone	comb		pin	ping		net	let
	dine	dime		ban	bang		noose	loose
	line	lime		tan	tang		not	lot
	gain	game		sun	sung		nip	lip
	ran	ram		run	rung		know	low
	clan	clam		stun	stung		never	lever
							nap	lap
							night	light
							seen	seal
							pain	pail
							fin	fill

C. PAIRED SENTENCES

The following paired sentences are identical, except that the final word in the first sentence contains /n/, and the final word in the second sentence contains one of the replacements. Complete instructions for this type of exercise are given in Chap. 5, 5-2C.

/n/ – /m/	/n/ – /ŋ/	/n/ – /l/
1. Do you like gin?	1. I think he ran.	1. He has a need
Do you like Jim?	I think he rang.	He has a lead.
2. Buy me a cone.	2. Did you hear the pin?	2. It's my knife.
Buy me a comb.	Did you hear the ping?	It's my life.
3. Throw me the line.	3. Did you sin?	3. It's my night.
Throw me the lime.	Did you sing?	It's my light.
4. Is it a gain?	4. Does it have a tan?	4. It's a knot.
Is it a game?	Does it have a tang?	It's a lot.
5. Is it tin?	5. Is it a win?	
Is it Tim?	Is it a wing?	

D. LISTENING FOR REPLACEMENTS IN FAMILIAR /n/ WORDS

You will hear a list of words containing /n/. Sometimes the words will be pronounced correctly with /n/; other times the words will be said incorrectly with your replacement. Complete instructions for this drill are found in Chap. 5, 5-2D.

22–3. A FEW REMINDERS ABOUT ORAL PRACTICE PROCEDURES

If this is the first practice chapter assigned to you by your instructor, you may wish to review the comments about beginning oral practice in Chap. 2, 2-4. Before you actually begin practicing each individual pronunciation drill, you may also desire to review the supplementary explanations about the exercise in Chap. 2, 2-5.

22–4. THE PRONUNCIATION OF /n/

A. PRONOUNCING ISOLATED /n/

In the event that you cannot pronounce /n/ through imitation alone, your instructor will help you with the following suggestions about placement. Should placement be required, you should review the definition of a nasal in Chap. 4, 4-4H, and the description of /n/ in Figure 5 in Chapter 4.

1. The Position of the Tongue on the Upper Gum Ridge

The position of the tongue is clearly visible when you pronounce /n/, and if you use a mirror, you should easily see what you are doing. Press your tongue tip slowly and firmly against your upper gum ridge. Concentrate on feeling your tongue tip in contact with the upper gum ridge as you pronounce /n/. This part of pronouncing /n/ is particularly important because of the nature of two of the replacements. When you substitute /m/ for /n/, you form /m/ by pressing your lips together; when you substitute /ŋ/ for /n/, you form /ŋ/ by pressing the back of your tongue against your soft palate. Note that /n/ commonly becomes dental—the tongue tip touches the upper, middle front teeth—before /θ/, as in mo**nth** and te**nth** and before /ð/ as in o**n the** and i**n th**is.

2. The Escaping Breath

The consonant /n/ is voiced, and the soft palate is lowered. When your tongue tip is pressed firmly against your upper gum ridge, force the voiced breath out through your nose in a smooth, steady stream. This part of pronouncing /n/ is especially important if your replacement is /l/, because when you pronounce /l/, your tongue tip touches the gum ridge as it does for /n/. However, the voiced breath stream is forced out of the mouth around one or both sides of your tongue. Check this aspect of your pronunciation by saying the target and lightly placing your fingers on your nostrils. If you pronounce /n/, you should feel some vibration as the breath escapes through your nose; if you pronounce /l/, you will not feel this vibration.

B.   PRONOUNCING SYLLABIC /ņ/

We noted earlier that the target may become syllabic when it has a common point of articulation with a preceding consonant such as /t/ or /d/. Syllabic /ņ/ always occurs in a weak-stressed syllable. It is formed by keeping the tongue tip on the upper gum ridge after the preceding /t/ or /d/, and then strongly exploding the /t/ or /d/ through the nose. Try saying the word **button** slowly. If you are successful in keeping your tongue tip pressed against your gum ridge for /t/ and /n/, you will pronounce syllabic /ņ/. If, however, you remove your tongue tip from the gum ridge after having pronounced /t/ and then bring it back up for /n/, you will produce /ən/. If this occurs, say **button** several times and concentrate on keeping your tongue tip pressed against your gum ridge until you can keep it there while exploding /t/ through your nose. You should be able to feel the explosive vibration passing through your nose.

C.   PRONOUNCING /n/ IN FAMILIAR WORDS

Pronounce each of the following words carefully. If you are either practicing with your instructor or listening to the exercise on tape, imitate your speech model as accurately as possible.

Beginning	Middle	End
1. new	1. sunny	1. again
2. not	2. honey	2. skin
3. know	3. money	3. began
4. never	4. piano	4. can
5. nice	5. any	5. grin
6. next	6. many	6. begin
7. niece	7. fancy	7. fine
8. nose	8. funny	8. down
9. north	9. beginner	9. line
10. nephew	10. peanuts	10. train
11. neighbor	11. goodnight	11. bargain
12. narrow	12. animal	12. stone
13. need	13. Chinese	13. throne
14. neck	14. Japanese	14. clean
15. neat	15. cannot	15. sun
16. navy	16. runner	16. one
		17. vine
		18. tin
		19. pan
		20. chicken

D. PRONOUNCING WORD PAIRS CONTAINING /n/ AND A REPLACEMENT

Select some of the words from the paired lists in Section 22-2B containing /n/ and your replacement. Read one pair of words at a time, pronouncing the word with the target first (e.g., **dine–dime**). Make sure that you are saying /n/ first and /m/ second. Reverse the procedure, and pronounce the replacement word first and the target word second, making certain that you use /m/ first and /n/ second. Try to develop speed and accuracy as you do the drill. If you are either practicing with your instructor or listening to the exercise on tape, imitate your speech model as accurately as possible. If you are listening to the taped exercise, listen *only* to the drill that compares the target with your replacement. You will find this drill more difficult than the word list in Section 22-4C because of the closeness of target and replacement.

E. PRONOUNCING SYLLABIC /n̩/ IN FAMILIAR WORDS

Pronounce each of the following words carefully. If you are either practicing with your instructor or listening to the exercise on tape, imitate your speech model as accurately as possible.

1. button	5. gotten	9. carton	13. ridden	17. wouldn't
2. cotton	6. bitten	10. garden	14. wooden	18. shouldn't
3. kitten	7. written	11. hidden	15. didn't[2]	19. hadn't
4. mitten	8. certain	12. sudden	16. couldn't	20. needn't

F. Pronouncing Familiar Words Containing Frequent /n/ Consonant Clusters

You may find this exercise the most difficult of all the drills dealing with the pronunciation of /n/ in single words. It is often much more difficult to pronounce a consonant target when it is combined with another consonant in a cluster. Pronounce each of the words carefully. If you are either practicing with your instructor or listening to the drill on tape, imitate your speech model as accurately as possible.

/sn/	/nz/	/ns/	/nt/	/nd/
1. snap	1. begins	1. glance	1. want	1. around
2. sneeze	2. grins	2. chance	2. went	2. behind
3. sniff	3. cleans	3. fence	3. pant	3. pond
4. snug	4. hens	4. dance	4. point	4. stand
5. snake	5. chins	5. announce	5. front	5. find
6. snow				

/ntʃ/	/ndʒ/	/nθ/	/nts/	/ndz/	/nst/
1. bench	1. orange	1. tenth	1. counts	1. islands	1. glanced
2. lunch	2. hinge	2. ninth	2. wants	2. stands	2. announced
3. bunch		3. eleventh	3. tents	3. ponds	3. fenced
4. inch		4. month	4. points	4. finds	4. danced
			5. paints	5. spends	

G. Pronouncing /n/ in Phrases

Pronounce each of the phrases carefully. If you mispronounce a word, say it over again several times and then repeat the entire phrase. If you are either practicing with your instructor or listening to the drill on tape, imitate your speech model as accurately as possible.

1. a **new crayon** of **mine**
2. **gotten seven** to **nine peanuts**
3. **didn't need** a **teaspoon** of **lemon** juice
4. **cannot clean** out a **certain pan**

---

[2]Instead of using /ə/, some students omit the medial /d/ in contracted forms so that words like **didn't** and **wouldn't** are pronounced as /dɪnt/ and /wʊnt/. Be careful to avoid this tendency.

5. a **nephew dining alone again in** the **garden**
6. **when** the **beginner** dropped the **melon** at **dinner**
7. **know** a **nice sunny** place for sugar **cane**
8. **never can** have a **sunny tone** of voice
9. **sneezed between noon** and **one**
10. **couldn't** stop **sniffing in** the **snow**
11. **want** from **eleven** to **fifteen chickens**
12. **wouldn't find** a **tin screen**

H. PRONOUNCING SHORT PHRASES
    CONTAINING /n/ AND /l/

This drill is similar to the exercise in Section 22-4D, except that your /l/ replacement precedes the target in each phrase. Pronounce each of the phrases carefully. If you are either practicing with your instructor or listening to the exercise on tape, imitate your speech model as accurately as possible. Although these phrases are shorter than those in the preceding drill, you may find this exercise more difficult, because your replacement precedes /n/ in each phrase.

/l/ – /n/

1. call now
2. fill next
3. real neat
4. cool nose
5. will never
6. feel narrow
7. roll north
8. still know

I. PRONOUNCING /n/ IN BEGINNING CONVERSATION

This exercise gives you an opportunity to begin using some of your previously learned /n/ words in beginning conversation. Complete instructions for this type of drill are given in Chap. 5, 5-4H. Read the instructions, and adapt them to practice with /n/.

1. "It **began snowing** at _____."
2. "He broke the _____ **when** he **snapped** it."
3. "My **new** _____ is **brown and green**."
4. "I **need** a **tablespoon** of _____ at **once**."
5. "Have you **been** to _____ ?"
6. "My **niece** bought some **honey** at _____."
7. "**Wouldn't Jane** take **one** of the _____ ?"
8. "They **began tennis lessons** _____."
9. "How **many** _____ **can** come next **month**?"

10. "**Couldn't Jean** have **seen** the _____?"

11. "**One** of the **signs** advertised _____."

12. "**Didn't** the **night train** leave **New** York at _____?"

22–5.   CONVERSATION PRACTICE

So far you have learned how to pronounce your target by reading various kinds of exercises which contain /n/ words. Now you are ready to move into the final and most important part of your training program—learning how to pronounce /n/ automatically while you are talking more or less spontaneously. If this is the first practice chapter assigned to you by your instructor, you may wish to review the introductory comments on conversation in Chap. 2, 2-6 to 2-7.

A.   CARRYING /n/ INTO SPONTANEOUS DAILY CONVERSATION

This exercise requires you to use /n/ in daily conversation, starting with key words and expanding to all the /n/ words in your particular vocabulary. Complete instructions for this type of drill are given in Chap. 5, 5-5A, and there are supplementary comments about the exercise in Chap. 2, 2-7A.

B.   GENERAL CLASSROOM EXERCISES IN SPEAKING

Your instructor will plan a series of classroom conversation activities, and each assignment will be discussed fully in class before you carry it out. When your instructor announces the first speaking activity, you may wish to review the introductory comments on classroom speaking in Chap. 2, 2-7B.

chapter twenty-three

The Consonant Target
/ŋ/ (thing)

COMMON SPELLINGS FOR /ŋ/

The most frequent spellings are found in the words thi**ng** and tha**n**k; less frequent spellings include: to**ngue** and ha**nd**kerchief.

23–1. EAR TRAINING FOR THE /ŋ/ TARGET

A. A FEW REMINDERS ABOUT EAR TRAINING

The following test exercise will help you learn to recognize your /ŋ/ target. If this is the first practice chapter assigned to you by your instructor, you may wish to review the discussion about listening practice in Chap. 2, 2-2B to 2-3C.

The ear training drill for /ŋ/ requires a few additional remarks. The target /ŋ/ is most frequently mispronounced in the suffix -**ing**, because the student substitutes /n/ as in **n**ot for /ŋ/ in a word like goi**ng**. Some students also become confused between /ŋ/ in a word like si**ng**er and /ŋg/ in a word like fi**ng**er. This problem, which is related to the spelling **ng** in English words, is taken up later in the chapter.

B.   RECOGNIZING /ŋ/ IN THE SUFFIX **-ing** IN WORDS

In the following test exercise, your instructor will help you learn to recognize /ŋ/ in the suffix **-ing**. You will hear a list of words containing the suffix **-ing**. Listen carefully to your instructor's pronunciation, and familiarize yourself with the pronunciation of the target in the suffix. This exercise is found in Appendix 1. If you have difficulty recognizing the target, you may find it worthwhile to review the test with somebody outside class.

23–2. DISCRIMINATING BETWEEN /ŋ/ AND /n/

The following exercises will help you learn to compare /ŋ/ with your /n/ replacement.

A.   PAIRED LISTS OF WORDS

The words in the following paired list are identical, except that the words in Column 1 contain the target, and the words in Column 2 contain the /n/ replacement. Complete instructions for this type of drill are given in Chap. 5, 5-2B.

Column 1 /ŋ/	Column 2 /n/
sing	sin
wing	win
Bing	been
ping	pin
king	kin

B.   LISTENING FOR REPLACEMENTS IN FAMILIAR SUFFIX **-ing** WORDS

You will hear a list of words containing /ŋ/ in the suffix **-ing**. Sometimes the words will be pronounced correctly with /ŋ/; other times the words will be said incorrectly with /n/. Complete instructions for this drill are found in Chap. 5, 5-2D.

23–3. RULES FOR WORDS CONTAINING THE **ng** SPELLING

Some students become confused between /ŋ/ and /ŋg/ (/g/ as in got) in words containing the **ng** spelling. These students either add /g/ in a word like singer or omit /g/ in a word like finger. Some general rules regarding the pronunciation of **ng** are helpful.

1. Only /ŋ/ can appear at the end of a word (e.g., sing, ring, and belong). The /ŋ/ does not change when inflectional endings are added to the stem or root word. This means that /g/ is *not* added to the pronunciation of the following inflected examples: singer, ringing, and belonged. There are certain exceptions to this rule. The comparative and superlative forms of root adjectives are pronounced /ŋg/: e.g., stronger, strongest; longer, longest; and younger, youngest.
2. When **ng** occurs in the middle of the stem or root word, the **ng** is pronounced /ŋg/: e.g., finger, single, angry, hungry, and mango.

Whenever you are in doubt regarding the pronunciation of a word containing the **ng** spelling, look up the word in your dictionary, and memorize its pronunciation.

23–4. A FEW REMINDERS ABOUT ORAL PRACTICE PROCEDURES

If this is the first practice chapter assigned to you by your instructor, you may wish to review the comments about beginning oral practice in Chap. 2, 2-4. Before you actually begin practicing each individual pronunciation drill, you may also desire to review the supplementary explanations about the exercise in Chap. 2, 2-5.

23–5. THE PRONUNCIATION OF /ŋ/

A. Pronouncing Isolated /ŋ/

In the event that you cannot pronounce /ŋ/ through imitation alone, your instructor will help you with the following suggestions about placement. Should placement be required, you should review the definition of a nasal in Chap. 4, 4-4H, and the description of /ŋ/ in Figure 5 of Chapter 4.

1. The Position of the Tongue on the Soft Palate

The position of the tongue is reasonably visible when you pronounce /ŋ/, and if you use a mirror, you should be able to see what you are doing. Press the back of your tongue slowly and firmly against your soft palate. Concentrate on feeling the back of your tongue in contact with your soft palate as you pronounce /ŋ/. This part of pronouncing the target is particularly important. When your substitute /n/ for /ŋ/, you form /n/ by pressing your tongue tip against your upper gum ridge.

2. The Escaping Breath

The consonant /ŋ/ is voiced, and the soft palate is lowered. When the back of your tongue is pressed firmly against your soft palate, force the voiced breath out through your nose in a smooth, steady stream.

B.   PRONOUNCING /ŋ/ IN
THE SUFFIX -ing IN FAMILIAR WORDS

Pronounce each of the following words carefully. If you are either practicing with your instructor or listening to the exercise on tape, imitate your speech model as accurately as possible.

1. asking	6. falling	11. fishing	16. licking
2. buying	7. feeding	12. pouring	17. lifting
3. calling	8. feeling	13. snowing	18. putting
4. catching	9. blowing	14. hugging	19. pulling
5. during	10. getting	15. hurting	20. letting

C.   PRONOUNCING FAMILIAR WORDS
CONTAINING /n/ FOLLOWED BY THE SUFFIX -ing

In this exercise the replacement /n/ precedes the target in each of the practice words. Make sure that you are saying /n/ first and /ŋ/ second, and try to develop speed and accuracy as you do the drill. If you are either practicing with your instructor or listening to the exercise on tape, imitate your speech model as accurately as possible. You may find this exercise more difficult than the word list in Section 23-5B because of the closeness of target and replacement.

$$/n/ - /ŋ/$$

1. running	4. yawning	7. cleaning	10. dining
2. training	5. warning	8. frowning	11. planning
3. winning	6. beginning	9. chinning	12. shining
			13. spinning

D.   PRONOUNCING /ŋ/ IN WORDS
CONTAINING THE ng SPELLING

In each of the following words the ng spelling is pronounced /ŋ/. Be careful to avoid the use of the /ŋg/ pronunciation. Note that /ŋ/ and /g/ are both pronounced with the back of your tongue pressed against the soft palate. However, the back of the tongue is more tense and is pressed more firmly against the soft palate for /g/. This is necessary to produce the explosive release associated with /g/. When you pronounce the target in the following words, concentrate on keeping the back of your tongue relaxed and on pulling it away from the soft palate without the explosive quality of /g/. Pronounce each of the words carefully. If you are either practicing with your instructor or listening to the exercise on tape, imitate your speech model as accurately as possible. If you have difficulty determining whether you are pronouncing /ŋ/ or /ŋg/, your instructor will give you some discrimination practice between /ŋ/ and /ŋg/ with the words in this exercise.

1. along	7. long	13. young	19. ringing	25. hanging
2. among	8. king	14. wrong	20. singing	26. wringer
3. bang	9. sing	15. wing	21. springing	27. stinger
4. belong	10. song	16. lung	22. stinging	28. singer
5. bring	11. thing	17. gang	23. belonging	
6. ring	12. tongue	18. string	24. bringing	

E. Pronouncing /ŋg/ in Words Containing the **ng** Spelling

In each of the following words the **ng** spelling is pronounced /ŋg/. Be careful to avoid the use of the /ŋ/ pronunciation. If you have difficulty producing the consonant /g/, note the comments above about pronouncing /g/. Further information about /g/ is found in Chapter 24.

1. stronger	6. longest	11. jungle
2. strongest	7. single	12. anger
3. younger	8. angrily	13. linger
4. youngest	9. hunger	14. tangle
5. longer	10. jingle	15. finger

F. Pronouncing /ŋ/ in the Suffix **-ing** and /ŋg/ Words in Sentences

Pronounce each of the sentences carefully. If you mispronounce a word, say it over again several times, and then repeat the entire sentence. If you are either practicing with your instructor or listening to the drill on tape, imitate your speech model as accurately as possible.

1. His **youngest** brother was **yawning** while **opening** his presents on Christmas **morning**.
2. He began **practicing** his **singing during** the early **evening**.
3. He was **sitting** in the **single rocking** chair that was **sitting** on the porch, and slowly **nodding** his head while **falling** asleep.
4. Mother became **angry** because the **youngest** boys kept **playing, laughing,** and **clapping** their hands.
5. The wind was **blowing** so hard **during** the **raging** storm that the windows kept **shaking, banging,** and **rattling.**

G.　Pronouncing /ŋ/ in the Suffix -ing in Beginning Conversation

This exercise gives you an opportunity to begin using some of your previously learned suffix -*ing* words in beginning conversation. Complete instructions for this type of drill are given in Chap. 5, 5-4H. Read the instructions, and adapt them to practice with /ŋ/.

1.　"Are you **buying** some _____?"
2.　"Are you **putting** the _____ down?"
3.　"Are you **cooking** _____ for dinner?"
4.　"Are you **going** to _____?"
5.　"Are you **getting** some _____ at the store?"
6.　"Are you **asking** him about the _____?"
7.　"Are you **driving** to _____?"
8.　"Are you **eating** _____ for dinner this **evening**?"
9.　"Are you **hoping** for _____ on Christmas **morning**?"

23–6.　CONVERSATION PRACTICE

So far you have learned how to pronounce your target by reading various kinds of exercises which contain /ŋ/ and /ŋg/ words. Now you are ready to move into the final and most important part of your training program—learning how to pronounce /ŋ/ and /ŋg/ automatically while you are talking more or less spontaneously. If this is the first practice chapter assigned to you by your instructor, you may wish to review the introductory comments on conversation in Chap. 2, 2-6 to 2-7.

A.　Carrying /ŋ/ and /ŋg/ into Spontaneous Daily Conversation

This exercise requires you to use /ŋ/ and /ŋg/ in daily conversation, starting with key words and expanding to all the /ŋ/ and /ŋg/ words in your particular vocabulary. Complete instructions for this type of drill are given in Chap. 5, 5-5A, and there are supplementary comments about the exercise in Chap. 2, 2-7A.

B.　General Classroom Exercises in Speaking

Your instructor will plan a series of classroom conversation activities, and each assignment will be discussed fully in class before you carry it out. When your instructor announces the first speaking activity, you may wish to review the introductory comments on classroom speaking in Chap. 2, 2-7B.

chapter twenty-four

The Consonant Target
/p/ (pie)

COMMON SPELLINGS FOR /p/

The most frequent spellings are found in the words **p**ie and su**pp**er.

24–1. EAR TRAINING FOR THE /p/ TARGET

A. A FEW REMINDERS ABOUT EAR TRAINING

The following test exercises will help you learn to recognize your /p/ target. If this is the first practice chapter assigned to you by your instructor, you may wish to review the discussion about listening practice in Chap. 2, 2-2B to 2-3C.

The ear training exercises for /p/ require a few additional special remarks, because the replacements differ so widely. Note the following types of replacements.

1. You substitute /f/ as in **f**un, for /p/.

2. You substitute a fricative /p/, symbolized by /ꝑ/, for /p/. This sound is formed when you tense your lips moderately, hold them very close together, and then blow breath steadily out of your mouth through the slit-like opening between your lips. The friction-like quality of the escaping breath is /p̶/.

3. You have a problem involving the aspirate characteristics of pronouncing /p/. The target /p/ is frequently said with a strong explosive puff of air known as *aspiration*. This strong puff of air is used when /p/ comes at the beginning of a word as in **p**ie or when /p/ comes at the beginning of an emphasized or stressed syllable as in a**pp**ear. This heavy puff of breath is essential to the correct pronunciation of /p/ in these kinds of words. You mispronounce /p/ in words like **p**ie and a**pp**ear because you pronounce the target *without* the strong puff of breath. This type of mispronunciation frequently suggests /b/ to the native speaker of English.

Because of these various types of replacement pronunciations, several kinds of ear training drills are used in this chapter. Your instructor will tell you which exercise he wants you to carry out. Regardless of which ear training drills you listen to, observe carefully the clear, precise quality associated with the pronunciation of /p/.

B. RECOGNIZING /p/ IN WORDS WHEN THE REPLACEMENT IS /f/ OR /p̶/

You will hear a list of words containing /p/. After listening to each word, write *B* if you heard /p/ at the beginning of the word, *M* if you heard /p/ in the middle, and *E* if you heard /p/ at the end of the word. The answers will be read to you at the end of the drill. This exercise is found in Appendix 1. If you have difficulty recognizing the target, you may find it worthwhile to review the test with somebody outside class.

C. RECOGNIZING /p/ IN SENTENCES WHEN THE REPLACEMENT IS /f/ OR /p̶/

You will listen to a series of sentences containing a number of /p/ words. Each sentence will be read to you several times. Try to locate the /p/ words in each sentence, and write them down. The /p/ words in each sentence will be read to you at the end of the drill. The sentences appear later in the chapter in Section 24-4H. If you have difficulty recognizing the target, you may find it worthwhile to review the test with somebody outside class.

D. RECOGNIZING /p/ IN WORDS WHEN THE TARGET IS SAID WITH A STRONG PUFF OF AIR

In the following test exercise, your instructor will help you learn to recognize the strong air puff of /p/. You will hear a list of words containing /p/ at the beginning of a word or at the beginning of a stressed syllable. Listen carefully to your instructor's pronunciation, and familiarize yourself with the strong puff of breath. This exercise is found in Appendix 1. If you have difficulty recognizing the strong air puff, you may find it worthwhile to review the drill with somebody outside class.

24-2. DISCRIMINATING BETWEEN /p/ AND THE VARIOUS REPLACEMENTS

A. PROBABLE TYPES OF REPLACEMENT

The following exercises will help you learn to compare /p/ with your replacement. Your instructor has already told you which of the more common replacements you are using. If you are not employing one of these more common replacements, your instructor will tell you exactly how you are mispronouncing /p/ and provide you with some discrimination drills.

B. PAIRED LISTS OF WORDS

The words in the following paired list are identical, except that the words in Column 1 contain the target, and the words in Column 2 words contain the /f/ replacement. Complete instructions for this type of drill are given in Chap. 5, 5-2B.

Column 1 /p/	Column 2 /f/[1]
pat	fat
peel	feel
pill	fill
pine	fine
pig	fig
pool	fool
pound	found
pan	fan
past	fast
peeled	field
paint	faint
puppy	puffy
leaping	leafing
cheap	chief
cap	calf
leap	leaf

[1] If your replacement is /ɸ/, your instructor will carry out this drill with you by changing the /p/–/f/ pairs to /p/–/ɸ/ pairs.

C. PAIRED SENTENCES[2]

The following paired sentences are identical, except that the key word in the first sentence contains /p/, and the key word in the second sentence contains /f/. Complete instructions for this type of exercise are given in Chap. 5, 5-2C.

/p/ – /f/

1. Did you peel it?
   Did you feel it?
2. I think it's pine.
   I think it's fine.
3. He bought a pig.
   He bought a fig.
4. I see the pan.
   I see the fan.
5. Did she paint yesterday?
   Did she faint yesterday?
6. The cap is very small.
   The calf is very small.

D. LISTENING FOR REPLACEMENTS IN FAMILIAR /p/ WORDS

You will hear a list of words containing /p/. Sometimes the words will be pronounced correctly with /p/; other times the words will be said incorrectly with your replacement. Complete instructions for this type of drill are found in Chap. 5, 5-2D.

24–3. A FEW REMINDERS ABOUT ORAL PRACTICE PROCEDURES

If this is the first practice chapter assigned to you by your instructor, you may wish to review the comments about beginning oral practice in Chap. 2, 2-4. Before you actually begin practicing each individual pronunciation drill, you may also desire to review the supplementary explanations about the exercise in Chap. 2, 2-5.

24–4. THE PRONUNCIATION OF /p/

A. PRONOUNCING ISOLATED /p/

In the event that you cannot pronounce /p/ through imitation alone, your instructor will help you with the following suggestions about placement. Should placement be required, you should review the definition of a stop in Chap. 4, 4-4H, and the description of /p/ in Figure 5 of Chapter 4.

1. The Position of the Lips

Press your lips firmly together, compressing some breath behind your lips and building up some air pressure. Hold your breath in your mouth behind your tightly closed lips. Note that if your lips are not firmly closed, you may pro-

[2]See footnote 1.

nounce the /p/ replacement. Be careful not to press your upper front teeth against your lower lip, because this will cause you to pronounce /f/. Use a mirror if you wish to see the clearly visible lip position.

2. *The Escaping Breath*

Open your mouth suddenly and explode the air out vigorously, saying /p/. The breath is actually pushed out of your mouth. You may check your pronunciation by feeling and seeing the puff of breath: (1) place your hand in front of your mouth, and see if you can feel the exploding air puff against your fingers, or (2) hold a piece of facial tissue in front of your mouth, and see if it jumps or bounces sharply because of the forceful impact of the exploding puff of breath. If you are unable to accomplish this, your instructor will help you feel the air puff by placing your hand close to his mouth while he pronounces /p/. He will also let you observe the air puff striking the facial tissue. Note that accurate pronunciation of /p/ gives a clear, precise quality to this explosive voiceless consonant.

B.   ADDITIONAL COMMENTS

A few additional comments are useful at this point regarding the explosive release of /p/.

1. *When* /p/ *Is Final Before a Pause*

When /p/ is the final sound in the speaker's conversation—that is, it is to be followed by a pause—the speaker has two forms of pronunciation available to him: (1) he has the option of pronouncing an exploded /p/ with a weak puff of breath, or (2) he has the option of pronouncing an unexploded /p/ by keeping his lips closed and completely avoiding any air puff. Some speakers believe that an exploded /p/ adds clarity and precision to the articulation of their speech. Use your own judgment in pronouncing /p/ before a pause.

2. *When* /p/ *Is Final and Occurs Before Another Stop*

When /p/ is final and is followed by a word starting with another stop, the explosion is modified. If a word ending in /p/ is followed by another word beginning with /p/ (e.g., ri**pe p**ear), the target is pronounced only *once*, and it is prolonged. In other words, there is one stop and a delayed explosion.

When a word ending in /p/ is followed by a word starting with any other plosive (e.g., sto**p t**alking), only the *stop* portion of the pronunciation of /p/ is said. The explosion is articulated as part of the following sound, and there is only *one* stop and *one* explosion. Let us look for a moment at the sample phrase sto**p** talking. The speaker brings his lips together for /p/, but he also simultaneously raises his tongue tip to his upper gum ridge for the following /t/. When he begins pronouncing /t/, his breath has been compressed behind his tongue tip—rather than behind his closed lips—and the explosion is heard as /t/ when the speaker removes his tongue tip from his upper gum ridge. The breath is blocked with /p/, but it is exploded with /t/. Other combinations of two stops are pronounced similarly.

C. PRONOUNCING /p/ IN FAMILIAR WORDS

Pronounce each of the following words carefully. If you are either practicing with your instructor or listening to the exercise on tape, imitate your speech model as accurately as possible.

Beginning			Middle	End
1. part	11. pine	21. pen	1. report	1. sleep
2. person	12. puff	22. pencil	2. appear	2. shop
3. pain	13. push	23. penny	3. suppose	3. ripe
4. public	14. pea	24. pillow	4. repeat	4. step
5. pearls	15. pile	25. pony	5. apart	5. stop
6. peace	16. poor	26. pie	6. depend	6. soup
7. pair	17. past	27. page	7. repair	7. soap
8. perfect	18. paper	28. pail	8. poppy	8. cup
9. perhaps	19. picture	29. pancake	9. leaping	9. cap
10. patch	20. party	30. piano	10. hoping	10. tulip
			11. stopping	11. top
			12. carpet	12. mop

D. PRONOUNCING WORD PAIRS
CONTAINING /p/ AND THE /f/ REPLACEMENT

Select some of the words from the paired list in Section 24-2B containing /p/ and your /f/ replacement. Read one pair of words at a time, pronouncing the word with the target first (e.g., **pat–fat**). Make sure that you are saying /p/ first and /f/ second. Reverse the procedure, and pronounce the replacement word first and the target word second, making certain that you use /f/ first and /p/ second. Try to develop speed and accuracy as you do the drill. If you are either practicing with your instructor or listening to the exercise on tape, imitate your speech model as accurately as possible. You will find this drill more difficult than the word list in Section 24-4C because of the closeness of target and replacement.

E. PRONOUNCING FAMILIAR WORDS
CONTAINING FREQUENT /p/ CONSONANT CLUSTERS

You may find this exercise the most difficult of all the drills dealing with the pronunciation of /p/ in single words. It is often much more difficult to pronounce a consonant target when it is combined with another consonant in a cluster. Pronounce each of the words carefully. If you are either practicing with your instructor or listening to the drill on tape, imitate your speech model as accurately as possible.

/pr/	/pl/	/sp/	/pt/	/ps/	/mp/
1. practice	1. place	1. special	1. crept	1. drops	1. jump
2. prepare	2. plain	2. spend	2. chopped	2. stops	2. lamp
3. promise	3. please	3. spoon	3. kept	3. tops	3. camp
4. proud	4. plan	4. spin	4. leaped	4. tips	4. bump
5. press	5. plump	5. spoke	5. slept	5. rips	5. lump
6. print	6. plant				6. stamp
7. prison	7. plate				
8. president	8. plum				

F.   PRONOUNCING /p/ IN PHRASES

Pronounce each of the phrases carefully. If you mispronounce a word, say it over again several times, and then repeat the entire phrase. If you are either practicing with your instructor or listening to the drill on tape, imitate your speech model as accurately as possible.

1. a **pile** of **plain paper** on the **porch**
2. a **pair** of **pens** and **pencils**
3. a **repeat appearance** in **public**
4. a **picture** at **Paul's party**
5. **pushed** the **pea** under the **pillow**
6. a **plate** of **plums**
7. some **ripe** fruit in the **shop**
8. **stop** to **mop up** the **soap**

G.   PRONOUNCING SHORT PHRASES CONTAINING /p/ AND THE /f/ REPLACEMENT

This drill is similar to the exercise in Section 24-4C, except that your /f/ replacement precedes the target in each phrase. Pronounce each of the phrases carefully. If you are either practicing with your instructor or listening to the exercise on tape, imitate your speech model as accurately as possible. Although these phrases are shorter than those in the preceding drill, you may find this exercise more difficult because your replacement directly precedes /p/ in each phrase.

/f/ – /p/

1. rough person	6. safe pony
2. if peace comes	7. half piled
3. life pair	8. calf pushed
4. roof past fixing	9. enough pages
5. chief party	10. a leaf perhaps

H. Pronouncing /p/ in Sentences

Pronounce each of the sentences carefully. If you use a replacement, say the word over again several times and then repeat the entire sentence. If you are either practicing with your instructor or listening to the exercise on tape, imitate your speech model as accurately as possible.

1. **Papa's package** had broken, and his **pound** of **peaches** and **pears** had **spilled**.
2. **Peter** took some **peanuts, potatoes**, rice **pudding**, and a **piece** of **pumpkin pie** to the **picnic**.
3. He said it **appeared possible** to **paint** the **steep pool** at the **palace**.
4. They **passed** some **happy** men trying to **pull** a **post** out of the **pond** in the **pasture**.
5. The **pleasant policeman politely** asked the **postman** not to **pick** the **poppies** and **tulips** in the **park**.

I. Pronouncing /p/ in Beginning Conversation

This exercise gives you an opportunity to begin using some of your previously learned /p/ words in beginning conversation. Complete instructions for this type of drill are given in Chap. 5, 5-4H. Read the instructions, and adapt them to practice with /p/.

1. "Did you **repair** the _____ ?"
2. "**Please pick** up some _____ at the store."
3. "Did you **complete** your **report** for _____ ?"
4. "Do you **suppose** your new _____ is **expensive**?"
5. "My **parents** told me to _____ ."
6. "Did he **attempt** to **keep** his _____ ?"
7. "Did you **plan** to bring the _____ ?"
8. "**Pack** some _____ for our **trip**."
9. "Did he **help** you with the _____ ?"
10. "Is the **puppy** _____ ?"
11. "Did you **put** _____ **stamps** on the **envelope**?"
12. "Did you **speak** to **Perry** about the _____ ?"

24–5. CONVERSATION PRACTICE

So far you have learned how to pronounce your target by reading various kinds of exercises which contain /p/ words. Now you are ready to move into the final and most important part of your training program—learning to pronounce /p/ automatically while you are talking more or less spontaneously. If this is the first practice chapter assigned to you by your instructor, you may wish to review the introductory comments on conversation practice in Chap. 2, 2-6 to 2-7.

A.   CARRYING /p/ INTO SPONTANEOUS DAILY CONVERSATION

This exercise requires you to use /p/ in daily conversation, starting with key words and expanding to all the /p/ words in your particular vocabulary. Complete instructions for this type of drill are given in Chap. 5, 5-5A, and there are supplementary comments about the exercise in Chap. 2, 2-7A.

B.   GENERAL CLASSROOM EXERCISES IN SPEAKING

Your instructor will plan a series of classroom conversation activities, and each assignment will be discussed fully in class before you carry it out. When your instructor announces the first speaking activity, you may wish to review the introductory comments on classroom speaking in Chap. 2, 2-7B.

chapter twenty-five

The Consonant Target
/b/ (buy)

COMMON SPELLINGS FOR /b/

The most frequent spellings are found in the words **buy** and **robber**.[1]

25–1. EAR TRAINING FOR THE /b/ TARGET

A. A FEW REMINDERS ABOUT EAR TRAINING

The following test exercises will help you learn to recognize your /b/ target. If this is the first practice chapter assigned to you by your instructor, you may wish to review the discussion about listening practice in Chap. 2, 2-B to 2-3C.

---

[1] Note that spelled **b** is silent in the following familiar words: comb, combing, dumb, numb, lamb, limb, womb, and plumber.

212

B.   Recognizing /b/ in Words

You will hear a list of words containing /b/. After listening to each word, write *B* if you heard /b/ at the beginning or the word, *M* if you heard /b/ in the middle, and *E* if you heard /b/ at the end of the word. Observe carefully the clear, precise quality associated with the pronunciation of /b/. The answers will be read to you at the end of the drill. This exercise is found in Appendix 1. If you have difficulty recognizing the target, you may find it worthwhile to review the test with somebody outside class.

C.   Recognizing /b/ in Sentences

You will listen to a series of sentences containing a number of /b/ words. Each sentence will be read several times. Try to locate the /b/ words in each sentence, and write them down. The /b/ words in each test sentence will be read to you at the end of the drill. The sentences appear later in the chapter in Section 25-4H. If you have difficulty recognizing the target, you may find it worthwhile to review the test with somebody outside class.

25–2.   DISCRIMINATING BETWEEN /b/ AND THE VARIOUS REPLACEMENTS

A.   Probable Types of Replacement

The following exercises will help you learn to compare /b/ with your replacement. You are probably substituting one of the following common replacements for /b/: (1) /p/ as in **pie**, (2) /v/ as in **vine**, or (3) a fricative /b/ which is symbolized by /ƀ/. This sound is formed when you tense your lips slightly, hold them very close together, and then blow voiced breath steadily out of your mouth through the slit-like opening between your lips. Your instructor will tell you which replacement you are using. If you are not employing one of the more common replacements, your teacher will tell you exactly how you are mispronouncing /b/ and provide you with some discrimination drills.

B.   Paired Lists of Words

The words in the following paired lists are identical, except that the words in Column 1 contain the target, and the words in Column 2 contain one of the replacements. Complete instructions for this type of exercise are given in Chap. 5, 5-2B.

1.

Column 1 /b/	Column 2 /p/	**2.**	Column 1 /b/	Column 2 /v/[2]
boast	post		ban	van
bee	pea		bury	very
bark	park		best	vest
bull	pull		bail	veil
bay	pay		bent	vent
bear	pear		cab	calve
bit	pit		robe	rove
buy	pie		dub	dove
Ben	pen			
beach	peach			
big	pig			
been	pin			
cab	cap			
robe	rope			
rib	rip			

C. PAIRED SENTENCES

The following paired sentences are identical, except that the final word in the first sentence contains /b/, and the final word in the second sentence contains one of the replacements. Complete instructions for this type of drill are given in Chap. 5, 5-2C.

/b/ – /p/		/b/ – /v/[3]
1. Is that a bee?	4. He slipped on the beach.	1. He needs the bail.
Is that a pea?	He slipped on the peach.	He needs the veil.
2. I like the bay.	5. Did you catch the cab?	2. Did you get the boat?
I like the pay.	Did you catch the cap?	Did you get the vote?
3. Is it a good buy?	6. Does it have a rib?	3. He has some new cabs.
Is it a good pie?	Does it have a rip?	He has some new calves.

D. LISTENING FOR REPLACEMENTS IN FAMILIAR /b/ WORDS

You will hear a list of words containing /b/. Sometimes the words will be pronounced correctly with /b/; other times the words will be said incorrectly with your replacement. Complete instructions for this type of drill are found in Chap. 5, 5-2D.

---

[2]If your replacement is /b̶/, your instructor will carry out this drill with you by changing the /b/–/v/ pairs to /b/–/b̶/ pairs.

[3]If your replacement is /b̶/, your instructor will carry out this drill with you by changing the /b/–/v/ pairs to /b/–/b̶/ pairs.

25–3.   A FEW REMINDERS ABOUT ORAL PRACTICE PROCEDURES

If this is the first practice chapter assigned to you by your instructor, you may wish to review the comments about beginning oral practice in Chap. 2, 2-4. Before you actually begin practicing each individual pronunciation drill, you may also desire to review the supplementary explanations about the exercise in Chap. 2, 2-5.

25–4.   THE PRONUNCIATION OF /b/

A.   PRONOUNCING /b/ IN A SIMPLE SYLLABLE

In the event that you cannot pronounce /b/ through imitation alone, your instructor will help you with the following suggestions about placement. Should placement be required, you should review the definition of a stop in Chap. 4, 4-4H, and the description of /b/ in Figure 5 of Chapter 4. Note that because of the nature of the consonant, the target cannot be pronounced in isolation.

1.   The Position of the Lips

Press your lips firmly together, compressing some breath behind your lips and building up some air pressure. Hold your breath in your mouth behind your tightly closed lips. Note that if your lips are not firmly closed, you may pronounce the /b/ replacement. Be careful not to press your upper front teeth against your lower lip, because this will cause you to pronounce /v/. Use a mirror if you wish to see the clearly visible lip position.

2.   The Escaping Breath

Open your mouth suddenly, and explode the air out vigorously, saying the syllable /bɑ/ (/ɑ/) as in **h**o**t** and **f**a**ther**. This consonant is voiced, and you must be certain that your vocal bands are vibrating as you explode the breath out of your mouth. Check for the vibration of the bands by placing your fingers on your larynx as you pronounce /bɑ/. If you are unable to feel the vibration from your own larynx, your instructor will place your fingers on his larynx and say /bɑ/. Keep practicing until you can feel the vibration from your own larynx while pronouncing /bɑ/. When that happens you can double-check your pronunciation of the target by placing your hands over your ears while saying /bɑ/. You should be able to hear the vibration. Keep in mind that the vowel /ɑ/ is voiced and that you are *not* likely to unvoice the vowel. When checking for vibration, make sure that what you feel and hear *begins* on /b/ and not on the vowel. If you are using the correct lip position for the target and you do not feel or hear the vibration of the bands, you are pronouncing /pɑ/ rather than /bɑ/. The primary difference between /b/ and /p/ is voicing. Note that accurate pronunciation of /b/ gives a clear, precise quality to this explosive voiced consonant.

B.   ADDITIONAL COMMENTS

A few additional comments are useful at this point regarding the explosive release of /b/. Read the comments in Chap. 24, 24-4B. Keep in mind that the pronunciation of /b/ generally parallels the pronunciation of /p/: (1) final /b/ before a pause may be exploded or unexploded, (2) final /b/ followed by initial /b/ is pronounced *once* and prolonged (e.g., ri**b b**roken), and (3) when final /b/ is followed by any other plosive, there is only *one* stop and *one* explosion (e.g., ca**b d**river).

C.   PRONOUNCING /b/ IN FAMILIAR WORDS

Pronounce each of the following words carefully. If you are either practicing with your instructor or listening to the exercise on tape, imitate your speech model as accurately as possible.

Beginning		Middle		End[4]
1. be	11. bite	1. maybe	11. about	1. rub
2. because	12. bone	2. nearby	12. November	2. scrub
3. bill	13. butter	3. obey	13. December	3. grab
4. boy	14. button	4. good-bye	14. October	4. gab
5. beside	15. bus	5. cabin	15. hobby	5. rob
6. bounce	16. balloon	6. doorbell	16. tobacco	6. cub
7. bang	17. bark	7. horseback	17. harbor	7. robe
8. bank	18. beach	8. number	18. somebody	8. doorknob
9. beard	19. banana	9. robber	19. ribbon	9. crab
10. boast	20. before	10. rainbow	20. rubber	10. rib
				11. web
				12. tub
				13. cab
				14. globe

D.   PRONOUNCING WORD PAIRS
CONTAINING /b/ AND A REPLACEMENT

Select some of the words from the paired lists in Section 25-2B containing /b/ and your replacement. Read one pair of words at a time, pronouncing the

---

[4]If you have difficulty pronouncing final /b/, read footnote 3 in Chapter 8, and adapt the comments to the pronunciation of final voiced /b/.

word with the target first (e.g., **boast–post**). Make sure that you are saying /b/ first and /p/ second. Reverse the procedure, and pronounce the replacement word first and the target word second, making certain that you use /p/ first and /b/ second. Try to develop speed and accuracy as you do the drill. If you are either practicing with your instructor or listening to the exercise on tape, imitate your speech model as accurately as possible. If you are listening to the taped exercise, listen *only* to the drill that compares the target with your particular replacement. You will find this drill more difficult than the word list in Section 25-4C because of the closeness of target and replacement.

E.   PRONOUNCING FAMILIAR WORDS
   CONTAINING FREQUENT /b/ CONSONANT CLUSTERS

You may find this exercise the most difficult of all the drills dealing with the pronunciation of /b/ in single words. It is often much more difficult to pronounce a consonant target when it is combined with another consonant in a cluster. Pronounce each of the words carefully. If you are either practicing with your instructor or listening to the drill on tape, imitate your speech model as accurately as possible.

/br/	/bl/	/bz/	/bd/
1. bring	1. bless	1. clubs	1. clubbed
2. bright	2. block	2. cubs	2. grabbed
3. brick	3. blossom	3. grabs	3. rubbed
4. brass	4. blink	4. rubs	4. scrubbed
5. branch	5. bloom	5. scrubs	
6. break	6. black		
7. brown	7. blood		
8. brook	8. blanket		

F.   PRONOUNCING /b/ IN PHRASES

Pronounce each of the phrases carefully. If you mispronounce a word, say it over again several times, and then repeat the entire phrase. If you are either practicing with your instructor or listening to the drill on tape, imitate your speech model as accurately as possible.

1.   a **tub** of **beets** on the **bench**
2.   **rub** and **scrub** the **doorknob**
3.   a **basket** of **boiled cabbage**
4.   **begin before somebody** else
5.   **maybe** it's **nearby** on the **beach**
6.   **broke** the **brown tube** with the **block**

G.   PRONOUNCING SHORT PHRASES
CONTAINING /b/ AND A REPLACEMENT

This drill is similar to the exercise in Section 25-4D, except that your replacement precedes the target in each phrase. Pronounce each of the phrases carefully. If you are either practicing with your instructor or listening to the exercise on tape, imitate your speech model as accurately as possible. If you are listening to the taped exercise, listen *only* to the drill that compares your target with your particular replacement. Although these phrases are shorter than those in the preceding drill, you may find this exercise more difficult, because your replacement directly precedes /b/ in each phrase. If your replacement is /p/, keep in mind the previous comments about pronouncing two consecutive plosive sounds with one stop and one explosion.

/p/ – /b/	/v/ – /b/
1. sleep back there	1. gave butter
2. mop beside me	2. leave bones
3. top bank	3. have because
4. soup bone	4. love bananas
5. step back	5. save bills
6. ripe banana	6. dive before lunch
7. stop before now	
8. drop because ready	

H.   PRONOUNCING /b/ IN SENTENCES

Pronounce each of the sentences carefully. If you use a replacement, say the word over again several times, and then repeat the entire sentence. If you are either practicing with your instructor or listening to the exercise on tape, imitate your speech model as accurately as possible.

1.   He wanted to **grab** a **cab** and **bring Barbara** to the **beach** at once.
2.   Our **neighbor,** Mr. **Roberts, celebrated** his **birthday** last **February by** eating a **broiled crab** dinner.
3.   **Nobody** could **possibly believe** that **somebody** wanted to **rob** the **band members.**
4.   **Bill remembered** to tie a **ribbon** around the **robe** and the **rubber** slippers **before** putting them into the **box.**
5.   The **busy baker** at the **nearby bakery** said he could **probably bake** enough sweet **bread** for the party.

I.   PRONOUNCING /b/ IN BEGINNING CONVERSATION

This exercise gives you an opportunity to begin using some of your previously learned /b/ words in beginning conversation. Complete instructions for this type of drill are given in Chap. 5, 5-4H. Read the instructions and adapt them to practice with /b/.

1. "Is it **possible** to get some _____?"
2. "My **hobby** is _____."
3. "The **doorknob** is _____."
4. "The **black** priest **blessed** the _____."
5. "Please **scrub** the _____."
6. "Did you ask **about** the _____?"
7. "There was **blood** on the _____."
8. "Can you **buy** the _____ **before** tomorrow?"
9. "Will you be **able** to go to the _____?"
10. "Take a **cab** to get the _____."
11. "Did you **borrow** some **bread** and **butter** from _____?"
12. "Was my _____ in the **bicycle basket**?"

25–5.   CONVERSATION PRACTICE

So far you have learned how to pronounce your target by reading various kinds of exercises which contain /b/ words. Now you are ready to move into the final and most important part of your training program—learning to pronounce /b/ automatically while you are talking more or less spontaneously. If this is the first practice chapter assigned to you by your instructor, you may wish to review the introductory comments on conversation practice in Chap. 2, 2-6 to 2-7.

A.   CARRYING /b/ INTO SPONTANEOUS DAILY CONVERSATION

This exercise requires you to use /b/ in daily conversation, starting with key words and expanding to all the /b/ words in your particular vocabulary. Complete instructions for this type of drill are given in Chap. 5, 5-5A, and there are supplementary comments about the exercise in Chap. 2, 2-7A.

B.   GENERAL CLASSROOM EXERCISES IN SPEAKING

Your instructor will plan a series of classroom conversation activities, and each assignment will be discussed fully in class before you carry it out. When your instructor announces the first speaking activity, you may wish to review the introductory comments on classroom speaking in Chap. 2, 2-7B.

chapter twenty-six

The Consonant Target
/t/ (tie)

COMMON SPELLINGS FOR /t/

The most frequent spellings are found in the following words: **tie**, **letter**, and wal**ked**.[1]

26–1. EAR TRAINING FOR THE /t/ TARGET

A. A FEW REMINDERS ABOUT EAR TRAINING

The following test exercises will help you learn to recognize your /t/ target. If this is the first practice chapter assigned to you by your instructor, you may wish to review the discussion about listening practice in Chap. 2, 2-2B to 2-3C.

The ear training exercises for /t/ require a few additional remarks, because the replacements differ so widely. Note the following types of replacements.

---

[1]A discussion of the pronunciation of /t/ and of /d/, as in **d**ie and in **ed** and **d** endings, is found in Chapter 27.

1. You substitute /θ/ as in thought for /t/.

2. You substitute a dental /t/ for the target; that is, your tongue tip touches the upper, middle front teeth rather than your upper gum ridge.[2]

3. You have a problem involving the aspirate characteristics of pronouncing /t/. The target /t/ is frequently said with a strong explosive puff of air known as aspiration. This strong puff of air is used when /t/ comes at the beginning of a word as in tie or when /t/ comes at the beginning of an emphasized or stressed syllable as in attack. This heavy puff of breath is essential to the correct pronunciation of /t/ in these kinds of words. You mispronounce the target in words like tie and attack because you pronounce the target *without* the strong puff of breath. This type of mispronunciation frequently suggests /d/ to the native speaker of English.

4. Another problem involving the aspirate characteristics of pronouncing /t/ occurs as the reverse of the previously described replacement. The target is *pronounced without* a strong puff of breath when it occurs in the following types of words: (a) between two vowels in words like letter and notice; (b) between /n/ and a weak-stressed vowel as in twenty; and /c/ before syllabic /l/ in a word like little[3] You mispronounce /t/ in words like these because you pronounce the target with *too much* of an air puff.

5. You substitute /d/ for /t/. This occurs primarily in words like letter and little, as well as before syllabic /n̩/ in cotton.[3]

6. You substitute a glottal stop for /t/ in words pronounced with syllabic /l/ and syllabic /n̩/.[3] A glottal stop is formed by closing the vocal bands firmly, and then opening them suddenly and exploding the breath from the glottis.

7. You omit /t/ in several different types of words: (a) in final consonant clusters, as in post, correct, lift, and guests; (b) before /l/ in words like costly and softly; and (c) after /n/ in words like twenty and center.

Because of these various types of replacement pronunciations, several kinds of ear training drills are used in this chapter. Your instructor will tell you which exercise he wants you to carry out. Regardless of which ear training drills you listen to, observe carefully the clear, precise quality associated with the pronunciation of /t/.

B.   RECOGNIZING /t/ IN WORDS WHEN THE REPLACEMENT IS /θ/, DENTAL /t/, OR A GLOTTAL STOP

You will hear a list of words containing /t/. After listening to each word, write *B* if you heard /t/ at the beginning of the word, *M* if you heard /t/ in the

[2]Note that dental /t/ is acceptable when the target precedes /θ/, or /ð/ as in them (e.g., right thought and at the store).

[3]/l/ and /n/ may become syllabic and replace a vowel when they have a common point of articulation with the preceding consonant. Thus /t/, /l/, and /n/ are all formed on the upper gum ridge. /l/ and /n/ become syllabic after /t/ in words like little and cotton. A description of syllabic /l/ is found in Chapter 16, and a description of syllabic /n̩/ is found in Chapter 22.

middle, and *E* if you heard /t/ at the end of the word. The answers will be read to you at the end of the drill. This exercise is found in Appendix 1. If you have difficulty recognizing the target, you may find it worthwhile to review the test with somebody outside class.

C.   RECOGNIZING /t/ IN SENTENCES WHEN
THE REPLACEMENT IS /θ/, DENTAL /t/, OR A GLOTTAL STOP

You will listen to a series of sentences containing a number of /t/ words. Each sentence will be read several times. Try to locate the /t/ words in each sentence, and write them down. The /t/ words in each test sentence will be read to you at the end of the drill. The sentences appear later in the chapter in Section 26-4H. If you have difficulty recognizing the target, you may find it worthwhile to review the test with somebody outside class.

D.   RECOGNIZING /t/ IN WORDS WHEN
THE TARGET IS SAID WITH A STRONG PUFF OF AIR

In the following test exercise your instructor will help you learn to recognize the strong air puff of /t/. You will hear a list of words containing /t/ at the beginning of a word or at the beginning of a stressed syllable. Listen carefully to your instructor's pronunciation, and familiarize yourself with the strong puff of breath. This exercise is found in Appendix 1. If you have difficulty recognizing the strong air puff, you may find it worthwhile to review the drill with somebody outside class.

E.   RECOGNIZING /t/ IN WORDS
WHEN THE TARGET IS SAID WITHOUT A STRONG PUFF OF AIR
OR WHEN THE REPLACEMENT IS /d/

In the following test exercise your instructor will help you learn to recognize the pronunciation of /t/ that is used in words like letter, twenty and little. Listen carefully to your instructor's pronunciation, and pay particular attention to the quality of /t/ in words of this type. This exercise is found in Appendix 1.[4]

F.   RECOGNIZING /t/ IN WORDS
IN WHICH THE TARGET IS TYPICALLY OMITTED

In the following test exercise your instructor will help you learn to recognize the pronunciation of /t/ when it is used in words like post, costly, and center.

---

[4]The pronunciation of /t/ in words like letter, twenty, and little varies in American English. Your instructor will demonstrate two common pronunciations. One pronunciation is a /t/ which is said with a weak puff of breath. The second pronunciation is called a one tap trill, and this sound is produced with a single stroke or tap of the tongue tip against the upper gum ridge. Words like latter and ladder or atom and Adam sound very much alike in the speech of the person who uses this second pronunciation. Use whichever pronunciation is easiest for you, unless there is a preference for one or the other in your area. If you have any questions about which pronunciation, if any, is the preferred one in your area, ask your instructor.

Listen carefully to your instructor's pronunciation, and pay particular attention to the presence of /t/ in these words. This exercise is found in Appendix 1. If you have difficulty recognizing /t/ in this drill, you may wish to review the exercise with somebody outside class.

26–2. DISCRIMINATING BETWEEN /t/ AND THE VARIOUS REPLACEMENTS

A. PROBABLE TYPES OF REPLACEMENT

The following exercises will help you learn to compare /t/ with your replacement. Your instructor has already told you which of the more common replacements you are using. If you are not employing one of these more common replacements, your instructor will tell you exactly how you are mispronouncing /t/ and provide you with some discrimination drills.

B. PAIRED LISTS OF WORDS

The words in the following paired lists are identical, except that the words in Column 1 contain the target, and the words in Column 2 contain one of the replacements. Complete instructions for this type of exercise are given in Chap. 5, 5-2B.

1. Column 1 /t/	Column 2 /θ/[5]	2. Column 1 /t/	Column 2 /d/
tank	thank	tie	die
torn	thorn	ten	den
true	through	to	do
tree	three	time	dime
tin	thin	matter	madder
pat	path	latter	ladder
boat	both	pat	pad
bat	bath	sat	sad
		sight	side
		seat	seed
		feet	feed
		beat	bead
		bit	bid

C. PAIRED SENTENCES

The following paired sentences are identical, except that the final word in the first sentence contains /t/, and the final word in the second sentence contains one of the replacements. Complete instructions for this type of drill are given in Chap. 5, 5-2C.

[5]If your replacement is dental /t/, your instructor will carry out this drill with you by changing the /t/–/θ/ pairs to /t/–dental /t/ pairs.

/t/ – /θ/[6]	/t/ – /d/
1. I think it's tin. I think it's thin.	1. Do you have the time? Do you have the dime?
2. Did you get a bat? Did you get a bath?	2. Give her a pat. Give her a pad.
3. Are you true? Are you through?	3. I found a seat. I found a seed.
4. It looks like a tree. It looks like a three.	4. Does he have the beat? Does he have the bead?

D.   LISTENING FOR REPLACEMENTS IN FAMILIAR /t/ WORDS

You will hear a list of words containing /t/. Sometimes the words will be pronounced correctly with /t/; other times the words will be said incorrectly with your replacement. Complete instructions for this type of drill are given in Chap. 5, 5-2D.

26–3.   A FEW REMINDERS ABOUT ORAL PRACTICE PROCEDURES

If this is the first practice chapter assigned to you by your instructor, you may wish to review the comments about beginning oral practice in Chap. 2, 2-4. Before you actually begin practicing each individual pronunciation drill, you may also desire to review the supplementary explanations about the exercise in Chap. 2, 2-5.

26–4.   THE PRONUNCIATION OF /t/

A.   PRONOUNCING ISOLATED /t/

In the event that you cannot pronounce /t/ through imitation alone, your instructor will help you with the following suggestions about placement. Should placement be required, you should review the definition of a stop in Chap. 4, 4-4H, and the description of /t/ in Figure 5 of Chapter 4.

1.   The Position of the Tongue on the Upper Gum Ridge

The position of the tongue is clearly visible when you pronounce /t/, and if you use a mirror, you should easily see what you are doing. Press your tongue tip slowly and firmly against your upper gum ridge, compressing some breath behind your tongue and building up some air pressure. Hold your breath in your mouth behind your tongue tip. Concentrate on feeling your tongue tip in contact with the upper gum ridge as you pronounce /t/. This part of pronouncing /t/ is

[6]See footnote 5.

particularly important because of the nature of several of the replacements. When you substitute a glottal stop for /t/, or omit the target, there is *no* contact between your tongue tip and your upper gum ridge. Definite contact between these articulators will help you avoid these replacements. The use of dental /t/ and /θ/ involves incorrect contact. In both instances your tongue tip is touching your teeth. Keeping your tongue tip *off* your teeth and *on* your gum ridge will help you avoid these replacements.

2. *The Escaping Breath*

Remove the tongue tip from your upper gum ridge suddenly, and explode the air out vigorously over the tip of your tongue saying /t/. You may check your pronunciation by feeling and seeing the puff of breath: (1) place your hand in front of your mouth, and see if you can feel the exploding air puff against your fingers, or (2) hold a piece of facial tissue in front of your mouth, and see if it jumps or bounces sharply because of the forceful impact of the exploding puff of breath. If you are unable to accomplish this, your instructor will help you feel the air puff by placing your hand close to his mouth while he pronounces /t/. He will also let you observe the air puff striking the facial tissue. If your replacement is too strong an air puff, concentrate on reducing the exploding breath. Pronounce the words *two* and *letter*, and compare the amount of breath you are employing for each /t/. If the explosive air puff appears the same for both targets, sharply reduce the amount of breath you are exploding for /t/ in *letter*. Check your progress by feeling and seeing the puff of breath as described earlier. Finally, remember that the essential difference between /t/ and /d/ is voicing. If your replacement is /d/, check your pronunciation by placing your fingers on your larynx, making certain that there is no vocal-band vibration. Note in all instances that accurate pronunciation of /t/ gives a clear, precise quality to this explosive voiceless consonant.

B.   ADDITIONAL COMMENTS

A few additional comments are useful at this point regarding the explosive release of /t/. Read the comments in Chap. 24, 24-4B. Keep in mind that the pronunciation of /t/ generally parallels the pronunciation of /p/: (1) final /t/ before a pause may be exploded or unexploded, (2) final /t/ followed by initial /t/ is pronounced *once* and prolonged (e.g., da**t**e **t**onight), and (3) when final /t/ is followed by any other plosive, there is only *one* stop and *one* explosion (e.g., bough**t c**ake).

C.   PRONOUNCING /t/ IN FAMILIAR WORDS

Pronounce each of the following words carefully. If you are either practicing with your instructor or listening to the exercise on tape, imitate your speech model as accurately as possible.

Beginning		Middle		End
1. ten	1. attend	21. getting	41. softly	1. date
2. taxi	2. attack	22. putting	42. mostly	2. eight
3. top	3. attach	23. beating	43. swiftly	3. peanut
4. tar	4. retake	24. lettuce	44. correctly	4. cigarette
5. tin	5. retype	25. sweater	45. perfectly	5. fruit
6. tail	6. detain	26. waiting	46. exactly	6. plate
7. take	7. return	27. exciting	47. battle	7. coat
8. talk	8. retain	28. hurting	48. kettle	8. cat
9. time	9. attain	29. letter	49. little	9. polite
10. tell	10. attention	30. pretty	50. cattle	10. seat
11. tailor	11. pretend	31. center	51. petal	11. right
12. television	12. guitar	32. ninety	52. rattle	12. bought
13. telegram	13. better	33. panting	53. metal	13. bright
14. tire	14. bitter	34. planted	54. settle	
15. toe	15. butter	35. renting	55. button	
16. tongue	16. invited	36. wanting	56. cotton	
17. turkey	17. notice	37. enter	57. kitten	
18. table	18. Betty	38. printed	58. rotten	
19. teacher	19. cutting	39. seventy	59. written	
20. tea	20. hotter	40. costly	60. certain	
			61. bitten	

D. Pronouncing Word Pairs Containing /t/ and a Replacement

Select some of the words from the paired lists in Section 26-2B containing /t/ and your replacement. Read one pair of words at a time, pronouncing the word with the target first (e.g., **tank–thank**). Make sure that you are saying /t/ first and /θ/ second. Reverse the procedure, and pronounce the replacement word first and the target word second, making certain that you use /θ/ first and /t/ second. Try to develop speed and accuracy as you do the drill. If you are either practicing with your instructor or listening to the exercise on tape, imitate your speech model as accurately as possible. If you are listening to the taped exercise, listen *only* to the drill that compares the target with your particular replacement. You will find this drill more difficult than the word list in Section 26-4C because of the closeness of target and replacement.

E. Pronouncing Familiar Words
Containing Frequent /t/ Consonant Clusters

You may find this exercise the most difficult of all the drills dealing with the pronunciation of /t/ in single words. It is often much more difficult to pronounce a consonant target when it is combined with another consonant in a cluster. Pronounce each of the words carefully. If you are either practicing with your instructor or listening to the drill on tape, imitate your speech model as accurately as possible.[7]

/tr/	/tw/	/lt/	/kt/	/nt/
1. trade	1. twelve	1. melt	1. protect	1. account
2. train	2. twenty	2. built	2. perfect	2. amount
3. travel	3. twins	3. felt	3. parked	3. bent
4. trip	4. twinkle	4. salt	4. expect	4. parent
5. tree		5. belt	5. backed	5. slant
6. truck			6. raked	
7. trunk			7. worked	
8. trouble			8. act	
			9. correct	

/pt/	/st/	/ft/	/ʃt/	/sts/	
1. clapped	1. almost	1. left	1. rushed	1. pests	7. beasts
2. dropped	2. against	2. lift	2. pushed	2. guests	8. rests
3. flipped	3. lost	3. draft	3. flashed	3. posts	9. forests
4. skipped	4. pest	4. swift	4. dashed	4. dentists	10. tastes
5. ripped	5. post	5. soft	5. mashed	5. priests	11. pastes
	6. biggest	6. sniffed	6. crashed	6. artists	12. wastes
	7. guest	7. gift			
	8. forest				
	9. rest				

/kts/	/fts/	/nts/	/skt/
1. protects	1. lifts	1. accounts	1. asked
2. perfects	2. drafts	2. amounts	2. masked
3. corrects	3. gifts	3. parents	3. risked
4. expects		4. slants	
5. acts			

F. PRONOUNCING /t/ IN PHRASES

Pronounce each of the phrases carefully. If you mispronounce a word, say it over again several times, and then repeat the entire phrase. If you are either practicing with your instructor or listening to the drill on tape, imitate your speech model as accurately as possible.

1. **eating mostly tangerines** and **tomatoes**
2. a **little plate** of **bitter lettuce**
3. **return** the **twenty tickets tomorrow**

---

[7]Although we have noted that final /t/ before a pause may be exploded or unexploded, it is suggested that you explode /t/ when it is final in a cluster before a pause. This should help you make certain that you do not omit the target in these difficult combinations.

4. **about wanting** a **guitar teacher**
5. **two guests at last** for the **party**
6. **took** the **post** for **certain** on **Tuesday**
7. **too** much **to expect** from the **guests**
8. **waiting to settle** the **rest**

G. PRONOUNCING SHORT PHRASES CONTAINING /t/ AND THE /θ/ OR DENTAL /t/ REPLACEMENT

This drill is similar to the exercise in Section 26-4D, except that your /θ/ replacement precedes the target in each phrase. Do this drill if your replacement is dental /t/, because the presence of /θ/ before /t/ is likely to make you change the target to a dental /t/. Pronounce each of the phrases carefully. If you are either practicing with your instructor or listening to the exercise on tape, imitate your speech model as accurately as possible. Although these phrases are shorter than those in the preceding drill, you may find this exercise more difficult, because your replacement directly precedes /t/ in each phrase.

/θ/ – /t/

1. path to school	5. mouth touched
2. cloth torn	6. both teachers
3. breath taken	7. underneath ten
4. bath time	8. earth turned

H. PRONOUNCING /t/ IN SENTENCES

Pronounce each of the sentences carefully. If you use a replacement, say the word over again several times, and then repeat the entire sentence. If you are either practicing with your instructor or listening to the exercise on tape, imitate your speech model as accurately as possible.

1. **Tom told** him **it** would **take too** much **time to telephone** the **city** police.
2. I saw **Tim** and **Betty parked** in the **lot** near **Times Supermarket** on **Saturday**.
3. They **told** him **to return** the **rest** of his **football tickets at** once.
4. **Patty** was **excitedly collecting bottle** caps so she could **enter** the **knit sweater contest**.
5. The **doctor** was **detained** and **took fifteen minutes to** reach the **Center Hotel**.

I. PRONOUNCING /t/ IN BEGINNING CONVERSATION

This exercise gives you an opportunity to begin using some of your previously learned /t/ words in beginning conversation. Complete instructions for this type of drill are given in Chap. 5, 5-5H. Read the instructions, and adapt them to practice with /t/.

1. "Is your _____ made of **cotton**?"
2. "Was the _____ **rotten**?"
3. "He **turned left** and drove **to** _____."
4. "Were your _____ **tests correct**?"
5. "He **dropped** the _____."
6. "Is the _____ very **costly**?"
7. "They **fought** the **battle** at _____."
8. "Did you **tell Betty about** her _____?"
9. "Did **Ted** buy the **better** _____?"
10. "Did you **attend** the _____ **last** week?"
11. "Please **put** some _____ on the **table**."
12. "**Tell** him **to** bring some _____ **tomorrow**."
13. "Did he **take** the _____ to the **tailor**?"
14. "Was he **teasing** the _____?"
15. "Did you **notice** the _____?"
16. "Your _____ is **torn**."
17. "Did the **waiter** give you some _____ for **dessert**?"

26–5. CONVERSATION PRACTICE

So far you have learned how to pronounce your target by reading various kinds of exercises which contain /t/ words. Now you are ready to move into the final and most important part of your training program—learning to pronounce /t/ automatically while you are talking more or less spontaneously. If this is the first practice chapter assigned to you by your instructor, you may wish to review the introductory comments on conversation practice in Chap. 2, 2-6 to 2-7.

A. CARRYING /t/ INTO SPONTANEOUS DAILY CONVERSATION

This exercise requires you to use /t/ in daily conversation, starting with key words and expanding to all the /t/ words in your particular vocabulary. Complete instructions for this type of drill are given in Chap. 5, 5-5A, and there are supplementary comments about the exercise in Chap. 2, 2-7A.

B. GENERAL CLASSROOM EXERCISES IN SPEAKING

Your instructor will plan a series of classroom conversation activities, and each assignment will be discussed fully in class before you carry it out. When your instructor announces the first speaking activity, you may wish to review the introductory comments on classroom speaking in Chap. 2, 2-7B.

chapter twenty-seven

The Consonant Target
/d/ (die)

COMMON SPELLINGS FOR /d/

The most frequent spellings are found in the words **d**ay, la**dd**er, and love**d**.
An explanation is necessary at this point about the past tense and the past participle of regular English verbs which are formed by adding an **ed** or **d** ending. The pronunciation of the **ed** or **d** spelling in these verb forms becomes /t/, /d/, or a syllable containing either /t/ or /d/. Some simple rules determine these pronunciations. The rules, which are given below, are based on the concept of voicing. You may wish to review the comments about voiced and voiceless consonants in Chap. 4, 4-3A. Pay particular attention to these rules if your instructor tells you that your replacement is the substitution of /t/ as in **t**ie for /d/.

1. When the sound preceding the **ed** or **d** ending is any one of the following voiceless sounds, the ending is pronounced /t/: /p/ (ho**p**ed), /f/ (sni**ff**ed), /ʃ/ (pu**sh**ed), /k/ (coo**k**ed), /s/ (ra**c**ed), /tʃ/ (pa**tch**ed), and /θ/ (fro**th**ed).

2. When the sound preceding the **ed** or **d** ending is any one of the following voiced sounds, the ending is pronounced /d/ (this includes all vowels, diphthongs, and the following voiced consonants): /b/ (robbed), /g/ (tagged), /v/ (lived), /ð/ (bathed), /l/ (failed), /m/ (ashamed), /n/ (cleaned), /ŋ/ (longed), /z/ (seized), /dʒ/ (changed), and /ʒ/ (rouged).

3. When the sound preceding the **ed** or **d** ending is either /t/ or /d/, the ending is pronounced with a syllable. The syllable may be said as /əd/ (/ə/ as in **a**bout), or /ɪd/ (/ɪ/ as in **i**t.). Examples include /d/ (flood**ed**) and /t/ (pant**ed**).

Certain English adjectives look like verb forms because of their *ed* endings (e.g., **ragged** and **naked**). The *ed* endings of these adjectives are pronounced either /əd/ or /ɪd/. Other adjectives function as either adjectives or verbs, depending upon usage. When the word is used as an adjective, the ending is pronounced with a syllable. When the word is used as a verb, the ending is said according to the previously described rules. An example of this type of word is **aged**.

1. He has aged /eɪdʒd/ greatly. (verb)
2. Her father is an aged /eɪdʒəd/ man. (adjective)

27–1. EAR TRAINING FOR THE /d/ TARGET

A. A Few Reminders About Ear Training

The following test exercises will help you learn to recognize your /d/ target. If this is the first practice chapter assigned to you by your instructor, you may wish to review the discussion about listening practice in Chap. 2, 2-2B to 2-3C.

B. Recognizing /d/ in Words

You will hear a list of words containing /d/. After listening to each word, write *B* if you heard /d/ at the beginning of the word, *M* if you heard /d/ in the middle, and *E* if you heard /d/ at the end of the word. Observe carefully the clear, precise quality associated with the pronunciation of /d/. The answers will be read to you at the end of the drill. This exercise is found in Appendix 1. If you have difficulty recognizing the target, you may find it worthwhile to review the test with somebody outside class.

C. Recognizing /d/ in Sentences

You will listen to a series of sentences containing a number of /d/ words. Each sentence will be read to you several times. Try to locate the /d/ words in each sentence, and write them down. The /d/ words in each test sentence will be read to you at the end of the drill. The sentences appear later in the chapter in Section 27-4H. If you have difficulty recognizing the target, you may find it worthwhile to review the test with somebody else outside class.

D.   RECOGNIZING /d/ IN WORDS IN WHICH THE TARGET IS TYPICALLY OMITTED

You will notice in Section 27-2A that one of the possible replacements is the omission of the target in words like **bold**, **behind**, **wonderful**, and **shoulder**. If this is one of your problems, your instructor will carry out this drill with you. In this test exercise your instructor will help you learn to recognize the pronunciation of /d/ when it is used in the word types mentioned earlier. Listen carefully to your instructor's pronunciation, and pay particular attention to the presence of /d/ in the test words. This exercise is found in Appendix 1. If you have difficulty recognizing /d/ in this drill, you may wish to review the exercise with somebody outside class.

27–2.   DISCRIMINATING BETWEEN /d/ AND THE VARIOUS REPLACEMENTS

A.   PROBABLE TYPES OF REPLACEMENT

The following exercises will help you learn to compare /d/ with your replacement. You are probably substituting one of the following common replacements for /d/: (1) /ð/ as in **the**m, (2) dental (d) — that is, your tongue touches the upper, middle front teeth rather than your upper gum ridge,[1] or (3) /t/ as in **tie**. You may also omit /d/ in the following types of words: (1) in final consonant clusters as in bo**ld** and behi**nd**, and (2) after /n/ or /l/ as in wo**nd**erful and shou**ld**er. Your instructor will tell you which replacement you are using. If you are not employing one of the more common replacements, your teacher will tell you exactly how you are mispronouncing /d/ and provide you with some discrimination drills.

B.   PAIRED LISTS OF WORDS

The words in the following paired lists are identical, except that the words in Column 1 contain the target, and the words in Column 2 contain one of the replacements. Complete instructions for this type of exercise are given in Chap. 5, 5-2B.

[1]Note that dental /d/ is acceptable when the target precedes /θ/ as in (**th**ought) or /ð/ as in ba**d th**ing, and ma**d**e **th**at.

1. Column 1 /d/	Column 2 /ð/[2]	2. Column 1 /d/	Column 2 /t/
dare	there	die	tie
doe	though	den	ten
day	they	do	to
Dan	than	dear	tear
doze	those	dime	time
den	then	madder	matter
fodder	father	ladder	latter
ladder	lather	pad	pat
laid	lathe	ride	right
breed	breathe	rode	wrote
		sad	sat
		side	sight
		seed	seat
		feed	feet
		bead	beat
		bid	bit
		hide	height

C.   PAIRED SENTENCES

The following paired sentences are identical, except that the final word in the first sentence contains /d/, and the final word in the second sentence contains one of the replacements. Complete instructions for this type of drill are given Chap. 5, 5-2C.

/d/ – /ð/[3]

1. Will it breed?
   Will it breathe?
2. Is it day?
   Is it they?
3. It's my father.
   It's my fodder.
4. I see the ladder.
   I see the lather.

/d/ – /t/

1. Do you have the dime?
   Do you have the time?
2. Give her a pad.
   Give her a pat.
3. Can he ride?
   Can he write?
4. I think he rode.
   I think he wrote.
5. I found three seeds.
   I found three seats.
6. Does he have the bead?
   Does he have the beat?

[2]If your replacement is dental /d/, your instructor will carry out this drill with you by changing the /d/–/ð/ pairs to /d/–dental /d/ pairs.
[3]See footnote 2.

D.   LISTENING FOR REPLACEMENTS IN FAMILIAR /d/ WORDS

You will hear a list of words containing /d/. Sometimes the words will be pronounced correctly with /d/; other times the words will be said incorrectly with your replacement. Complete instructions for this type of drill are given in Chap. 5, 5-2D.

27–3.   A FEW REMINDERS ABOUT ORAL PRACTICE PROCEDURES

If this is the first chapter assigned to you by your instructor, you may wish to review the comments about beginning oral practice in Chap. 2, 2-4. Before you actually begin practicing each individual pronunciation drill, you may also desire to review the supplementary explanations about the exercise in Chap. 2, 2-5.

27–4.   THE PRONUNCIATION OF /d/

A.   PRONOUNCING /d/ IN A SIMPLE SYLLABLE

In the event that you cannot pronounce /d/ through imitation alone, your instructor will help you with the following suggestions about placement. Should placement be required, you should review the definition of a stop in Chap. 4, 4-4H and the description of /d/ in Figure 5 of Chapter 4. Note that because of the nature of the consonant, the target cannot be pronounced in isolation.

1.   The Position of the Tongue on the Upper Gum Ridge

The position of the tongue is clearly visible when you pronounce /d/, and if you use a mirror, you should easily see what you are doing. Press your tongue tip slowly and firmly against your upper gum ridge, compressing some breath behind your lips and building up some air pressure. Hold your breath in your mouth behind your tongue tip. Concentrate on feeling your tongue tip in contact with the upper gum ridge as you pronounce /d/. This part of pronouncing /d/ is particularly important because of the nature of the replacements. When you use /ð/ or dental /d/, there is incorrect contact, because your tongue tip is touching your teeth. Keeping your tongue tip *off* your teeth and *on* your gum ridge will help you avoid these replacements. When you omit the target after /n/ or /l/, there is *no* contact between your tongue tip and your upper gum ridge. Definite contact between these articulators will help you avoid omitting /d/.

2. The Escaping Breath

Remove the tongue tip from your upper gum ridge suddenly, and explode the air out vigorously, saying the syllable /dɑ/ (/ɑ/) as in (hot) and (father). This consonant is voiced, and you must be certain that your vocal bands are vibrating as you explode the breath out of your mouth. Check for the vibration of the bands by placing your fingers on your larynx as you pronounce /dɑ/. If you are unable to feel the vibration from your own larynx, your instructor will place your fingers on his larynx and say /dɑ/. Keep practicing until you can feel the vibration from your own larynx while pronouncing /dɑ/. When that happens, you can double-check your pronunciation of the target by placing your hands over your ears while saying /dɑ/. You should be able to hear the vibration. Keep in mind that the vowel /ɑ/ is voiced and that you are *not* likely to unvoice the vowel. When checking for vibration, make sure that what you feel and hear *begins* on /d/ and not on the vowel. If you are using the correct tongue position for the target, and you do not feel or hear the vibration of the bands, you are pronouncing /tɑ/ rather than /dɑ/. The primary difference between /d/ and /t/ is voicing. Note that accurate pronunciation of /d/ gives a clear, precise quality to this explosive voiced consonant.

B. ADDITIONAL COMMENTS

A few additional comments are useful at this point regarding the explosive release of /d/. Read the comments in Chap. 24, 24-4B. Keep in mind that the pronunciation of /d/ generally parallels the pronunciation of /p/: (1) final /d/ before a pause may be exploded or unexploded, (2) final /d/ followed by initial /d/ is pronounced *once* and prolonged (e.g., brea**d d**ropped), and (3) when final /d/ is followed by any other plosive there is only *one* stop and *one* explosion (e.g., sai**d g**aily).

C. PRONOUNCING /d/ IN FAMILIAR WORDS

Pronounce each of the following words carefully. If you are either practicing with your instructor or listening to the exercise on tape, imitate your speech model as accurately as possible.

Beginning

1. deer	8. dog	15. does
2. donkey	9. duck	16. doing
3. dime	10. daisy	17. done
4. dock	11. day	18. double
5. door	12. dial	19. dare
6. dinner	13. down	20. dust
7. desk	14. dig	

Middle			End[4]	
1. sidewalk	11. nobody	21. winding	1. paid	11. red
2. ladder	12. reading	22. thunder	2. proud	12. said
3. spider	13. Monday	23. shoulder	3. period	13. mud
4. pudding	14. Sunday	24. children	4. bad	14. parade
5. Thursday	15. window	25. colder	5. bird	15. seed
6. idea	16. sandwich	26. bolder	6. add	16. road
7. feeding	17. laundry	27. building	7. ahead	17. head
8. guiding	18. hundred	28. older	8. crowd	18. flood
9. lady	19. wondering		9. good	19. bread
10. leading	20. standing		10. need	20. bed

D.   PRONOUNCING WORD PAIRS CONTAINING /d/ AND A REPLACEMENT

Select some of the words from the paired lists in Section 27-2B containing /d/ and your replacement. Read one pair of words at a time, pronouncing the word with the target first (e.g., **die–tie**). Make sure that you are saying /d/ first and /t/ second. Reverse the procedure, and pronounce the replacement word first and the target word second, making certain that you use /t/ first and /d/ second. Try to develop speed and accuracy as you do the drill. If you are either practicing with your instructor or listening to the exercise on tape, imitate your speech model as accurately as possible. If you are listening to the taped exercise, listen *only* to the drill that compares the target with your particular replacement. You will find this drill more difficult than the word list in Section 27-4C because of the closeness of target and replacement.

E.   PRONOUNCING FAMILIAR WORDS CONTAINING
FREQUENT /d/ CONSONANT CLUSTERS

You may find this exercise the most difficult of all the drills dealing with the pronunciation of /d/ in single words. It is often much more difficult to pronounce a consonant target when it is combined with another consonant in a cluster. Pronounce each of the words carefully. If you are either practicing with your instructor or listening to the drill on tape, imitate your speech model as accurately as possible.[5]

---

[4]If you have difficulty pronouncing final /d/, read footnote 3 in Chapter 8, and adapt the comments to the pronunciation of final voiced /d/.

[5]Although we have noted that final /d/ before a pause may be exploded or unexploded, it is suggested that you explode /d/ when it is final in a cluster before a pause. This should help make certain that you do not omit the target in these difficult combinations.

/dr/	/ld/	/nd/	/md/	/ŋd/
1. dream	1. airfield	1. behind	1. ashamed	1. banged
2. drag	2. build	2. beyond	2. alarmed	2. belonged
3. drive	3. bold	3. found	3. aimed	
4. drop	4. failed	4. fond	4. climbed	
5. dry	5. cold	5. round		
6. dress	6. world	6. blind		
7. drinking	7. gold	7. husband		
	8. hold	8. ground		
	9. sold			
	10. told			

/gd/	/dʒd/	/vd/	/zd/	/dz/	/ndʒd/
1. begged	1. caged	1. arrived	1. gazed	1. reads	1. changed
2. hugged	2. judged	2. dived	2. blazed	2. leads	2. arranged
3. tagged	3. edged		3. raised	3. beads	3. sponged
4. drugged	4. raged			4. seeds	
5. jogged	5. managed			5. needs	
6. wagged					
7. sagged					

F.   PRONOUNCING /d/ IN PHRASES

Pronounce each of the phrases carefully. If you mispronounce a word, say it over again several times, and then repeat the entire phrase. If you are either practicing with your instructor or listening to the drill on tape, imitate your speech model as accurately as possible.

1. a **need** for a **third period**
2. **advance ahead** of the **crowd**
3. **hiding under** the **older bed**
4. **glad** he was not **rude** with the **candy**

5. a **parade** of **ducks ending** on the **road**
6. a **bad tide caused** a **flood**
7. **doing double** time in the **meadow**
8. **wondering** about a **damp stadium**

G.   PRONOUNCING SHORT PHRASES
CONTAINING /d/ AND THE /t/ REPLACEMENT

This drill is similar to the exercise in Section 27-4D, except that your /t/ replacement precedes the target in each phrase. Pronounce each of the phrases carefully. If you are either practicing with your instructor or listening to the exercise on tape, imitate your speech model as accurately as possible. Although these phrases are shorter than those in the preceding drill, you may find this exercise more difficult, because your replacement directly precedes /d/ in each phrase. Keep in mind the previous comments about pronouncing two consecutive plosive sounds with one stop and one explosion.

$$/t/ - /d/$$

1. bright day	5. bought dinner
2. polite doings	6. right downtown
3. peanut dip	7. eight deer
4. seat dented	8. put down

H.   PRONOUNCING /d/ IN SENTENCES

Pronounce each of the words carefully. If you use a replacement, say the word over again several times, and then repeat the entire sentence. If you are either practicing with your instructor or listening to the exercise on tape, imitate your speech model as accurately as possible.

1. They **had** some **delicious** roast **duck** with **homemade pudding** for **dinner** last **Monday.**
2. **Judy wanted** to give **everybody** some **good candy** for **dessert** in **December.**
3. The **Dutch doctor** was **discovered wandering** about on the **docks** at the **end** of the **day.**
4. **Eddie** is **driving** home **today and** he **should** arrive in **Denver** at **dawn.**
5. The **delivery** boy was **paid** a **dollar** for **dropping** off the **medicine** for the sick **lady.**

I.   PRONOUNCING /d/ IN BEGINNING CONVERSATION

This exercise gives you an opportunity to begin using some of your previously learned /d/ words in beginning conversation. Complete instructions for this type of drill are given in Chap. 5, 5-4H. Read the instructions, and adapt them to practice with /d/.

1. "**Did** you have a _____ **sandwich** for **dinner**?"
2. "Are you **wondering** about the _____?"
3. "Was the _____ **sold**?"
4. "Was **Dan glad** to get a **ride** to _____?"
5. "Is your new _____ **red**?"
6. "**Did** you like the _____ **pudding yesterday**?"
7. "**Did** you **deliver** the _____?"
8. "**Do** the **children need** the _____?"
9. "Was he **standing** near the _____?"
10. "**Dad** wants a _____ for his **birthday**."
11. "Was he **ashamed** about the _____?"

12. "Was he **reading** the _____?"

13. "**Did** you buy some _____ at the **drugstore**?"

14. "Did **somebody order** the _____?"

27–5.   CONVERSATION PRACTICE

So far you have learned how to pronounce your target by reading various kinds of exercises which contain /d/ words. Now you are ready to move into the final and most important part of your training program—learning to pronounce /d/ automatically while you are talking more or less spontaneously. If this is the first practice chapter assigned to you by your instructor, you may wish to review the introductory comments on conversation practice in Chap. 2, 2-6 to 2-7.

A.   CARRYING /d/ INTO SPONTANEOUS DAILY CONVERSATION

This exercise requires you to use /d/ in daily conversation, starting with key words and expanding to all the /d/ words in your particular vocabulary. Complete instructions for this type of drill are given in Chap. 5, 5-5A, and there are supplementary comments about the exercise in Chap. 2, 2-7A.

B.   GENERAL CLASSROOM EXERCISES IN SPEAKING

Your instructor will plan a series of classroom conversation activities, and each assignment will be discussed fully in class before you carry it out. When your instructor announces the first speaking activity, you may wish to review the introductory comments on classroom speaking in Chap. 2, 2-7B.

chapter twenty-eight

The Consonant Target
/k/ (key)

COMMON SPELLINGS FOR /k/

The most frequent spellings are found in the following words: **key** and **c**ome; less frequent spellings include ti**ck**, s**q**uare, **Ch**ristmas, a**cc**ount, the first sound of the letter **x** when it is equal to /ks/, as in box, and the first sound of the letters **cc** when they are equal to /ks/, as in accept.[1]

28–1. EAR TRAINING FOR THE /k/ TARGET

A. A FEW REMINDERS ABOUT EAR TRAINING

The following test exercises will help you learn to recognize your /k/ target. If this is the first practice chapter assigned to you by your instructor, you may wish to review the discussion about listening practice in Chap. 2, 2-2B to 2-3C.

---

[1] Note that spelled **k** is silent in the following familiar words: know, knot, knuckle, knit, knock, knife, knew, knee, and doorknob.

The ear training exercises for /k/ require a few additional special remarks, because the replacements differ so widely. Note the following types of replacements.

1. You have a problem involving the aspirate characteristics of pronouncing /k/. The target /k/ is frequently said with a strong explosive puff of air known as *aspiration*. This strong puff of air is used when /k/ comes at the beginning of a word, as in **key**, or when /k/ comes at the beginning of an emphasized or stressed syllable, as in **account**. This heavy puff of breath is essential to the correct pronunciation of /k/ in these kinds of words. You mispronounce the target in words like **key** and **account**, because you pronounce the target *without* the strong puff of breath. This type of mispronunciation frequently suggests /g/ to the native speaker of English.
2. The pronunciation of /k/ requires firm contact between the back of the tongue and the soft palate. Without this type of contact the target lacks its typically clear and precise quality. You may have difficulty developing the proper contact between your tongue and soft palate, and either pronounce /k/ with a fuzzy, sometimes friction-like, quality or omit the target.
3. Some students have omission problems in certain types of final consonant clusters: for example, they omit /k/ in words like desk, asked, and risks.

Because of these various types of replacement pronunciations, several kinds of ear training drills are used in this chapter. Your instructor will tell you which exercise he wants you to carry out. Regardless of which ear training drills you listen to, observe carefully the preciseness used in pronouncing /k/.

B. Recognizing /k/ in Words
   When the Replacement Is Caused by Poor Contact

In the following test exercise, your instructor will help you learn to identify the clear, precise quality that is associated with pronouncing /k/. You will hear a list of /k/ words in various positions. Listen carefully to your instructor's pronunciation, and familiarize yourself with the clarity of the target. This exercise is found in Appendix 1. If you have difficulty recognizing the preciseness of /k/, you may find it worthwhile to review the drill with somebody outside class.

C. Recognizing /k/ in Words
   When the Target Is Said with a Strong Puff of Air

In the following test exercise your instructor will help you learn to recognize the strong air puff of /k/. You will hear a list of words containing /k/ at the beginning of a word or at the beginning of a stressed syllable. Listen carefully to your instructor's pronunciation, and familiarize yourself with the strong puff of breath. This exercise is found in Appendix 1. If you have difficulty recognizing the strong air puff, you may find it worthwhile to review the drill with somebody outside class.

D. RECOGNIZING /k/ IN WORDS WHEN THE TARGET IS OMITTED IN CERTAIN FINAL CONSONANT CLUSTERS

In the following test exercise, your instructor will help you learn to recognize the pronunciation of /k/ when it is used in words like desk, asked, and risks. Listen carefully to your instructor's pronunciation, and pay particular attention to the presence of /k/ in these words. This exercise is found in Appendix 1. If you have difficulty recognizing /k/ in this drill, you may wish to review the exercise with somebody outside class.

28–2. DISCRIMINATING BETWEEN /k/ AND THE VARIOUS REPLACEMENTS

A. PROBABLE TYPES OF REPLACEMENT

The following exercise will help you learn to compare /k/ with your replacement. Your instructor has already told you which one of the more common replacements you are using. If you are not employing one of these more common replacements, your instructor will tell you exactly how you are mispronouncing /k/ and provide you with some discrimination drills.

B. LISTENING FOR REPLACEMENTS IN FAMILIAR /k/ WORDS

You will hear a list of words containing /k/. Sometimes the words will be pronounced correctly with /k/; other times the words will be said incorrectly with your replacement. Complete instructions for this type of drill are given in Chap. 5, 5-2D.

28–3. A FEW REMINDERS ABOUT ORAL PRACTICE PROCEDURES

If this is the first practice chapter assigned to you by your instructor, you may wish to review the comments about beginning oral practice in Chap. 2, 2-4. Before you actually begin practicing each individual pronunciation drill, you may also desire to review the supplementary explanations about the exercise in Chap. 2, 2-5.

28–4. THE PRONUNCIATION OF /k/

A. PRONOUNCING ISOLATED /k/

In the event that you cannot pronounce /k/ through imitation alone, your instructor will help you with the following suggestions about placement. Should placement be required, you should review the definition of a stop in Chap. 4, 4-4H and the description of /k/ in Figure 5 of Chapter 4.

1. The Position of the Back of the Tongue on the Soft Palate

Press the back of your tongue slowly and firmly against your soft palate, compressing some breath behind your tongue and building up some air pressure. Hold your breath in your mouth behind the back of your tongue. Concentrate on feeling the back of your tongue in contact with your soft palate. This part of pronouncing /k/ is particularly important if you omit the target or have a contact problem. When you omit /k/, there is *no* contact between the back of the tongue and the soft palate. When you produce a fuzzy or friction-like /k/, you are failing to press your tongue against the soft palate with sufficient tension or pressure. This quality may also be heard if you move your tongue up to the soft palate too slowly. A tongue that is firmly placed against your soft palate will help you avoid these replacements. Note that the exact point of contact between the tongue and the soft palate varies according to the kind of vowel that follows /k/. The contact tends to be further forward before front vowels than before back vowels. Compare the words **keep** and **cool**, and observe the difference in contact position. The /k/ in **cool**—before the back vowel /u/—is made much further back on the soft palate than is the /k/ in **keep** before the front vowel /i/. If you have difficulty noting the difference in position, try the series **kill**, **cool**, and **call**. Observe how your tongue moves progressively further back on your soft palate from the first word to the last word in the sequence. Normally most speakers make these contact adjustments automatically. Do not be concerned about placing your tongue in the exact same place on your soft palate for every pronunciation of /k/, unless your instructor indicates that you have a problem in this area.

2. The Escaping Breath

Remove the back of your tongue from your soft palate suddenly, and explode the air vigorously over your tongue and out through your mouth, saying /k/. You may check your pronunciation by feeling and seeing the puff of breath: (1) place your hand in front of your mouth, and see if you can feel the exploding air puff against your fingers, and (2) hold a piece of facial tissue in front of your mouth, and see if it jumps or bounces sharply because of the forceful impact of the exploding puff of breath. If you are unable to accomplish this, your instructor will help you feel the air puff by placing your hand close to his mouth while he pronounces /k/. He will also let you observe the air puff striking the facial tissue.

B. Additional Comments

A few additional comments are useful at this point regarding the explosive release of /k/. Read the comments in Chap. 24, 24-4B. Keep in mind that the pronunciation of /k/ generally parallels the pronunciation of /p/: (1) final /k/ before a pause may be exploded or unexploded, (2) final /k/ followed by initial

/k/ is pronounced *once* and prolonged (e.g., spea**k c**arefully), and (3) when final /k/ is followed by any other plosive, there is only *one* stop and *one* explosion (e.g., la**ke t**rout).

C. PRONOUNCING /k/ IN FAMILIAR WORDS

Pronounce each of the following words carefully. If you are either practicing with your instructor or listening to the exercise on tape, imitate your speech model as accurately as possible.

Beginning		Middle	End
1. keep	15. corn	1. require	1. lake
2. kind	16. cow	2. became	2. brook
3. kiss	17. cup	3. because	3. dock
4. can	18. candle	4. raccoon	4. tack
5. could	19. coal	5. mechanic	5. snack
6. cousin	20. canoe	6. account	6. like
7. candy	21. coffee	7. acquire	7. speak
8. cap	22. camera	8. accent	8. work
9. car	23. key	9. accept	9. week
10. careful	24. comb	10. accident	10. took
11. call	25. copper	11. package	11. talk
12. cover	26. color	12. except	12. sick
13. king	27. cabbage	13. excuse	13. lock
14. cave	28. chorus	14. excite	14. back
		15. explain	15. sack
		16. extra	16. rock
		17. ticket	17. luck
		18. working	18. cook
		19. picking	19. attack
		20. packing	20. pancake

D. PRONOUNCING FAMILIAR WORDS CONTAINING FREQUENT /k/ CONSONANT CLUSTERS

You may find this exercise more difficult than the preceding drill. It is often much more difficult to pronounce a consonant target when it is combined with another consonant in a cluster. Pronounce each of the words carefully. If you are either practicing with your instructor or listening to the drill on tape, imitate your speech model as accurately as possible.[2]

---

[2]Although we have noted that final /k/ before a pause may be exploded or unexploded, it is suggested that you explode /k/ when it is final in a cluster before a pause. This should help make certain that you do not omit the target in these difficult combinations.

/kr/	/kl/	/kw/	/sk/	/skw/
1. cracker	1. clean	1. question	1. school	1. squeak
2. cream	2. climb	2. quit	2. skin	2. squeeze
3. crack	3. clever	3. quick	3. sky	3. squeal
4. crash	4. class	4. quite	4. skate	4. square
5. cry	5. clock	5. queen	5. skirt	5. squash
6. crayon	6. cloud	6. quarter	6. scared	
7. crowd	7. clay	7. quart	7. scold	
8. crown	8. cloth	8. quiet	8. scoop	

/skr/	/kt/	/ks/	/ŋk/	/lk/	/sk/
1. scream	1. object	1. fix	1. drank	1. silk	1. desk
2. scrap	2. ached	2. six	2. wink	2. milk	2. ask
3. scratch	3. protect	3. mix	3. bank		3. task
4. screen	4. looked	4. hooks	4. trunk		4. risk
5. screw	5. smoked	5. pecks	5. pink		5. tusk
	6. barked	6. ax	6. sink		6. mask
	7. subject	7. wax	7. blink		
	8. act	8. box			

/kts/	/kst/	/ŋks/	/lks/	/sks/	/skt/
1. objects	1. next	1. winks	1. silks	1. desks	1. asked
2. protects	2. mixed	2. banks	2. milks	2. asks	2. risked
3. perfects	3. fixed	3. trunks		3. tasks	3. masked
4. directs		4. blinks		4. risks	
5. acts		5. sinks		5. tusks	
				6. masks	

E.   PRONOUNCING /k/ IN PHRASES

Pronounce each of the phrases carefully. If you mispronounce a word, say it over again several times, and then repeat the entire phrase. If you are either practicing with your instructor or listening to the drill on tape, imitate your speech model as accurately as possible.

1. a **cow** and a **calf** by the **king's lake**
2. **candy canes** on the **Christmas** tree
3. a **cold** ice **cream cone** on the **corner**
4. **like** to **bake** a **cream cake**
5. **asked** to **make** a **kite** for the **kid**
6. **asks** of **Kenneth** in the **cafeteria**
7. an **extra mask** on his **desk** at **school**

F.   PRONOUNCING /k/ IN SENTENCES

Pronounce each of the words carefully. If you use a replacement, say the word over again several times, and then repeat the entire sentence. If you are either practicing with your instructor or listening to the exercise on tape, imitate your speech model as accurately as possible.

1. The **crabby cook** was **excited because** the **company** didn't **like** the **pumpkin** pie.
2. They **drank** some **coffee** from the **copper kettle** in the **kitchen** while **packing**.
3. The **class** took their **crayons** and began **coloring** the **lake carefully**.
4. The **clerk called quickly** and said the **pink candles** would **cost** too much.
5. The **mechanic came** for the **car because** my **cousin called** him.

G.   PRONOUNCING /k/ IN BEGINNING CONVERSATION

This exercise gives you an opportunity to begin using some of your previously learned /k/ words in beginning conversation. Complete instructions for this type of drill are given in Chap. 5, 5-4H. Read the instructions, and adapt them to practice with /k/.

1. "My favorite **subject** is _____ _____."
2. "Was your _____ test **correct**?"
3. "Did you **come across** the _____ at **camp**?"
4. "**Could** they put the _____ in the **car**?"
5. "I **caught** a **cold** last **week** at _____."
6. "**Can** you **clean** the _____?"
7. "**Can** you **count** all of the _____?"
8. "I **picked** out my **skirt** and **coat** at _____."
9. "Did you **call** _____ last **week** and **explain**?
10. "I have an **account** at the _____ **bank**."
11. "I'm going to **California** in _____."

28–5.   CONVERSATION PRACTICE

So far you have learned how to pronounce your target by reading various kinds of exercises which contain /k/ words. Now you are ready to move into the final and most important part of your training program—learning to pronounce /k/ automatically while you are talking more or less spontaneously. If this is the first practice chapter assigned to you by your instructor, you may wish to review the introductory comments on conversation practice in Chap. 2, 2-6 to 2-7.

A.   CARRYING /k/ INTO SPONTANEOUS DAILY CONVERSATION

This exercise requires you to use /k/ in daily conversation, starting with key words and expanding to all the /k/ words in your particular vocabulary. Complete instructions for this type of drill are given in Chap. 5, 5-5A, and there are supplementary comments about the exercise in Chap. 2, 2-7A.

B.   GENERAL CLASSROOM EXERCISES IN SPEAKING

Your instructor will plan a series of classroom conversation activities, and each assignment will be discussed fully in class before you carry it out. When your instructor announces the first speaking activity, you may wish to review the introductory comments on classroom speaking in Chap. 2, 2-7B.

chapter twenty-nine

The Consonant Target
/g/ (get)

COMMON SPELLINGS FOR /g/

The most frequent spelling is found in the word **g**o: less frequent spellings include **gu**est, e**gg**, **gh**ost, and the first sound of the letter **x** when it is equal to /gz/ as in e**x**it.

29–1. EAR TRAINING FOR THE /g/ TARGET

A. A Few Reminders About Ear Training

The following test exercises will help you learn to recognize your /g/ target. If this is the first practice chapter assigned to you by your instructor, you may wish to review the discussion about listening practice in Chap. 2, 2-2B to 2-3C.

B.   RECOGNIZING /g/ IN WORDS

You will hear a list of words containing /g/. After listening to each word, write *B* if you heard /g/ at the beginning of the word, *M* if you heard /g/ in the middle, and *E* if you heard /g/ at the end of the word. Observe carefully the clear, precise quality associated with the pronunciation of /g/. The answers will be read to you at the end of the drill. This exercise is found in Appendix 1. If you have difficulty recognizing the target, you may find it worthwhile to review the test with somebody outside class.

C.   RECOGNIZING /g/ IN SENTENCES

You will listen to a series of sentences containing a number of /g/ words. Each sentence will be read several times. Try to locate the /g/ words in each sentence, and write them down. The /g/ words in each test sentence will be read to you at the end of the drill. The sentences appear later in the chapter in Section 29-4H. If you have difficulty recognizing the target, you may find it worthwhile to review the test with somebody outside class.

29–2.   DISCRIMINATING BETWEEN /g/ AND THE VARIOUS REPLACEMENTS

A.   PROBABLE TYPES OF REPLACEMENT

The following exercises will help you learn to compare /g/ with your replacement. You are probably substituting one of the following common replacements for /g/: (1) /k/ as in **k**ey, or (2) a fricative /g/, which is symbolized by /g̶/. This sound is formed by raising the back of your tongue close to your soft palate, and then blowing voiced breath steadily through the narrowed space between the arched back of the tongue and your soft palate. The tongue is relaxed. Your instructor will tell you which replacement you are using. If you are not employing one of the more common replacements, your teacher will tell you exactly how you are mispronouncing /g/ and provide you with some discrimination drills.[1]

B.   PAIRED LISTS OF WORDS

The words in the following paired list are identical, except that Column 1 words contain the target and Column 2 words contain the /g/ replacement. Complete instructions for this type of exercise are given in Chap. 5, 5-2B.

---

[1]Your instructor may tell you that you are adding /g/ in a word like singer and omitting /g/ in a word like finger. This type of problem is typically related to the spelling of **ng** in English words and is discussed in Chapter 23.

Column 1 /g/	Column 2 /k/[2]
gain	cane
game	came
gate	Kate
gold	cold
guard	card
gave	cave
glass	class
glue	clue
grow	crow
grab	crab
tagging	tacking
logging	locking
bagging	backing
tag	tack
pig	pick
log	lock
dig	Dick
bug	buck
bag	back
rag	rack
nag	nack
sag	sack

C. PAIRED SENTENCES[3]

The following paired sentences are identical, except that the final word in the first sentence contains /g/, and the final word in the second sentence contains /k/. Complete instructions for this type of drill are given in Chap. 5, 5-2C.

/g/ – /k/

1. I saw the guard.   4. Is that a log?
   I saw the card.   Is that a lock?
2. Where's the glass?   5. It's in the bag.
   Where's the class?   It's in the back.
3. Did you find the pig?   6. The rooster is growing.
   Did you find the pick?   The rooster is crowing.

D. LISTENING FOR REPLACEMENTS IN FAMILIAR /g/ WORDS

You will hear a list of words containing /g/. Sometimes the words will be pronounced correctly with /g/; other times the words will be said incorrectly

---

[2]If your replacement is /ɡ/, your instructor will carry out this drill with you by changing the /g/–/k/ pairs to /g/–/ɡ/ pairs.
[3]See footnote 2.

with your replacement. Complete instructions for this type of drill are given in Chap. 5, 5-2D.

29–3. A FEW REMINDERS ABOUT ORAL PRACTICE PROCEDURES

If this is the first practice chapter assigned to you by your instructor, you may wish to review the comments about beginning oral practice in Chap. 2, 2-4. Before you actually begin practicing each individual pronunciation drill, you may also desire to review the supplementary explanations about the exercise in Chap. 2, 2-5.

29–4. THE PRONUNCIATION OF /g/

A. PRONOUNCING /g/ IN A SIMPLE SYLLABLE

In the event that you cannot pronounce /g/ through imitation alone, your instructor will help you with the following suggestions about placement. Should placement be required, you should review the definition of a stop in Chap. 4, 4-4H and the description of /g/ in Figure 5 of Chapter 4. Note that because of the nature of the consonant, the target cannot be pronounced in isolation.

1. *The Position of the Back of the Tongue on the Soft Palate*

Press the back of your tongue slowly and firmly against your soft palate, compressing some breath behind your tongue and building up some air pressure. Hold your breath in your mouth behind the back of your tongue. Concentrate on feeling the back of your tongue in contact with your soft palate. Note that if the back of your tongue is not pressed firmly against the soft palate, you may produce the /g/ replacement.

2. *The Escaping Breath*

Remove the back of your tongue from your soft palate suddenly, and explode the air vigorously over your tongue and out through your mouth, saying the syllable /gɑ/ (/ɑ/) as in (hot) and (father). This consonant is voiced, and you must be certain that your vocal bands are vibrating as you explode the breath out of your mouth. Check for the vibration of the bands by placing your fingers on your larynx as you pronounce /gɑ/. If you are unable to feel the vibration from your own larynx, your instructor will place your fingers on his larynx and say /gɑ/. Keep practicing until you can feel the vibration from your own larynx while pronouncing /gɑ/. When that happens, you can double-check your pronunciation of the target by placing your hands over your ears while saying /gɑ/. You should be able to hear the vibration. Keep in mind that the vowel /ɑ/ is voiced, and that you are *not* likely to unvoice the vowel. When checking for vibration, make sure that what you feel and hear *begins* on /g/ and not on the vowel. If you are using the correct tongue position for the target and you do not feel or hear the vibration of the bands, you are pronouncing /kɑ/ rather than /gɑ/. The primary difference between /g/ and /k/ is voicing. Note that accurate pronunciation of /g/ gives a clear, precise quality to this explosive voiced consonant. Finally, observe that the exact point of contact between the tongue and the soft palate varies according to the kind of vowel that follows /g/. The contact tends to be further forward before front vowels than before back vowels. Compare the words **geese** and **goose**, and observe the difference in contact position. The /g/ in **goose**—before the back vowel /u/—is made much further back on the soft palate than is the /g/ in **geese** before the front vowel /i/. Normally most speakers make these contact adjustments automatically. Do not be concerned about placing your tongue in the exact same place on your soft palate for every pronunciation of /g/, unless your instructor indicates that you have a problem in this area.

B. ADDITIONAL COMMENTS

A few additional comments are useful at this point regarding the explosive release of /g/. Read the comments in Chap. 24, 24-4B. Keep in mind that the pronunciation of /g/ generally parallels the pronunciation of /p/: (1) final /g/ before a pause may be exploded or unexploded, (2) final /g/ followed by initial /g/ is pronounced *once* and prolonged (e.g., bi**g g**oose), (3) when final /g/ is followed by any other plosive there is only *one* stop and *one* explosion (e.g., bi**g d**oor).

C. PRONOUNCING /g/ IN FAMILIAR WORDS

Pronounce each of the following words carefully. If you are either practicing with your instructor or listening to the exercise on tape, imitate your speech model as accurately as possible.

Beginning

1. gain
2. game
3. gather
4. going
5. guess
6. give
7. get
8. got
9. gift
10. gay
11. gallop
12. gaily
13. gave
14. guest
15. goose
16. gun
17. gaze
18. girl
19. gone
20. gas

Middle		**End**[4]	
1. against	14. eagle	1. bag	11. fog
2. ago	15. mango	2. beg	12. frog
3. agree	16. eagerly	3. big	13. leg
4. wagon	17. cigarette	4. bug	14. log
5. bargain	18. cigar	5. egg	15. rug
6. began	19. vinegar	6. hug	16. flag
7. begin	20. exit	7. snug	17. fig
8. Chicago	21. exact	8. rag	18. hog
9. forget	22. example	9. tag	19. dug
10. hunger	23. exam	10. wig	20. wag
11. signal	24. examination		
12. single	25. exist		
13. tiger			

D.   PRONOUNCING WORD PAIRS
CONTAINING /g/ AND THE /k/ REPLACEMENT

Select some of the words from the paired list in Section 29-2B containing /g/ and your /k/ replacement. Read one pair of words at a time, pronouncing the word with the target first (e.g., **gain–cane**). Make sure that you are saying /g/ first and /k/ second. Reverse the procedure, and pronounce the replacement word first and the target word second, making certain that you use /k/ first and /g/ second. Try to develop speed and accuracy as you do the drill. If you are either practicing with your instructor or listening to the exercise on tape, imitate your speech model as accurately as possible. You will find this drill more difficult than the word list in Section 29-4C because of the closeness of target and replacement.

E.   PRONOUNCING FAMILIAR WORDS
CONTAINING FREQUENT /g/ CONSONANT CLUSTERS

You may find this exercise the most difficult of all the drills dealing with the pronunciation of /g/ in single words. It is often much more difficult to pronounce a consonant target when it is combined with another consonant in a cluster. Pronounce each of the words carefully. If you are either practicing with your instructor or listening to the drill on tape, imitate your speech model as accurately as possible

[4]If you have difficulty pronouncing final /g/, read footnote 3 in Chapter 8, and adapt the comments to the pronunciation of final voiced /g/.

/gr/	/gl/	/gz/	/gd/
1. grass	1. glass	1. bags	1. begged
2. gray	2. gloves	2. bugs	2. hugged
3. green	3. glue	3. eggs	3. tagged
4. grape	4. globe	4. hugs	4. drugged
5. grin	5. glad	5. begs	5. jogged
6. grapefruit	6. glance	6. drugs	6. wagged
7. grocer	7. glare	7. rags	7. sagged
8. grow		8. rugs	

F. Pronouncing /g/ in Phrases

Pronounce each of the phrases carefully. If you mispronounce a word, say it over again several times, and then repeat the entire phrase. If you are either practicing with your instructor or listening to the drill on tape, imitate your speech model as accurately as possible.

1. **going** to **guide** the **single girl**
2. **begin growing big figs**
3. **agree** to **guess** if its a **wig**
4. **beg** a **gallon** of **good gas**
5. **digging** up **grass** in the **fog**
6. **glad** to wipe the **guitar** with a **rag**
7. **got** the **cigar** off the **rug**

G. Pronouncing Short Phrases Containing /g/ and the /k/ Replacement

This drill is similar to the exercise in Section 29-4D, except that your /k/ replacement precedes the target in each phrase. Pronounce each of the phrases carefully. If you are either practicing with your instructor or listening to the exercise on tape, imitate your speech model as accurately as possible. Although these phrases are shorter than those in the preceding drill, you may find this exercise more difficult, because your replacement directly precedes /g/ in each phrase. Keep in mind the previous comments about pronouncing two consecutive plosive sounds with one stop and one explosion.

/k/ – /g/

1. bank guard
2. brick garage
3. back gate
4. silk gift
5. pink gardenia
6. magic garden
7. week gone
8. check guests
9. speak gaily
10. like gum
11. ask guides
12. black gun

H. Pronouncing /g/ in Sentences

Pronounce each of the words carefully. If you use a replacement, say the word over again several times, and then repeat the entire sentence. If you are

either practicing with your instructor or listening to the exercise on tape, imitate your speech model as accurately as possible.

1. He **gladly agreed** to **give** Mr. **Gordon** the **egg**.
2. The **gardener gathered** up some **mangoes** and **grapes** and **gave** them to the **grocer**.
3. The **big dog** stopped **growling** and **began wagging** his tail.
4. **Gary forgot** to put the **gaily** painted **green** and **gold flag** in the **playground**.
5. They said "**good-bye**" **gaily** and **eagerly agreed** to meet in **Chicago** in **August**.

I.   PRONOUNCING /g/ IN BEGINNING CONVERSATION

This exercise gives you an opportunity to begin using some of your previously learned /g/ words in beginning conversation. Complete instructions for this type of drill are given in Chap. 5, 5-4H. Read the instructions, and adapt them to practice with /g/.

1. "He **goes jogging** _____ miles daily."
2. "The **tag** fell off the _____."
3. "Did he **give** you the **exam** on _____?"
4. "Please **glue** the _____."
5. "Please **begin** washing your _____."
6. "I need a **gallon** of _____."
7. "Please **drag** the _____ into the **garage**."
8. "Did you **grin** when you **forgot** the _____?"
9. "**Get** a pack of **cigarettes** at _____."
10. "Are you **eager** to **give** him the _____?"
11. "Was the _____ **gray** or **green**?"
12. "Did you buy a **wig** for _____?"
13. "I **gave** her a _____ for a birthday **gift**."
14. "I think the use of **drugs** is _____."
15. "The **guide** is taking the **guests** to _____."

29–5.   CONVERSATION PRACTICE

So far you have learned how to pronounce your target by reading various kinds of exercises which contain /g/ words. Now you are ready to move into the final and most important part of your training program—learning to pronounce /g/ automatically while you are talking more or less spontaneously. If this is the first practice chapter assigned to you by your instructor, you may wish to review the introductory comments on conversation practice in Chap. 2, 2-6 to 2-7.

A.   CARRYING /g/ INTO SPONTANEOUS DAILY CONVERSATION

This exercise requires you to use /g/ in daily conversation, starting with key words and expanding to all the /g/ words in your particular vocabulary. Complete instructions for this type of drill are given in Chap. 5, 5-5A, and there are supplementary comments about the exercise in Chap. 2, 2-7A.

B.   GENERAL CLASSROOM EXERCISES IN SPEAKING

Your instructor will plan a series of classroom conversation activities, and each assignment will be discussed fully in class before you carry it out. When your instructor announces the first speaking activity, you may wish to review the introductory comments on classroom speaking in Chap. 2, 2-7B.

part III

THE PRONUNCIATION
OF THE
VOWEL
AND DIPHTHONG TARGETS
OF
AMERICAN ENGLISH

chapter thirty

The Vowel Target
/i/ (bead)

COMMON SPELLINGS FOR /i/

The most frequent spellings are found in the words **equal, feet, east, seize,** and **field**; less frequent spellings include **people, key,** and **policemen.**

30-1. EAR TRAINING FOR THE /i/ TARGET

A. A FEW REMINDERS ABOUT EAR TRAINING

The following test exercises will help you learn to recognize your /i/ target. If this is the first practice chapter assigned to you by your instructor, you may wish to review the discussion about listening practice in Chap. 2, 2-2B to 2-3C.

B. RECOGNIZING /i/ IN WORDS

You will hear a list of words containing /i/. After listening to each word, write *B* if you heard /i/ at the beginning of the word, *M* if you heard /i/ in the middle, and *E* if you heard /i/ at the end of the word. The answers will be read

to you at the end of the drill. This exercise is found in Appendix 1. If you have difficulty recognizing the target, you may find it worthwhile to review the test with somebody outside class.

C. RECOGNIZING /i/ IN SENTENCES

You will listen to a series of sentences containing a number of /i/ words. Each sentence will be read several times. Try to locate the /i/ words in each sentence, and write them down. The /i/ words in each test sentence will be read to you at the end of the drill. The sentences appear later in the chapter in Section 30-4E. If you have difficulty recognizing the target, you may find it worthwhile to review the test with somebody else outside class.

30–2. DISCRIMINATING BETWEEN /i/ AND THE /ɪ/ REPLACEMENT

A. PROBABLE TYPES OF REPLACEMENT

The following exercises will help you learn to compare /i/ with your probable replacement of /ɪ/ as in bid. If you are not employing this common replacement, your instructor will tell you exactly how you are mispronouncing /i/ and provide you with some discrimination drills.

B. PAIRED LISTS OF WORDS

The words in the following paired list are identical, except that the words in Column 1 contain the target, and the words in Column 2 contain the /ɪ/ replacement. Complete instructions for this type of exercise are given in Chap. 5, 5-2B.

Column 1 /i/	Column 2 /ɪ/
each	itch
bean	bin
beaten	bitten
feet	fit
green	grin
least	list
team	Tim
field	filled
heat	hit
seat	sit
sleep	slip
heel	hill
deep	dip
meal	mill
sheep	ship

C. Paired Sentences

The following paired sentences are identical except that the final word in the first sentence contains /i/, and the final word in the second sentence contains the /ɪ/ replacement. Complete instructions for this type of exercise are given in Chap. 5, 5-2C.

/i/ – /ɪ/

1. Has he been beaten?
   Has he been bitten?
2. Where's the sheep?
   Where's the ship?

3. I like the meal.
   I like the mill.
4. He found the peel.
   He found the pill.

5. Did you sleep?
   Did you slip?

D. Listening for Replacements in Familiar /i/ Words

You will hear a list of words containing /i/. Sometimes the words will be pronounced correctly with /i/; other times the words will be said incorrectly with your replacement. Complete instructions for this type of drill are found in Chap. 5, 5-2D.

30–3. A FEW REMINDERS ABOUT ORAL PRACTICE PROCEDURES

If this is the first practice chapter assigned to you by your instructor, you may wish to review the comments about beginning oral practice in Chap. 2, 2-4. Before you actually begin practicing each individual pronunciation drill, you may also desire to review the supplementary explanations about the exercise in Chap. 2, 2-5.

30–4. THE PRONUNCIATION OF /i/

A. Pronouncing Isolated /i/

In the event that you cannot pronounce /i/ through imitation alone, your instructor will help you with the following suggestions about placement. Should placement be required, you should review the explanatory comments about front vowels in Chap. 4, 4-4F, and the description of /i/ in Figure 3 of Chapter 4.

1. The Position of the Lips

The target /i/ is considered unround. Spread your lips as if you were smiling. The narrow slit-like appearance of the lips is the usual lip position for the pronunciation of /i/.

2. The Position of the Tongue

Press the edges of your tongue firmly against the bottoms of your upper back teeth. Arch the blade of your tongue so that it is steep and close to the front of the hard palate, and keep your tongue tip low and pointed toward the biting edges of your lower, middle front teeth. You may or may not touch your teeth with your tongue tip. Your jaws are close together. It is very difficult to place your tongue in the correct position for the target for two reasons: (1) you cannot see what you are doing, and (2) the difference between the position of the tongue for /i/ and the position for the replacement /ɪ/ is very small. Note that when you pronounce /ɪ/ your tongue arch is slightly lower and flatter than for /i/. The lower jaw also drops slightly so that the mouth is open a bit wider for /ɪ/ than for /i/. Thus if you place your tongue too low—and open your mouth too much—you may pronounce /ɪ/ rather than the target.

3. Vowel Length and Muscular Tension

Two more suggestions may simplify the pronunciation of /i/ for you. The target is frequently heard as a long sound, and you will pronounce /i/ more accurately if you prolong the vowel while saying it. The target is also said with strong tensing of the muscles, and this muscular tension may be felt. Place your thumb under the fleshy part of your instructor's chin, and listen to his pronunciation of the target. You should be able to feel a definite sensation of pressure against your thumb as your instructor pronounces /i/. This pressure is caused primarily by the muscles of his tongue pushing themselves against your thumb as he says the target. Keep your thumb against his chin, and listen to his pronunciation of /ɪ/. There should be little or no sensation of pressure against your thumb, because the replacement is pronounced with much less muscular tension than /i/. Note that if you use too little muscular tension while pronouncing /i/, you may pronounce /ɪ/ rather than the target.

4. Pronouncing the Target

Place your thumb under the fleshy part of your chin, and pronounce /i/, keeping in mind the suggestions given earlier. Because of the difficulty you may have in placing your tongue in the proper position for /i/, listen intently to your instructor's pronunciation as he helps you pronounce the target. Use a mirror if you wish to check your lip position.

B. Pronouncing /i/ in Familiar Words

Pronounce each of the following words carefully. If you are either practicing with your instructor or listening to the exercise on tape, imitate your speech model as accurately as possible.

Beginning		Middle		End
1. either	1. between	11. bead	21. machine	1. see
2. even	2. feel	12. dream	22. meet	2. degree
3. east	3. keep	13. secret	23. please	3. free
4. easy	4. mean	14. tease	24. steep	4. tree
5. equal	5. need	15. asleep	25. steel	5. bee
6. eagle	6. real	16. peace	26. wheel	6. agree
7. Easter	7. reason	17. creep	27. meal	7. three
8. Egypt	8. seem	18. reached	28. heal	8. tea
9. eat	9. speak	19. weeds		9. knee
10. each	10. deep	20. complete		10. key

C. PRONOUNCING WORD PAIRS CONTAINING /i/ AND THE /ɪ/ REPLACEMENT

Select some of the words from the paired list in Section 30-2B containing /i/ and your /ɪ/ replacement. Read one pair of words at a time, pronouncing the word with the target first (e.g., **each–itch**). Make sure that you are saying /i/ first and /ɪ/ second. Reverse the procedure, and pronounce the replacement word first and the target word second, making certain that you use /ɪ/ first and /i/ second. Try to develop speed and accuracy as you do the drill. If you are either practicing with your instructor or listening to the exercise on tape, imitate your speech model as accurately as possible. You will find this drill more difficult than the word list in Section 30-4B because of the closeness of target and replacement.

D. PRONOUNCING /i/ IN PHRASES

Pronounce each of the phrases carefully. If you mispronounce a word, say it over again several times, and then repeat the entire phrase. If you are either practicing with your instructor or listening to the drill on tape, imitate your speech model as accurately as possible.

1. **eating sweet peaches** and **cream cheese**
2. **dreaming** of ice **cream** at **Halloween**
3. **meet either speech teacher** at **Easter**
4. **easy** to **sweep** the **green leaves**
5. **seaweed** on the **beach** in the **evening**
6. **even** spilled **tea** on his **knee**
7. a **meal** of **beans** and **cheap** roast **beef**

E. PRONOUNCING /i/ IN SENTENCES

Pronounce each of the sentences carefully. If you use a replacement, say the word over again several times, and then repeat the entire sentence. If you are

either practicing with your instructor or listening to the exercise on tape, imitate your speech model as accurately as possible.

1. There were **seals** and **greasy seaweed** all over the **beach east** of the **airfield**.
2. The **people** had **reason** to **believe** there was enough **meat** left to **eat** for one **week**.
3. The **speaker** at **each meeting** said the **Peace** Corps **needed eager** workers.
4. **Peter seemed extremely sleepy** and finally fell **asleep** by early **evening**.
5. The **three** construction **machines reached** high above the **freezing street**.

F. PRONOUNCING /i/ IN BEGINNING CONVERSATION

This exercise gives you an opportunity to begin using some of your previously learned /i/ words in beginning conversation. Complete instructions for this type of drill are given in Chap. 5, 5-4H. Read the instructions and adapt them to practice with /i/.

1. "Do you **need** a _____?"
2. "Is playing _____ **easy**?"
3. "Do you like to **eat** _____?"
4. "Did you **receive** a _____?"
5. "Do you **see** the _____?"
6. "Did they **keep** the _____?"
7. "Did they **seem** to like the _____?"
8. "Did the _____ **freeze**?"
9. "Did you **agree** to **speak** to _____?"
10. "**Please** give us the _____."
11. "Put the _____ in the **freezer**."
12. "My _____ is made of **steel**."
13. "My **team** was **beaten** last _____."
14. "I **believe these green leaves** come from a _____ **tree**."
15. "The **heel** on my _____ is worn out."

30–5. CONVERSATION PRACTICE

So far you have learned how to pronounce your target by reading various kinds of exercises which contain /i/ words. Now you are ready to move into the final and most important part of your training program—learning to pronounce /i/ automatically while you are talking more or less spontaneously. If this is the first practice chapter assigned to you by your instructor, you may wish to review the introductory comments on conversation practice in Chap. 2, 2-6 to 2-7.

A.   Carrying /i/ into Spontaneous Daily Conversation

This exercise requires you to use /i/ in daily conversation, starting with key words and expanding to all the /i/ words in your particular vocabulary. Complete instructions for this type of drill are given in Chap. 5, 5-5A, and there are supplementary comments about the exercise in Chap. 2, 2-7A.

B.   General Classroom Exercises in Speaking

Your instructor will plan a series of classroom conversation activities, and each assignment will be discussed fully in class before you carry it out. When your instructor announces the first speaking activity, you may wish to review the introductory comments on classroom speaking in Chap. 2, 2-7B.

chapter thirty-one

The Vowel Target
/ɪ/ (bid)

COMMON SPELLINGS FOR /ɪ/

The most frequent spelling is found in the word big; less frequent spellings include built, business, pretty, been, and women.

31–1. EAR TRAINING FOR THE /ɪ/ TARGET

A. A Few Reminders About Ear Training

The following test exercises will help you learn to recognize your /ɪ/ target. If this is the first practice chapter assigned to you by your instructor, you may wish to review the discussion about listening practice in Chap. 2, 2-2B to 2-3C.

B. Recognizing /ɪ/ in Words

You will hear a list of words containing /ɪ/. After listening to each word, write *B* if you heard /ɪ/ at the beginning of the word or *M* if you heard /ɪ/ in the middle of the word. The answers will be read to you at the end of the drill. This exercise is found in Appendix 1. If you have difficulty recognizing the target, you may find it worthwhile to review the test with somebody outside class.

C. Recognizing /ɪ/ in Sentences

You will listen to a series of sentences containing a number of /ɪ/ words. Each sentence will be read several times. Try to locate the /ɪ/ words in each sentence, and write them down. The /ɪ/ words in each test sentence will be read to you at the end of the drill. The sentences appear later in the chapter in Section 31-4F. If you have difficulty recognizing the target, you may find it worthwhile to review the test with somebody outside class.

31–2. DISCRIMINATING BETWEEN /ɪ/ AND THE /i/ REPLACEMENT

A. Probable Types of Replacement

The following exercises will help you learn to compare /ɪ/ with your probable replacement of /i/ as in (bead). If you are not employing this common replacement, your instructor will tell you exactly how you are mispronouncing /ɪ/ and provide you with some discrimination drills.[1]

B. Paired Lists of Words

The words in the following paired list are identical, except that the words in Column 1 contain the target, and the words in Column 2 contain the /i/ replacement. Complete instructions for this type of exercise are given in Chap. 5, 5-2B.

---

[1] The vowel /ɪ/ is frequently pronounced with weak stress or emphasis in a variety of different kinds of words. For example, *only* /ɪ/ should be pronounced in words like invite and going. However, in a number of other words the weak-stressed vowel may *vary*: (1) in words like event and enough the speaker may pronounce the initial vowel with /i/, with /ə/ as in about, or with /ɪ/; (2) in words like remain, delight, believe, and select, the speaker may pronounce the second sound with /i/, /ə/, or /ɪ/; (3) in words like coffee, honey, hurry, and Monday, the speaker may pronounce the last sound with /i/ or /ɪ/; and (4) in words like telephone, passes, boasted, and market, the speaker may pronounce the middle or final weak-stressed syllable with /ɪ/ or /ə/. Additional examples of this latter variation are given in footnote 2 of Chapter 41. In all the preceding examples where variation is possible, no one of the demonstrated pronunciations is considered better or more acceptable than another one of the pronunciations. Use whatever pronunciation is easiest for you in words like these, unless there is a preference for some particular pronunciation in your area. If you have any questions about which pronunciation, if any, is the preferred one in your area, ask your instructor. The stressed vowels in the practice words in this unit *must* all be pronounced with /ɪ/. A few words contain weak-stressed vowels that *must* be pronounced with /ɪ/. Some additional practice words contain weak-stressed vowels that may vary between /ɪ/ and /ə/, as indicated above. Finally, note that the frequent use of weak-stressed /ɪ/ in one-syllable words is explained in Chapter 48 as part of the discussion and practice of weak stress.

Column 1 /ɪ/	Column 2 /i/
itch	each
bin	bean
bitten	beaten
fit	feet
grin	green
list	least
Tim	team
filled	field
hit	heat
sit	seat
slip	sleep
hill	heel
dip	deep
mill	meal
ship	sheep

C. PAIRED SENTENCES

The following paired sentences are identical, except that the final word in the first sentence contains /ɪ/, and the final word in the second sentence contains the /i/ replacement. Complete instructions for this type of exercise are given in Chap. 5, 5-2C.

1. Has he been bitten?
   Has he been beaten?
2. Where's the ship?
   Where's the sheep?
3. I like the mill.
   I like the meal.
4. He found the pill.
   He found the peel.
5. Did you slip?
   Did you sleep?

D. LISTENING FOR REPLACEMENTS IN FAMILIAR /ɪ/ WORDS

You will hear a list of words containing /ɪ/. Sometimes the words will be pronounced correctly with /ɪ/; other times the words will be said incorrectly with your replacement. Complete instructions for this type of drill are found in Chap. 5, 5-2D.

31–3. A FEW REMINDERS ABOUT ORAL PRACTICE PROCEDURES

If this is the first practice chapter assigned to you by your instructor, you may wish to review the comments about beginning oral practice in Chap. 2, 2-4. Before you actually begin practicing each individual pronunciation drill, you may also desire to review the supplementary explanations about the exercise in Chap. 2, 2-5.

31–4. THE PRONUNCIATION OF /ɪ/

A. PRONOUNCING ISOLATED /ɪ/

In the event that you cannot pronounce /ɪ/ through imitation alone, your instructor will help you with the following suggestions about placement. Should placement be required, you should review the explanatory comments about front vowels in Chap. 4, 4-4F, and the description of /ɪ/ in Figure 3 of Chapter 4.

1. The Position of the Lips

The target /ɪ/ is considered unround. Spread your lips as if you were smiling. The narrow slit-like appearance of the lips is the usual lip position for the pronounciation of /ɪ/.

2. The Position of the Tongue

Press the edges of your tongue firmly against the bottoms of your upper back teeth. Arch the blade of your tongue so that it is steep and close to the front of the hard palate, and keep your tongue tip low and pointed toward the biting edges of your lower, middle front teeth. You may or may not touch your teeth with your tongue tip. Your jaws are close together. It is very difficult to place your tongue in the correct position for the target for two reasons: (1) you cannot see what you are doing, and (2) the difference between the position of the tongue for /ɪ/ and the position for the replacement /i/ is very small. Note that when you pronounce /i/ your tongue arch is slightly higher and steeper than for /ɪ/. The lower jaw also rises slightly so that the mouth is slightly more closed for /i/ than for /ɪ/. Thus if you place your tongue too high—and close your mouth too much—you may pronounce /i/ rather than the target.

3. Muscular Tension

The target is said with little tensing of the muscles, while the replacement /i/ is said with strong muscular tension. This difference in tension may be felt and will aid you in avoiding the replacement. Place your thumb under the fleshy part of your instructor's chin and listen to his pronunciation of the target. There should be little or no sensation of pressure against your thumb as your instructor pronounces /ɪ/. Keep your thumb against his chin, and listen to his pronunciation of /i/. You should be able to feel a definite sensation of pressure against your thumb as your instructor pronounces /i/. This pressure is caused primarily by the muscles of his tongue pushing themselves against your thumb as he says /i/. Note that if you use too much muscular tension while pronouncing /ɪ/, you may pronounce /i/ rather than the target.

4. *Pronouncing the Target*

Place your thumb under the fleshy part of your chin, and pronounce /ɪ/, keeping in mind the suggestions given earlier. Because of the difficulty you may have in placing your tongue in the proper position for /ɪ/, listen intently to your instructor's pronunciation as he helps you pronounce the target. Use a mirror if you wish to check your lip position.

B.   PRONOUNCING /ɪ/ IN FAMILIAR WORDS

Pronounce each of the following words carefully. If you are either practicing with your instructor or listening to the exercise on tape, imitate your speech model as accurately as possible.

Beginning		Middle		
1. is	7. instant	1. little	8. since	15. gift
2. it	8. interested	2. sit	9. give	16. wish
3. in	9. isn't	3. did	10. until	17. lift
4. if	10. into	4. his	11. pillow	18. minute
5. ink	11. ill	5. will	12. miss	19. bring
6. inch		6. him	13. admit	20. sing
		7. live	14. fix	

C.   PRONOUNCING WORD PAIRS CONTAINING /ɪ/ AND THE /i/ REPLACEMENT

Select some of the words from the paired list in Section 31-2B containing /ɪ/ and your /i/ replacement. Read one pair of words at a time, pronouncing the word with the target first (e.g., **itch–each**). Make sure that you are saying /ɪ/ first and /i/ second. Reverse the procedure, and pronounce the replacement word first and the target word second, making certain that you use /i/ first and /ɪ/ second. Try to develop speed and accuracy as you do the drill. If you are either practicing with your instructor or listening to the exercise on tape, imitate your speech model as accurately as possible. You will find this drill more difficult than the word list in Section 31-4B because of the closeness of target and replacement.

D.   PRONOUNCING /ɪ/ IN PHRASES

Pronounce each of the phrases carefully. If you mispronounce a word, say it over again several times, and then repeat the entire phrase. If you are either practicing with your instructor or listening to the drill on tape, imitate your speech model as accurately as possible.

1. **chicken** and **fish** for **dinner**
2. **six tickets** for **Christmas**
3. **kitten** on the **kitchen window**
4. a **nickel** for **his little sister**
5. a **brick bridge** over the **river**
6. a **liver sandwich in** school

E. PRONOUNCING SHORT PHRASES CONTAINING /ɪ/ AND /i/

This drill is similar to the exercise in Section 31-4C, except that your /i/ replacement precedes the target in each phrase. Pronounce each of the phrases carefully. If you are either practicing with your instructor or listening to the exercise on tape, imitate your speech model as accurately as possible. Although these phrases are shorter than those in the preceding drill, you may find this exercise more difficult, because your replacement directly precedes /ɪ/ in each phrase.

/i/ – /ɪ/

1. see into
2. knee is hurt
3. three inches
4. key isn't
5. free invitation
6. ski invention
7. bee is flying
8. agree it isn't
9. tea instantly

F. PRONOUNCING /ɪ/ IN SENTENCES

Pronounce each of the sentences carefully. If you use a replacement, say the word over again several times, and then repeat the entire sentence. If you are either practicing with your instructor or listening to the exercise on tape, imitate your speech model as accurately as possible.

1. Tommy **will visit** the **city if his** father **will** let **him** go.
2. **Jill is** about to **bring** the hot **fig** pie to the **children.**
3. He **didn't** thank **him** when he **fixed** the **big picture.**
4. Joe **instantly filled** the pan **with** water **until it** was full.
5. **Jim is going** to walk home **since** he **lives** over **this hill.**

G. PRONOUNCING /ɪ/ IN BEGINNING CONVERSATION

This exercise gives you an opportunity to begin using some of your previously learned /ɪ/ words in beginning conversation. Complete instructions for this type of drill are given in Chap. 5, 5-4H. Read the instructions, and adapt them to practice with /ɪ/.

1. "**Is this** the _____?"
2. "**Is it** a _____?"

   3. "Do you **think this** _____ **is pretty**?"

   4. "**Will** you **give him** the _____ ?"

   5. "Do you **think** you can **pick** up the _____ ?"

   6. "**Will** you **bring** the _____ to **Dick**?"

   7. "Are you **interested in** _____ ?"

   8. "**Did** he **fix** the _____ ?"

   9. "**Did** he go **skin diving** _____ ?"

   10. "Do you want **this ticket** for the _____ ?"

31–5. CONVERSATION PRACTICE

So far you have learned how to pronounce your target by reading various kinds of exercises which contain /ɪ/ words. Now you are ready to move into the final and most important part of your training program—learning to pronounce /ɪ/ automatically while you are talking more or less spontaneously. If this is the first practice chapter assigned to you by your instructor, you may wish to review the introductory comments on conversation practice in Chap. 2, 2-6 to 2-7.

A. CARRYING /ɪ/ INTO SPONTANEOUS DAILY CONVERSATION

This exercise requires you to use /ɪ/ in daily conversation, starting with key words and expanding to all the /ɪ/ words in your particular vocabulary. Complete instructions for this type of drill are given in Chap. 5, 5-5A, and there are supplementary comments about the exercise in Chap. 2, 2-7A.

B. GENERAL CLASSROOM EXERCISES IN SPEAKING

Your instructor will plan a series of classroom conversation activities, and each assignment will be discussed fully in class before you carry it out. When your instructor announces the first speaking activity, you may wish to review the introductory comments on classroom speaking in Chap. 2, 2-7B.

chapter thirty-two

The Diphthong Target
/eɪ/ (cave)[1]

COMMON SPELLINGS FOR /eɪ/

The most frequent spellings are found in the words c**a**ve, b**ay**, and m**ai**l; less frequent spellings include br**ea**k, **eigh**t, r**ei**ndeer, and th**ey**.

32–1.   EAR TRAINING FOR THE /eɪ/ TARGET

A.   A FEW REMINDERS ABOUT EAR TRAINING

The following test exercises will help you learn to recognize your /eɪ/ target. If this is the first practice chapter assigned to you by your instructor, you may wish to review the discussion about listening practice in Chap. 2, 2-2B to 2-3C.

---

[1] I have used the diphthong symbol /eɪ/, because the target is pronounced as a diphthong by a large majority of American English speakers in syllables containing primary and secondary stress (e.g., play and playmate). The single vowel /e/ is only heard in syllables containing weak stress (e.g., vacation and chaotic). See C. M. Wise, *Applied Phonetics* (Englewood Cliffs, N.J.: Prentice-Hall, Inc., 1957), p. 99.

B. Recognizing /eɪ/ in Words

You will hear a list of words containing /eɪ/. After listening to each word, write *B* if you heard /eɪ/ at the beginning of the word, *M* if you heard /eɪ/ in the middle, and *E* if you heard /eɪ/ at the end of the word. The answers will be read to you at the end of the drill. This exercise is found in Appendix 1. If you have difficulty recognizing the target, you may find it worthwhile to review the test with somebody outside class.

C. Recognizing /eɪ/ in Sentences

You will listen to a series of sentences containing a number of /eɪ/ words. Each sentence will be read several times. Try to locate the /eɪ/ words in each test sentence, and write them down. The /eɪ/ words in each test sentence will be read to you at the end of the drill. The sentences appear later in the chapter in Section 32-4E. If you have difficulty recognizing the target, you may find it worthwhile to review the test with somebody outside class.

32–2. DISCRIMINATING BETWEEN /eɪ/ AND THE VARIOUS REPLACEMENTS

A. Probable Types of Replacement

The following exercises will help you learn to compare /eɪ/ with your replacement. You are probably substituting one of the following common replacements for /eɪ/: (1) /ɛ/ as in bed, or (2) the single or pure vowel /e/ as in chaotic. Your instructor will tell you which replacement you are using. If you are not employing one of the more common replacements, your teacher will tell you exactly how you are mispronouncing /eɪ/ and provide you with some discrimination drills.

B. Paired Lists of Words

The words in the following paired list are identical, except that the words in Column 1 contain the target, and the words in Column 2 contain the /ɛ/ replacement. Complete instructions for this type of exercise are given in Chap. 5, 5-2B.

Column 1 /eɪ/	Column 2 /ɛ/[2]	Column 1 /eɪ/	Column 2 /ɛ/[2]
aid	Ed	mate	met
age	edge	paper	pepper
fail	fell	pain	pen
gate	get	sail	sell
late	let	taste	test
laid	lead	tail	tell
main	men	weight	wet

[2]If your replacement is /e/, your instructor will carry out this drill with you by changing the /eɪ/ – /ɛ/ pairs to /eɪ/ – /e/ pairs.

C.   PAIRED SENTENCES

The following paired sentences are identical, except that the final word in the first sentence contains /eɪ/, and the final word in the second sentence contains the /ɛ/ replacement. Complete instructions for this type of exercise are given in Chap. 5, 5-2C.

/eɪ/ – /ɛ/[3]

1. Do you need aid?
   Do you need Ed?
2. He dropped the paper.
   He dropped the pepper.
3. It's the right age.
   It's the right edge.
4. Will it sail?
   Will it sell?
5. I have a new pain.
   I have a new pen.
6. Do you like the taste?
   Do you like the test?

D.   LISTENING FOR REPLACEMENTS IN FAMILIAR /eɪ/ WORDS

You will hear a list of words containing /eɪ/. Sometimes the words will be pronounced correctly with /eɪ/; other times the words will be said incorrectly with your replacement. Complete instructions for this type of drill are found in Chap. 5, 5-2D.

32–3.   A FEW REMINDERS
ABOUT ORAL PRACTICE PROCEDURES

If this is the first practice chapter assigned to you by your instructor, you may wish to review the comments about beginning oral practice in Chap. 2, 2-4. Before you actually begin practicing each individual pronunciation drill, you may also desire to review the supplementary explanations about the exercise in Chap. 2, 2-5.

32–4.   THE PRONUNCIATION OF /eɪ/

A.   PRONOUNCING ISOLATED /eɪ/

In the event that you cannot pronounce /eɪ/ through imitation alone, your instructor will help you with the following suggestions about placement. Should placement be required, you should review the explanatory comments about front vowels in Chap. 4, 4-4F, the comments about diphthongs in Chap. 4, 4-4G, and the description of /eɪ/ in Figure 4 of Chapter 4.

1.   The Position of the Lips

The target /eɪ/ is considered unround, and your lips are spread as in a smile for both vowels. As the articulators glide from /e/ up to /ɪ/ as in bid, your

[3]See footnote 2.

lips gradually close and become more narrowed and slit-like. Note that your lips are spread farther apart for /ɛ/ than for /eɪ/.

2. Tongue Position, Length, and Muscular Tension

Press the edges of your tongue firmly against the bottoms of your upper back teeth. Keep your tongue tip low and pointed toward the biting edges of your lower, middle front teeth. You may or may not touch your teeth with your tongue tip. Note that your upper and lower front teeth are farther apart for /ɛ/ that for /eɪ/. Arch the blade of your tongue in the direction of the front of the hard palate, remembering that the arch is higher for the first sound /e/ than for /ɛ/. If you place your tongue too low—and open your mouth too much—you may pronounce /ɛ/ rather than the target.

The most important thing to remember about the arched tongue position for the target is its movement. The tongue moves from the initial arched position for /e/ up to the arched tongue position for /ɪ/, traveling with a smooth, continuous gliding movement. This causes your mouth to close slightly, because your lower jaw is simultaneously rising with your tongue. Watch your instructor pronounce /eɪ/ for you several times, and observe the closing movements of his lips and lower jaw. Because of the lip, tongue, and jaw movements associated with the pronunciation of /eɪ/, the target is heard as a long sound; you will pronounce the target more accurately if you prolong it. The length is especially important if your replacement is /e/, because you eliminate the diphthongal gliding movements up to /ɪ/ when you produce the single vowel. The target is also pronounced with fairly strong tensing of the tongue muscles. Tense your tongue when you pronounce the target; this will also help you acquire the required gliding movements of tongue and jaw. Remember that it is very difficult to place your tongue in the correct beginning position of the target for two reasons: (1) the difference between the tongue positions of the target and /ɛ/ is very small, and (2) the tongue positions are not clearly visible for either /eɪ/ or /ɛ/.

3. Pronouncing the Target

Try pronouncing /eɪ/, keeping in mind the suggestions given above. Because of the difficulty you may have in placing your tongue in the proper beginning position for the target, listen intently to your instructor's pronunciation as he helps you pronounce the target. Try to feel the movements of your tongue, lips, and lower jaw while pronouncing /eɪ/. Use a mirror to observe your lip and jaw movements.

B. PRONOUNCING /eɪ/ IN FAMILIAR WORDS

Pronounce each of the following words carefully. If you are either practicing with your instructor or listening to the exercise on tape, imitate your speech model as accurately as possible.

Beginning		Middle			End
1. aim	1. safe	11. awake	21. behave		1. away
2. age	2. lazy	12. make	22. remain		2. stay
3. able	3. snake	13. afraid	23. became		3. pay
4. aid	4. made	14. naked	24. change		4. may
5. apron	5. bake	15. jail	25. same		5. day
6. April	6. name	16. bail	26. complain		6. bay
7. ace	7. page	17. fail	27. save		7. clay
8. ate	8. obtain	18. sale	28. great		8. gray
	9. place	19. male	29. trade		9. pray
	10. plate	20. trail	30. game		10. obey

C.   PRONOUNCING WORD PAIRS CONTAINING /eɪ/ AND THE /ɛ/ REPLACEMENT

Select some of the words from the paired list in Section 32-2B containing /eɪ/ and your /ɛ/ replacement. Read one pair of words at a time, pronouncing the word with the target first (e.g., **fail–fell**). Make sure that you are saying /eɪ/ first and /ɛ/ second. Reverse the procedure, and pronounce the replacement word first and the target word second, making certain that you use /ɛ/ first and /eɪ/ second. Try to develop speed and accuracy as you do the drill. If you are either practicing with your instructor or listening to the exercise on tape, imitate your speech model as accurately as possible. You will find this drill more difficult than the word list in Section 32-4B because of the closeness of target and replacement.

D.   PRONOUNCING /eɪ/ IN PHRASES

Pronounce each of the phrases carefully. If you mispronounce a word, say it over again several times, and then repeat the entire phrase. If you are either practicing with your instructor or listening to the drill on tape, imitate your speech model as accurately as possible.

1. **race** the **gray waves** into the **bay**
2. **able** to **wade** or **sail**
3. **ate bacon** and **grapefruit** on the **plane**
4. **baker's apron** on the **maple table**
5. **take** the blue **jay** off the **highway**
6. a **way** of drag **racing** all **day**
7. **chain** the **gate** at the **playground**

E.   PRONOUNCING /eɪ/ IN SENTENCES

Pronounce each of the sentences carefully. If you use a replacement, say the word over again several times, and then repeat the entire sentence. If you are either practicing with your instructor or listening to the exercise on tape, imitate your speech model as accurately as possible.

1. The **rainbow came** at **daybreak** during the **rain** and **hail** storm.
2. The **sailor's suitcase** was **taken** by **mistake** from the **train** in the **station**.
3. **Elaine's baby** was well-**behaved** and **lay patiently** in the **cradle** most of the day.
4. **Jay explained** that he **may** spend his **vacation raking hay** and picking **grapes** at his **favorite** farm.
5. **They gave** him **eight** pictures of **famous baseball players**.

F.   Pronouncing /eɪ/ in Beginning Conversation

This exercise gives you an opportunity to begin using some of your previously learned /eɪ/ words in beginning conversation. Complete instructions for this type of drill are given in Chap. 5, 5-4H. Read the instructions, and adapt them to practice with /eɪ/.

1. "My **grade** in _____ was excellent."
2. "Did you **pay** for the _____ ?"
3. "Did he **break** the _____ ?"
4. "Will you **wait** while I **mail** my _____ ?"
5. "I'm **sailing** for _____ in **April**."
6. "I **weighed** _____ **today** on my new **scale**."
7. "Did **Fay take** her _____ home?"
8. "Did **James explain** the _____ problem?"
9. "My **favorite state** in the United **States** is _____."

32–5.   CONVERSATION PRACTICE

So far you have learned how to pronounce your target by reading various kinds of exercises which contain /eɪ/ words. Now you are ready to move into the final and most important part of your training program—learning to pronounce /eɪ/ automatically while you are talking more or less spontaneously. If this is the first practice chapter assigned to you by your instructor, you may wish to review the introductory comments on conversation practice in Chap. 2, 2-6 to 2-7.

A.   Carrying /eɪ/ into Spontaneous Daily Conversation

This exercise requires you to use /eɪ/ in daily conversation, starting with key words and expanding to all the /eɪ/ words in your particular vocabulary. Complete instructions for this type of drill are given in Chap. 5, 5-5A, and there are supplementary comments about this exercise in Chap. 2, 2-7A.

B.   GENERAL CLASSROOM EXERCISES IN SPEAKING

Your instructor will plan a series of classroom conversation activities, and each assignment will be discussed fully in class before you carry it out. When your instructor announces the first speaking activity, you may wish to review the introductory comments on classroom speaking in Chap. 2, 2-7B.

chapter thirty-three

The Vowel Target
/ɛ/ (bed)

COMMON SPELLINGS FOR /ɛ/

The most frequent spellings are found in the words beg and meadow; less frequent spellings include friend, says, again, guest, and many.

33–1. EAR TRAINING FOR THE /ɛ/ TARGET

A. A FEW REMINDERS ABOUT EAR TRAINING

The following test exercises will help you learn to recognize your /ɛ/ target. If this is the first practice chapter assigned to you by your instructor, you may wish to review the discussion about listening practice in Chap. 2, 2-2B to 2-3C.

B. RECOGNIZING /ɛ/ IN WORDS

You will hear a list of words containing /ɛ/. After listening to each word, write *B* if you heard /ɛ/ at the beginning of the word or *M* if you heard /ɛ/ in the middle of the word. The answers will be read to you at the end of the drill. This exercise is found in Appendix 1. If you have difficulty recognizing the target, you may find it worthwhile to review the test with somebody outside class.

C. RECOGNIZING /ɛ/ IN SENTENCES

You will listen to a series of sentences containing a number of /ɛ/ words. Each sentence will be read several times. Try to locate the /ɛ/ words in each sentence, and write them down. The /ɛ/ words in each test sentence will be read to you at the end of the drill. The sentences appear later in the chapter in Section 33-4E. If you have difficulty recognizing the target, you may find it worthwhile to review the test with somebody outside class.

33–2. DISCRIMINATING BETWEEN /ɛ/ AND THE VARIOUS REPLACEMENTS

A. PROBABLE TYPES OF REPLACEMENT

The following exercises will help you learn to compare /ɛ/ with your replacement. You are probably substituting one of the following common replacements for /ɛ/: (1) /ae/ as in **bad**, (2) /ɪ/ as in **bid**, or (3) /eɪ/ as in **cave**. Your instructor will tell you which replacement you are using. If you are not employing one of the more common replacements, your teacher will tell you exactly how you are mispronouncing /ɛ/ and provide you with some discrimination drills.[1]

B. PAIRED LISTS OF WORDS

The words in the following paired lists are identical, except that the words in Column 1 contain the target, and the words in Column 2 contain one of the replacements. Complete instructions for this type of exercise are given in Chap. 5, 5-2B.

[1]Certain words may be pronounced with either /ɛ/ or /ae/. In these words the vowel letters combine with **r**: **chair, pear, care, their,** and **there.** Use whatever pronunciation is easiest for you in words like these, unless there is a preference for one particular pronunciation in your area. Words of this type are not included in this chapter. However, if you have any questions about which pronunciation, if any, is the preferred one in your area, ask your instructor.

1. Column 1	Column 2	2. Column 1	Column 2	3. Column 1	Column 2
/ɛ/	/ae/	/ɛ/	/ɪ/	/ɛ/	/eɪ/
any	Annie	etch	itch	Ed	aid
Ellen	Allan	Ben	been	edge	age
end	and	set	sit	fell	fail
Ed	add	better	bitter	get	gate
bed	bad	bell	bill	let	late
beg	bag	bet	bit	lead	laid
bend	band	dead	did	men	main
guess	gas	fell	fill	met	mate
left	laughed	left	lift	pepper	paper
led	lad	peck	pick	pen	pain
men	man	pets	pits	sell	sail
met	mat	sled	slid	test	taste
pen	pan	meant	mint	tell	tail
peck	pack	pen	pin	wet	weight
pet	pat	ten	tin	red	raid
said	sad	send	sinned	fed	fade
set	sat				
send	sand				

C. Paired Sentences

The following paired sentences are identical, except that the final word in the first sentence contains /ɛ/, and the final word in the second sentence contains one of the replacements. Complete instructions for this type of exercise are given in Chap. 5, 5-2C.

/ɛ/ – /ae/	/ɛ/ – /ɪ/	/ɛ/ – /eɪ/
1. Did you see any?	1. Did she start to etch?	1. Do you need Ed?
Did you see Annie?	Did she start to itch?	Do you need aid?
2. I like Ellen.	2. Does it taste better?	2. He dropped the pepper.
I like Allan.	Does it taste bitter?	He dropped the paper.
3. I think he left.	3. I saw the bell.	3. It's the right edge.
I think he laughed.	I saw the bill.	It's the right age.
4. I saw the men.	4. I found the pets.	4. Will it sell?
I saw the man.	I found the pits.	Will it sail?
5. He dropped the pen.		5. I have a new pen.
He dropped the pan.		I have a new pain.
		6. Do you like the test?
		Do you like the taste?

D. Listening for Replacements in Familiar /ɛ/ Words

You will hear a list of words containing /ɛ/. Sometimes the words will be pronounced correctly with /ɛ/; other times the words will be said incorrectly with your replacement. Complete instructions for this type of drill are found in Chap. 5, 5-2D.

33–3.   A FEW REMINDERS ABOUT ORAL PRACTICE PROCEDURES

If this is the first practice chapter assigned to you by your instructor, you may wish to review the comments about beginning oral practice in Chap. 2, 2-4. Before you actually begin practicing each individual pronunciation drill, you may also desire to review the supplementary explanations about the exercise in Chap. 2, 2-5.

33–4.   THE PRONUNCIATION OF /ɛ/

A.   PRONOUNCING ISOLATED /ɛ/

In the event that you cannot pronounce /ɛ/ through imitation alone, your instructor will help you with the following suggestions about placement. Should placement be required, you should review the explanatory comments about front vowels in Chap. 4, 4-4F, and the description of /ɛ/ in Figure 3 of Chapter 4.

1.   *The Position of the Lips*

The target /ɛ/ is considered unround. Your lips are spread farther apart for the target than for /eɪ/ and /ɪ/. However, your lips are spread farther apart for the /ae/ replacement than for /ɛ/.

2.   *The Position of the Tongue and Muscular Tension*

Press the edges of your tongue loosely against the bottoms of your upper back teeth. Arch the blade of your tongue in the direction of the front of the hard palate, and keep your tongue tip low and pointed toward the bottoms of your lower, middle front teeth. You may or may not touch your teeth with your tongue tip. Note that your jaws are farther apart for the target than for /eɪ/ and /ɪ/. However, the jaws are opened wider for the /ae/ replacement than for /ɛ/. The tongue arch is lower and flatter for the target than for /eɪ/ and /ɪ/. However, the tongue arch is lower and flatter for the /ae/ replacement than for /ɛ/. You will notice in Figure 3 of Chapter 4 that /ɛ/ is positioned between /e/ and /ae/. If you place your tongue too high—and close your mouth too much—you may pronounce one of the higher positioned replacements; conversely if you place your tongue too low—and open your mouth too much—you may pronounce the lower /ae/ replacement. It is very difficult to place your tongue in the correct position for the target for two reasons: (1) the difference between the tongue position of the target and the positions of the various replacements is very small, and (2) you cannot see the tongue position of /ɪ/, and it is difficult to see the tongue position for either /eɪ/ or the target, The tongue position for /ae/ is easily seen. The target is pronounced with little muscular tension. Keep your tongue fairly relaxed when you pronounce /ɛ/.

3. Pronouncing the Target

Try pronouncing /ɛ/, keeping in mind the suggestions given above. Because of the difficulty you may have in placing your tongue in the proper position for /ɛ/, listen intently to your instructor's pronunciation as he helps you pronounce the target. Note how much he opens his mouth, and use a mirror if it helps you with your own pronunciation.

B.   PRONOUNCING /ɛ/ IN FAMILIAR WORDS

Pronounce each of the following words carefully. If you are either practicing with your instructor or listening to the exercise on tape, imitate your speech model as accurately as possible.

Beginning   **Middle**

Beginning		Middle		
1. every	1. already	11. myself	21. friend	31. penny
2. ever	2. America	12. next	22. center	32. rent
3. any	3. ahead	13. present	23. bend	33. bless
4. edge	4. better	14. rest	24. attend	34. pest
5. else	5. says	15. ready	25. against	35. beg
6. empty	6. electric	16. well	26. general	36. leg
7. errand	7. fresh	17. sentence	27. length	37. bread
8. Ellen	8. held	18. spend	28. strength	38. measure
9. enemy	9. less	19. many	29. benefit	39. treasure
10. excellent	10. pen	20. meant	30. bench	40. leisure

C.   PRONOUNCING WORD PAIRS CONTAINING /ɛ/ AND A REPLACEMENT

Select some of the words from the paired lists in Section 33-2B containing /ɛ/ and your replacement. Read one pair of words at a time, pronouncing the word with the target first (e.g., **Ellen–Allan**). Make sure that you are saying /ɛ/ first and /ae/ second. Reverse the procedure, and pronounce the replacement word first and the target word second, making certain that you say /ae/ first and /ɛ/ second. Try to develop speed and accuracy as you do the drill. If you are either practicing with your instructor or listening to the exercise on tape, imitate your speech model as accurately as possible. If you are listening to the taped exercise, listen *only* to the drill that compares the target with your particular replacement. You will find this drill more difficult than the word list in Section 33-4B because of the closeness of target and replacement.

D.   PRONOUNCING /ɛ/ IN PHRASES

Pronounce each of the phrases carefully. If you mispronounce a word, say it over again several times, and then repeat the entire phrase. If you are either practicing with your instructor or listening to the exercise on tape, imitate your speech model as accurately as possible.

1.   buying **seven heads** of **excellent lettuce**
2.   **ten** ripe **yellow lemons**
3.   **mend** the **desk** in the **hotel**
4.   **Ellen's second red dress** in **November**
5.   **pressing** the **bell** for the **elevator**
6.   an **American election** in **November**
7.   an **excellent question** from the **secretary**
8.   a **penny** in the **center** of the **bench**

E.   PRONOUNCING /ɛ/ IN SENTENCES

Pronounce each of the sentences carefully. If you use a replacement, say the word over again several times, and then repeat the entire sentence. If you are either practicing with your instructor or listening to the exercise on tape, imitate your speech model as accurately as possible.

1.   **Betty** received the **second special** delivery **letter yesterday,** and it needed **eleven cents extra** postage.
2.   The **smell** of **eggs** for **breakfast** was **getting everybody** hungry.
3.   "**Yes,**" the man **said,** "We want **plenty** of **help** in **checking** the **fence.**
4.   **Helen said** she wanted a new **pen** and **pencil set** for her birthday **present.**
5.   He **says** you will **never get wet** in bad **weather** with an **umbrella** over your **head.**

F.   PRONOUNCING /ɛ/ IN BEGINNING CONVERSATION

This exercise gives you an opportunity to begin using some of your previously learned /ɛ/ words in beginning conversation. Complete instructions for this type of drill are given in Chap. 5, 5-5H. Read the instructions, and adapt them to practice with /ɛ/.

1.   "Is the _____ **red** or **yellow**?"
2.   "Will you **lend** me the _____ ?"
3.   "Can you **get several** _____ ?"
4.   "Did you **forget** the _____ ?"

5. "Do you **smell** the _____ **again**?"

6. "Did you **remember** to get the _____?"

7. "Did you **send** the **second telegram** to _____?"

8. "Did you **guess** that it was _____?"

9. "The **best** show on **television** is _____."

10. "Is **every** _____ **empty**?"

11. "**When** is _____ coming?"

12. "I **spent** _____ dollars **yesterday**."

13. "Did you **measure** the _____?"

14. "My **rent** is _____."

15. "Do you have **any** _____?"

16. "My **best friend** lives in _____."

17. "I **meant** to **get** a **better** _____ at the store."

33–5. CONVERSATION PRACTICE

So far you have learned how to pronounce your target by reading various kinds of exercises which contain /ɛ/ words. Now you are ready to move into the final and most important part of your training program—learning to pronounce /ɛ/ automatically while you are talking more or less spontaneously. If this is the first practice chapter assigned to you by your instructor, you may wish to review the introductory comments on conversation practice in Chap. 2, 2-6, to 2-7.

A. CARRYING /ɛ/ INTO SPONTANEOUS DAILY CONVERSATION

This exercise requires you to use /ɛ/ in daily conversation, starting with key words and expanding to all the /ɛ/ words in your particular vocabulary. Complete instructions for this type of drill are given in Chap. 5, 5-5A, and there are supplementary comments about this exercise in Chap. 2, 2-7A.

B. GENERAL CLASSROOM EXERCISES IN SPEAKING

Your instructor will plan a series of classroom conversation activities, and each assignment will be discussed fully in class before you carry it out. When your instructor announces the first speaking activity, you may wish to review the introductory comments on classroom speaking in Chap. 2, 2-7B.

chapter thirty-four

The Vowel Target
/ae/ (**bad**)[1]

COMMON SPELLINGS FOR /ae/

The most frequent spelling is found in the word **cat**; a less frequent spelling is found in the word **laugh**.

34–1. EAR TRAINING FOR THE /ae/ TARGET

A. A FEW REMINDERS ABOUT EAR TRAINING

The following test exercises will help you learn to recognize your /ae/ target. If this is the first practice chapter assigned to you by your instructor, you

[1]Keep in mind that while /ae/ is the typical General American pronunciation of the words in this chapter, certain of these words are pronounced differently in Eastern New England and in New York City. The standard pronunciation in these areas may be /a/, /ɑ/, or /ae/ in the following types of words: (1) before /θ/ as in **path**, (2) before /s/ as in **ask** and **class**, (3) before /f/ as in **laugh** and **half**, and (4) before /n/ plus another consonant as in **aunt** and **branch**. The vowel /a/ is the lowest front vowel in American English, and /a/ is typically *not* heard in General American speech as a single vowel. It does appear in General American as part of the diphthongs /aɪ/ as in **ride** and /aʊ/ as in **out**. The vowel /ɑ/ as in **father** is the frequently heard low back General American vowel. If the dialectal preference in your area is for either /a/ or /ɑ/ in certain words, your instructor will help you determine which words should be learned with /ae/ and which words should be pronounced with /a/ or /ɑ/.

may wish to review the discussion about listening practice in Chap. 2, 2-2B to 2-3C.

B.   RECOGNIZING /ae/ IN WORDS

You will hear a list of words containing /ae/. After listening to each word, write *B* if you heard /ae/ at the beginning of the word or *M* if you heard /ae/ in the middle of the word. The answers will be read to you at the end of the drill. This exercise is found in Appendix 1. If you have difficulty recognizing the target, you may find it worthwhile to review the test with somebody outside class.

C.   RECOGNIZING /ae/ IN SENTENCES

You will listen to a series of sentences containing a number of /ae/ words. Each sentence will be read several times. Try to locate the /ae/ words in each sentence, and write them down. The /ae/ words in each test sentence will be read to you at the end of the drill. The sentences appear later in the chapter in Section 34-4E. If you have difficulty recognizing the target, you may find it worthwhile to review the test with somebody outside class.

34–2.   DISCRIMINATING BETWEEN /ae/ AND THE VARIOUS REPLACEMENTS

A.   PROBABLE TYPES OF REPLACEMENT

The following exercises will help you learn to compare /ae/ with your replacement. You are probably substituting one of the following common replacements for /ae/: (1) /ɛ/ as in bed, (2) /ɑ/ as in father, or (3) /eɪ/ as in cave. Your instructor will tell you which replacement you are using. If you are not employing one of the more common replacements, your teacher will tell you exactly how you are mispronouncing /ae/ and provide you with some discrimination drills.[2]

B.   PAIRED LISTS OF WORDS

The words in the following paired lists are identical, except that the words in Column 1 contain the target, and the words in Column 2 contain one of the replacements. Complete instructions for this type of exercise are given in Chap. 5, 5-2B.

---

[2]Certain words may be pronounced with either /ae/ or /ɛ/. In these words the vowel letters combine with r: chair, pear, care, their, and there. Use whatever pronunciation is easiest for you in words like these, unless there is a preference for one particular pronunciation in your area. Words of this type are not included in this chapter. However, if you have any questions about which pronunciation, if any, is the preferred one in your area, ask your instructor.

1.

Column 1 /ae/	Column 2 /ɛ/
Annie	any
Allan	Ellen
and	end
add	Ed
bad	bed
bag	beg
band	bend
gas	guess
laughed	left
lad	led
man	men
mat	met
pan	pen
pack	peck
pat	pet
sad	said
sat	set
sand	send

2.

Column 1 /ae/	Column 2 /ɑ/
Ann	on
add	odd
battle	bottle
Dan	Don
hat	hot
pat	pot
stack	stock
tap	top
cat	cot
map	mop
sack	sock
lack	lock
rack	rock

3.

Column 1 /ae/	Column 2 /eɪ/
add	aid.
lad	laid
mat	mate
pan	pain
hat	hate
stack	steak
tap	tape
cat	Kate
lack	lake
rack	rake

C. PAIRED SENTENCES

The following paired sentences are identical, except that the final word in the first sentence contains /ae/, and the final word in the second sentence contains one of the replacements. Complete instructions for this type of exercise are given in Chap. 5, 5-2C.

/ae/ – /ɛ/
1. Did you see Annie?
   Did you see any?
2. I like Allan.
   I like Ellen.
3. I think he laughed.
   I think he left.
4. I saw the man.
   I saw the men.
5. He dropped the pan.
   He dropped the pen.

/ae/ – /ɑ/
1. Did you see the battle?
   Did you see the bottle?
2. Is his name Dan?
   Is his name Don?
3. Did he give you a pat?
   Did he give you a pot?
4. I have a wet map.
   I have a wet mop.
5. There's a hole in my sack.
   There's a hole in my sock.

/ae/ – /eɪ/
1. I see the mat.
   I see the mate.
2. I have a pan.
   I have a pain.
3. I found the stack.
   I found the steak.
4. He has a rack.
   He has a rake.

D. LISTENING FOR REPLACEMENTS IN FAMILIAR /ae/ WORDS

You will hear a list of words containing /ae/. Sometimes the words will be pronounced correctly with /ae/; other times the words will be said incorrectly with your replacement. Complete instructions for this type of drill are found in Chap. 5, 5-2D.

34–3. A FEW REMINDERS
ABOUT ORAL PRACTICE PROCEDURES

If this is the first practice chapter assigned to you by your instructor, you may wish to review the comments about beginning oral practice in Chap. 2, 2-4. Before you actually begin practicing each individual pronunciation drill, you may also desire to review the supplementary explanations about the exercise in Chap. 2, 2-5.

34–4. THE PRONUNCIATION OF /ae/

A. PRONOUNCING ISOLATED /ae/

In the event that you cannot pronounce /ae/ through imitation alone, your instructor will help you with the following suggestions about placement. Should placement be required, you should review the explanatory comments about front vowels in Chap. 4, 4-4F and the description of /ae/ in Figure 3 of Chapter 4.

1. *The Position of the Lips*

The target is considered unround, and your lips are spread into a rather oval shape for the target. Your lips are spread farther apart for the target than for /ɛ/ and /eɪ/. However, your lips are spread farther apart for the /ɑ/ replacement than for /ae/.

2. *The Position of the Tongue and Muscular Tension*

Arch the blade of your tongue in the direction of the front of the hard palate, and keep your tongue tip low and pointed toward the bottoms of your lower, middle front teeth. You may or may not touch your teeth with your tongue tip. You may or may not also press the edges of your tongue very loosely against the bottoms of your upper back teeth. Note that your jaws are farther apart for the target than for /ɛ/ and /eɪ/. However, the jaws are opened wider for the /ɑ/ replacement than for /ae/. The tongue arch is lower and flatter for the target than for /ɛ/ and /eɪ/. However, the tongue arch is lower and flatter for the /ɑ/ replacement than for /ae/. Actually the tongue is almost flat in the mouth for /ɑ/. If you place your tongue too high—and close your mouth too much—you may pronounce one of the higher positioned replacements; conversely if you place your tongue too low—and open your mouth too much—you may pronounce the lower /ɑ/ replacement. It is very difficult to place your tongue in the correct position for the target for two reasons: (1) the difference between the tongue position of the target and the positions of the various replacements is very small, and (2) the tongue positions are not clearly visible for either /ɛ/ or /eɪ/. However, the tongue positions for /ɑ/ and the target are easily seen. The target is usually pronounced with little muscular tension. Keep your tongue fairly relaxed when you pronounce /ae/.

3. Pronouncing the Target

Try pronouncing /ae/, keeping in mind the suggestions given above. Because of the difficulty you may have in placing your tongue in the proper position for /ae/, listen intently to your instructor's pronunciation as he helps you pronounce the target. Note how much he opens his mouth, and use a mirror to aid you with your own pronunciation.

B. Pronouncing /ae/ in Familiar Words

Pronounce each of the following words carefully. If you are either practicing with your instructor or listening to the exercise on tape, imitate your speech model as accurately as possible.

Beginning		Middle		
1. add	1. back	11. happy	21. demand	31. jacket
2. after	2. battle	12. fast	22. branch	32. pasture
3. answer	3. camp	13. mad	23. matter	33. January
4. ask	4. lap	14. dance	24. flag	34. land
5. angry	5. chance	15. man	25. nap	35. ranch
6. animal	6. family	16. last	26. half	36. manage
7. accident	7. crack	17. handle	27. natural	37. rapidly
8. apple	8. class	18. bass	28. happen	38. satisfy
9. ashes	9. drag	19. pass	29. narrow	39. thank
10. ax	10. drank	20. sad	30. package	40. began

C. Pronouncing Word Pairs Containing /ae/ and a Replacement

Select some of the words from the paired lists in Section 34-2B containing /ae/ and your replacement. Read one pair of words at a time, pronouncing the word with the target first (e.g., **Annie–any**). Make sure that you are saying /ae/ first and /ɛ/ second. Reverse the procedure, and pronounce the replacement word first and the target word second, making certain that you say /ɛ/ first and /ae/ second. Try to develop speed and accuracy as you do the drill. If you are either practicing with your instructor or listening to the exercise on tape, imitate your speech model as accurately as possible. If you are listening to the taped exercise, listen *only* to the drill that compares the target with your particular replacement. You will find this drill more difficult than the word list in Section 34-4B because of the closeness of target and replacement.

D.   PRONOUNCING /ae/ IN PHRASES

Pronounce each of the phrases carefully. If you mispronounce a word, say it over again several times, and then repeat the entire phrase. If you are either practicing with your instructor or listening to the exercise on tape, imitate your speech model as accurately as possible.

1. a **black cat** crossed his **path**
2. **apple salad** and a **ham sandwich**
3. threw his **cap** and **bat** on the **grass**
4. give the **fat lamb** a **bath** at **last**
5. **accidentally** spilled **ashes** on the **blanket**
6. **glad** to **hand** him the **scrapbook**
7. a **hammer** and a **ladder** in the **Captain's wagon**
8. **demand** to **stand** with **Jack** at **camp**

E.   PRONOUNCING /ae/ IN SENTENCES

Pronounce each of the sentences carefully. If you use a replacement, say the word over again several times, and then repeat the entire sentence. If you are either practicing with your instructor or listening to the exercise on tape, imitate your speech model as accurately as possible.

1. **Dad** took the **family** to the **Pancake Palace last Saturday.**
2. **Sam wrapped** up some **crackers** and **jam** with the **mangoes** and **bananas.**
3. The **valley** was **planted** with **carrots, radishes,** and **cabbages.**
4. **Jack** used a **damp rag** to take his **math answer** off the **blackboard.**
5. He **happily began** to light the **tan candle** in the old-**fashioned lamp** with a **match.**

F.   PRONOUNCING /ae/ IN BEGINNING CONVERSATION

This exercise gives you an opportunity to begin using some of your previously learned /ae/ words in beginning conversation. Complete instructions for this type of drill are given in Chap. 5, 5-4H. Read the instructions, and adapt them to practice with /ae/.

1. "Did you **ask** for the _____?"
2. "Were you **glad** to get the _____?"
3. "Is the _____ in the **back** yard?"
4. "Will you **pass** the _____ to **Ann**?

5. "Did you **catch** the _____?"

6. "I **plan** to **travel** to _____."

7. "The _____ **accidentally** fell and was **smashed**."

8. "My favorite **candy** is _____."

9. "Did you **thank** him for the _____?"

10. "Did you **answer** your _____ teacher's question?"

11. "My favorite **class** is _____."

12. "Did you **manage** to get the _____ on **Saturday**?"

34–5. CONVERSATION PRACTICE

So far you have learned how to pronounce your target by reading various kinds of exercises which contain /ae/ words. Now you are ready to move into the final and most important part of your training program—learning to pronounce /ae/ automatically while you are talking more or less spontaneously. If this is the first practice chapter assigned to you by your instructor, you may wish to review the introductory comments on conversation practice in Chap. 2, 2-6 to 2-7.

A.   CARRYING /ae/ INTO SPONTANEOUS DAILY CONVERSATION

This exercise requires you to use /ae/ in daily conversation, starting with key words and expanding to all the /ae/ words in your particular vocabulary. Complete instructions for this type of drill are given in Chap. 5, 5-5A, and there are supplementary comments about this exercise in Chap. 2, 2-7A.

B.   GENERAL CLASSROOM EXERCISES IN SPEAKING

Your instructor will plan a series of classroom conversation activities, and each assignment will be discussed fully in class before you carry it out. When your instructor announces the first speaking activity, you may wish to review the introductory comments on classroom speaking in Chap. 2, 2-7B.

chapter thirty-five

The Vowel Target
/u/ (pool)

COMMON SPELLINGS FOR /u/

The most frequent spellings are found in the words m**oo**n, gr**ew**, tr**u**ce, and l**o**se; less frequent spellings include tw**o**, thr**ou**gh, fr**ui**t, sh**oe**, and gr**ou**p.[1]

35–1. EAR TRAINING FOR THE /u/ TARGET

A.   A FEW REMINDERS ABOUT EAR TRAINING

The following test exercises will help you learn to recognize your /u/ target. If this is the first practice chapter assigned to you by your instructor, you

---

[1]Certain words are always pronounced with /ju/, combining the consonant /j/ as in yellow with the vowel /u/. Examples include beauty, few, view, music, human, and cue. Words of this type are not included in this chapter, but they are found in Chapter 18. Other words may be pronounced with /u/, /ju/, or /ɪu/ (/ɪ/) as in bid, depending upon the speaker. However, there seems to be a preference for /u/. Examples include tune, new, student, due, and suit. Still other words are pronounced /ɪu/ or /u/, depending upon the speaker. Again, there seems to be a preference for /u/. Examples include shoe, chew, blue, and June. If you have difficulty pronouncing words in either of the last two groups, use the pronunciation that is easier for you, unless there is a preference for one particular pronunciation in your area. If you have any questions about which pronunciation, if any, is the preferred one in your area, ask your instructor.

may wish to review the discussion about listening practice in Chap. 2, 2-2B to 2-3C.

B. RECOGNIZING /u/ IN WORDS

You will hear a list of words containing /u/. After listening to each word, write *M* if you heard /u/ in the middle of the word or *E* if you heard /u/ at the end of the word. The answers will be read to you at the end of the drill. This exercise is found in Appendix I. If you have difficulty recognizing the target, you may find it worthwhile to review the test with somebody outside class.

C. RECOGNIZING /u/ IN SENTENCES

You will listen to a series of sentences containing a number of /u/ words. Each sentence will be read several times. Try to locate the /u/ words in each sentence, and write them down. The /u/ words in each test sentence will be read to you at the end of the drill. The sentences appear later in the chapter in Section 35-4E. If you have difficulty recognizing the target, you may find it worthwhile to review the test with somebody outside class.

35–2. DISCRIMINATING BETWEEN /u/ AND THE /ʊ/ REPLACEMENT

A. PROBABLE TYPES OF REPLACEMENT

The following exercises will help you learn to compare /u/ with your probable replacement of /ʊ/ as in pull. If you are not employing this common replacement, your instructor will tell you exactly how your are mispronouncing /u/ and provide you with some discrimination drills.

B. PAIRED LISTS OF WORDS

The words in the following paired list are identical, except that the words in Column 1 contain the target, and the words in Column 2 contain the /ʊ/ replacement. Complete instructions for this type of exercise are given in Chap. 5, 5-2B.

Column 1 /u/	Column 2 /ʊ/
pool	pull
fool	full
who'd	hood
shooed	should
cooed	could
wooed	would

C. Listening for Replacements in Familiar /u/ Words

You will hear a list of words containing /u/. Sometimes the words will be pronounced correctly with /u/; other times the words will be said incorrectly with your replacement. Complete instructions for this type of drill are found in Chap. 5, 5-2D.

35-3. A FEW REMINDERS ABOUT ORAL PRACTICE PROCEDURES

If this is the first practice chapter assigned to you by your instructor, you may wish to review the comments about beginning oral practice in Chap. 2, 2-4. Before you actually begin practicing each individual pronunciation drill, you may also desire to review the supplementary explanations about the exercise in Chap. 2, 2-5.

35-4. THE PRONUNCIATION OF /u/

A. Pronouncing Isolated /u/

In the event that you cannot pronounce /u/ through imitation alone, your instructor will help you with the following suggestions about placement. Should placement be required, you should review the explanatory comments about back vowels in Chap. 4, 4-4F, and the description of /u/ in Figure 3 of Chapter 4.

1. The Position of the Lips

The target /u/ is considered round, and your lips should be well-rounded for the target.

2. The Position of the Tongue

Press the edges of your tongue firmly against the bottoms of your upper back teeth. Arch the back of the tongue so that it is steep and close to your soft palate, and keep your tongue tip low and pointed toward the biting edges of your lower, middle front teeth. You may or may not touch your teeth with your tongue tip. Your jaws are close together. It is very difficult to place your tongue in the correct position for the target for two reasons: (1) you cannot see what you are doing, and (2) the difference between the position of the tongue for /u/ and the position for the replacement /ʊ/ is very small. Note that when you pronounce /ʊ/ your tongue arch is slightly lower and flatter than for /u/. The lower jaw also drops slightly so that the mouth is open a bit wider for /ʊ/ than for /u/. Thus if you place your tongue too low—and open your mouth too much—you may pronounce /ʊ/ rather than the target.

3.   Vowel Length and Muscular Tension

Two more suggestions may simplify the pronunciation of /u/ for you. The target is frequently heard as a long sound, and you will pronounce /u/ more accurately if you prolong the vowel while saying it. Because of the prolongation of the target, there is also a tendency for the lips to close slightly as you pronounce /u/. Watch your instructor pronounce /u/ for you several times, and observe how his lips close slightly as he says the target. Observe the difference when he pronounces /ʊ/ for you. The target is also said with strong tensing of the muscles, and this muscular tension may be felt. Place your thumb under the fleshy part of your instructor's chin and listen to his pronunciation of the target. You should be able to feel a definite sensation of pressure against your thumb as your instructor pronounces /u/. This pressure is caused primarily by the muscles of his tongue pushing themselves against your thumb as he says the target. Keep your thumb against his chin, and listen to his pronunciation of /ʊ/. There should be little or no sensation of pressure against your thumb, because the replacement is pronounced with much less muscular tension than /u/. Note that if you use too little muscular tension while pronouncing /u/, you may pronounce /ʊ/ rather than the target.

4.   Pronouncing the Target

Place your thumb under the fleshy part of your chin, and pronounce /u/, keeping in mind the suggestions given earlier. Because of the difficulty you may have in placing your tongue in the proper position for /u/, listen intently to your instructor's pronunciation as he helps you pronounce the target. Try to feel the slight closing movement of your lips, and use a mirror to observe your pronunciation.

B.   Pronouncing /u/ in Familiar Words

Pronounce each of the following words carefully. If you are either practicing with your instructor or listening to the exercise on tape, imitate your speech model as accurately as possible.

Middle				End
1. spool	8. truce	15. loop	22. choose	1. who
2. shoot	9. doing	16. loose	23. produce	2. too
3. moving	10. spoon	17. lose	24. scooping	3. zoo
4. juice	11. fool	18. smooth	25. student	4. canoe
5. stoop	12. group	19. sooner	26. tune	5. shoe
6. salute	13. afternoon	20. whom	27. June	6. blue
7. boots	14. food	21. rule	28. school	7. glue

C. PRONOUNCING WORD PAIRS
CONTAINING /u/ AND THE /ʊ/ REPLACEMENT

Select some of the words from the paired list in Section 35-2B containing /u/ and your /ʊ/ replacement. Read one pair of words at a time, pronouncing the word with the target first (e.g., **pool–pull**). Make sure that you are saying /u/ first and /ʊ/ second. Reverse the procedure and pronounce the replacement word first and the target word second, making certain that you use /ʊ/ first and /u/ second. Try to develop speed and accuracy as you do the drill. If you are either practicing with your instructor or listening to the exercise on tape, imitate your speech model as accurately as possible. You will find this drill more difficult than the word list in Section 35-4B because of the closeness of target and replacement.

D. PRONOUNCING /u/ IN PHRASES

Pronounce each of the phrases carefully. If you mispronounce a word, say it over again several times, and then repeat the entire phrase. If you are either practicing with your instructor or listening to the drill on tape, imitate your speech model as accurately as possible.

1. a **tablespoon** of **prunes** in the **room**[2]
2. roast **goose** and **noodle soup**
3. a **poodle** barking at the **moon**
4. broke a **tooth** at the zoo
5. a **blue ruler** on the **stool**
6. **doing** things with the **group** at the **movies**
7. drinking **fruit juice** in the **afternoon**

E. PRONOUNCING /u/ IN SENTENCES

Pronounce each of the sentences carefully. If you use a replacement, say the word over again several times, and then repeat the entire sentence. If you are either practicing with your instructor or listening to the exercise on tape, imitate your speech model as accurately as possible.

1. The **loose tools** were scattered **throughout** the **workroom** that **afternoon**.
2. The **cool** wind tossed the **balloon through** the **gloomy** park.

---

[2]Words like **roof, root, broom,** and **room**—and compounds formed with **room**—may be pronounced with either /u/ or /ʊ/. However, there seems to be a preference for /u/ in these words. Use the pronunciation that is easier for you, unless there is a preference for one particular pronunciation in your area. If you have any questions about which pronunciation, if any, is the preferred one in your area, ask your instructor.

3. **Whose** bag of **fruit** did **Susan** find in the **schoolroom** at **noon**?

4. They **soon** saw the **raccoon moving** slowly across the **smooth schoolyard** in the **moonlight**.

5. It was **foolish moving** the **two loosely glued broom** handles.

F.   PRONOUNCING /u/ IN BEGINNING CONVERSATION

This exercise gives you an opportunity to begin using some of your previously learned /u/ words in beginning conversation. Complete instructions for this type of drill are given in Chap. 5, 5-4H. Read the instructions, and adapt them to practice with /u/.

1. "I'll measure the _____ with the **ruler**."

2. "I like _____ **juice** in the morning."

3. "How **soon** is Mr. _____ coming to **school**?"

4. "He bought **new boots** last _____."

5. "Is **Ruth** buying some _____?"

6. "**Whose** _____ fell in the **pool**?"

7. "My favorite **food** is _____."

8. "Did he **lose** his _____ in **June**?"

9. "Are they **doing** something about the _____?"

10. "Does she like _____ **soup**?"

11. "He **threw** the _____ at me."

12. "Which _____ did he **choose**?"

35–5.   CONVERSATION PRACTICE

So far you have learned how to pronounce your target by reading various kinds of exercises which contain /u/ words. Now you are ready to move into the final and most important part of your training program—learning to pronounce /u/ automatically while you are talking more or less spontaneously. If this is the first practice chapter assigned to you by your instructor, you may wish to review the introductory comments on conversation practice in Chap. 2, 2-6 to 2-7.

A.   CARRYING /u/ INTO SPONTANEOUS DAILY CONVERSATION

This exercise requires you to use /u/ in daily conversation, starting with key words and expanding to all the /u/ words in your particular vocabulary. Complete instructions for this type of drill are given in Chap. 5, 5-5A, and there are supplementary comments about the exercise in Chap. 2, 2-7A.

B.   GENERAL CLASSROOM EXERCISES IN SPEAKING

Your instructor will plan a series of classroom conversation activities, and each assignment will be discussed fully in class before you carry it out. When your instructor announces the first speaking activity, you may wish to review the introductory comments on classroom speaking in Chap. 2, 2-7B.

chapter thirty-six

The Vowel Target
/ʊ/ (pull)

COMMON SPELLINGS FOR /ʊ/

The most frequent spellings are found in the words **cook** and **full**; less frequent spellings include w**ou**ld and w**o**man.

36–1.   EAR TRAINING FOR THE /ʊ/ TARGET

A.   A Few Reminders About Ear Training

The following test exercises will help you learn to recognize your /ʊ/ target. If this is the first practice chapter assigned to you by your instructor, you may wish to review the discussion about listening practice in Chap. 2, 2-2B to 2-3C.

B.   Recognizing /ʊ/ in Phrases and Sentences

You will listen to a series of phrases and sentences containing a number of /ʊ/ words. Each phrase or sentence will be read several times. Try to locate the

/ʊ/ words in each phrase or sentence, and write them down. The /ʊ/ words in each phrase or sentence will be read to you at the end of the drill. The materials appear later in the chapter in Sections 36-4D and E. If you have difficulty recognizing the target, you may find it worthwhile to review the test with somebody outside class.

36–2. DISCRIMINATING BETWEEN /ʊ/ AND THE VARIOUS REPLACEMENTS

A. PROBABLE TYPES OF REPLACEMENT

The following exercises will help you learn to compare /ʊ/ with your replacement. You are probably substituting one of the following common replacements for /ʊ/: (1) /u/, as in (pool) or (2) /ʌ/ as in (rub). Your instructor will tell you which replacement you are using. If you are not employing one of the more common replacements, your teacher will tell you exactly how you are mispronouncing /ʊ/ and provide you with some discrimination drills.

B. PAIRED LISTS OF WORDS

The words in the following paired lists are identical, except that the words in Column 1 contain the target, and the words in Column 2 contain one of the replacements. Complete instructions for this type of exercise are given in Chap. 5, 5-2B.

1.	Column 1 /ʊ/	Column 2 /u/	2.	Column 1 /ʊ/	Column 2 /ʌ/
	pull	pool		look	luck
	full	fool		put	putt
	hood	who'd		took	tuck
	should	shooed		book	buck
	could	cooed		could	cud
	would	wooed			

C. LISTENING FOR REPLACEMENTS IN FAMILIAR /ʊ/ WORDS

You will hear a list of words containing /ʊ/. Sometimes the words will be pronounced correctly with /ʊ/; other times the words will be said incorrectly with your replacement. Complete instructions for this type of drill are found in Chap. 5, 5-2D.

36–3. A FEW REMINDERS ABOUT ORAL PRACTICE PROCEDURES

If this is the first practice chapter assigned to you by your instructor, you may wish to review the comments about beginning oral practice in Chap. 2, 2-4.

Before you actually begin practicing each individual pronunciation drill, you may also desire to review the supplementary explanations about the exercise in Chap. 2, 2-5.

36–4. THE PRONUNCIATION OF /ʊ/

A. PRONOUNCING /ISOLATED /ʊ/

In the event that you cannot pronounce /ʊ/ through imitation alone, your instructor will help you with the following suggestions about placement. Should placement be required, you should review the explanatory comments about back vowels in Chap. 4, 4-4F, and the description of /ʊ/ in Figure 3 of Chapter 4.

1. The Position of the Lips

The target /ʊ/ is considered round, but your lips are not as round as for the /u/ replacement. Although there is a tendency for the lips to close slightly as you pronounce /u/, this movement does not occur when you pronounce the target. Watch your instructor pronounce /ʊ/ and /u/ several times for you, and observe the difference between lip positions. The /ʌ/ replacement has an unrounded lip position.

2. The Position of the Tongue

Press the edges of your tongue firmly against the bottoms of your upper back teeth. Arch the back of the tongue so that it is steep and close to the soft palate, and keep your tongue tip low and pointed toward the biting edges of your lower, middle front teeth. You may or may not touch your teeth with your tongue tip. Your jaws are close together. It is very difficult to place your tongue in the correct position for the target for two reasons: (1) you cannot see what you are doing, and (2) the difference between the position of the tongue for /u/ and the position for the /ʊ/ and /v/ replacements is very small. Note that when you pronounce /u/ your tongue arch is slightly higher and steeper than for /ʊ/. The lower jaw also rises slightly so that the mouth is slightly more closed for /u/ than for /ʊ/. Thus if you place your tongue too high—and close your mouth too much—you may pronounce /u/ rather than the target. The position for the /ʌ/ replacement requires a very slight arching of the middle of the tongue. Review Figure 3 of Chapter 4, and observe the difference in position between /ʊ/ and /ʌ/.

3. Muscular Tension

The target is said with little tensing of the muscles, while the replacement /u/ is said with strong muscular tension. This difference in tension may be felt and will aid you in avoiding this replacement. Place your thumb under the fleshy part of your instructor's chin, and listen to his pronunciation of the target. There should be little or no sensation of pressure against your thumb as your instructor pronounces /ʊ/. Keep your thumb against his chin and listen to his pronunciation of /u/. You should be able to feel a definite sensation of pressure against your thumb as your instructor pronounces /u/. This pressure is caused primarily by the muscles of his tongue pushing themselves against your thumb as he says /u/. Note that if you use too much muscular tension while pronouncing /ʊ/ you may pronounce /u/ rather than the target.

4. Pronouncing the Target

Place your thumb under the fleshy part of your chin, and pronounce /ʊ/, keeping in mind the suggestions given earlier. Because of the difficulty you may have in placing your tongue in the proper position for /ʊ/, listen intently to your instructor's pronunciation as he helps you pronounce the target. Use a mirror if you wish to check your lip position.

B.   Pronouncing /u/ in Familiar Words

Pronounce each of the following words carefully. If you are either practicing with your instructor or listening to the exercise on tape, imitate your speech model as accurately as possible.

Middle

1. cookbook	11. careful	21. woman
2. bushes	12. during	22. put
3. took	13. understood	23. stood
4. bullet	14. goodnight	24. shouldn't
5. hood	15. sure	25. should
6. good-bye	16. hooks	26. shook
7. wonderful	17. wouldn't	27. pull
8. could	18. look	28. crooked
9. shook	19. would	29. sugar
10. couldn't	20. poor	30. full

C.   Pronouncing Word Pairs Containing /u/ and a Replacement

Select some of the words from the paired lists in Section 36-2B containing /ʊ/ and your replacement. Read one pair of words at a time, pronouncing the word with the target first (e.g., **pull–pool**). Make sure that you are saying /ʊ/ first and /u/ second. Reverse the procedure, and pronounce the replacement word first and the target word second, making certain that you say /u/ first and /ʊ/ second. Try to develop speed and accuracy as you do the drill. If you are either practicing with your instructor or listening to the exercise on tape, imitate your speech model as accurately as possible. If you are listening to the taped exercise, listen *only* to the drill that compares the target with your particular replacement. You will find this drill more difficult than the word list in Section 36-4B because of the closeness of target and replacement.

D.   PRONOUNCING /ʊ/ IN PHRASES

Pronounce each of the phrases carefully. If you mispronounce a word, say it over again several times, and then repeat the entire phrase. If you are either practicing with your instructor or listening to the drill on tape, imitate your speech model as accurately as possible.

1. **sugar cookies** for the **cook**
2. a **crooked brook** in the **woods**
3. a **notebook** on the **bookcase**
4. threw a **football** at the **bull**
5. **pushed** a **bushel** of **wool**
6. **full** of **good** rice **pudding**

E.   PRONOUNCING /ʊ/ IN SENTENCES

Pronounce each of the sentences carefully. If you use a replacement, say the word over again several times, and then repeat the entire sentence. If you are either practicing with your instructor or listening to the exercise on tape, imitate your speech model as accurately as possible.

1. He **carefully pulled** the strange-**looking wooden** box out of the **brook**.
2. The **woodcutters took** the best-**looking bushes** for **firewood**.
3. They **looked** for the **wolf's crooked footprints** in the snow.
4. The **woman stood** up and **put** on the **wonderful-looking woolen hood**.
5. The **butcher wouldn't** trim his **bushy** beard **carefully**.

F.   PRONOUNCING /ʊ/ IN BEGINNING CONVERSATION

This exercise gives you an opportunity to begin using some of your previously learned /ʊ/ words in beginning conversation. Complete instructions for this type of drill are given in Chap. 5, 5-4H. Read the instructions, and adapt them to practice with /ʊ/.

1. "Is the _____ **good** to eat?"
2. "The **cookbook** had a recipe for _____."
3. "**Put** the picture of the _____ on the **bulletin** board."
4. "**Could** you place the _____ on the **bookcase**?"
5. "Did you **look** at the _____?"
6. "**Would** you like the _____?"
7. "Are you **sure** you were **careful** with the _____?"
8. "**Should** you give him the _____?"
9. "I'd like some **sugar** on my _____."
10. "My new _____ is made of **wool**."
11. "I need a **notebook** for my _____ class."

36–5. CONVERSATION PRACTICE

So far you have learned how to pronounce your target by reading various kinds of exercises which contain /ʊ/ words. Now you are ready to move into the final and most important part of your training program—learning to pronounce /ʊ/ automatically while you are talking more or less spontaneously. If this is the first practice chapter assigned to you by your instructor, you may wish to review the introductory comments on conversation practice in Chap. 2, 2-6 to 2-7.

A.   CARRYING /ʊ/ INTO SPONTANEOUS DAILY CONVERSATION

This exercise requires you to use /ʊ/ in daily conversation, starting with key words and expanding to all the /ʊ/ words in your particular vocabulary. Complete instructions for this type of drill are given in Chap. 5, 5-5A, and there are supplementary comments about the exercise in Chap. 2, 2-7A.

B.   GENERAL CLASSROOM EXERCISES IN SPEAKING

Your instructor will plan a series of classroom conversation activities, and each assignment will be discussed fully in class before you carry it out. When your instructor announces the first speaking activity, you may wish to review the introductory comments on classroom speaking in Chap. 2, 2-7B.

chapter thirty-seven

The Diphthong Target
/ou/ (post)[1]

COMMON SPELLINGS FOR /ou/

The most frequent spelling is found in the word **post**; less frequent spellings include kn**ow**, th**ough**, c**oa**l, **oh**, **owe**, s**ou**l, and g**oe**s.

37–1.   EAR TRAINING FOR THE /ou/ TARGET

A.   A Few Reminders About Ear Training

The following test exercises will help you learn to recognize your /ou/ target. If this is the first practice chapter assigned to you by your instructor, you may wish to review the discussion about listening practice in Chap. 2, 2-B to 2-3C.

---

[1] I have used the diphthong symbol /ou/, because the target is pronounced as a diphthong by a large majority of American English speakers in syllables containing primary and secondary stress (e.g., post and rowboat). The single vowel /o/ is only heard in syllables containing weak stress (e.g., window and obey). See C. M. Wise, *Applied Phonetics* (Englewood Cliffs, N.J.: Prentice-Hall, Inc., 1957), p. 99.

B. Recognizing /oʊ/ in Words

You will hear a list of words containing /oʊ/. After listening to each word, write *B* if you heard /oʊ/ at the beginning of the word, *M* if you heard /oʊ/ in the middle, and *E* if you heard /oʊ/ at the end of the word. The answers will be read to you at the end of the drill. This exercise is found in Appendix 1. If you have difficulty recognizing the target, you may find it worthwhile to review the test with somebody outside class.

C. Recognizing /oʊ/ in Sentences

You will listen to a series of sentences containing a number of /oʊ/ words. Each sentence will be read several times. Try to locate the /oʊ/ words in each test sentence, and write them down. The /oʊ/ words in each test sentence will be read to you at the end of the drill. The sentences appear later in the chapter in Section 37-4F. If you have difficulty recognizing the target, you may find it worthwhile to review the test with somebody outside class.

37–2. DISCRIMINATING BETWEEN /oʊ/ AND THE VARIOUS REPLACEMENTS

A. Probable Types of Replacement

The following exercises will help you learn to compare /oʊ/ with your replacement. You are probably substituting one of the following common replacements for /oʊ/: (1) /ɔ/ as in call,[2] (2) /ʌ/ as in rub, (3) the single or pure vowel /o/ as in obey, or (4) /ə/ as in papᴈr, for final weak-stressed /o/, as in potato and yellow.[3] Your instructor will tell you which replacement you are using.

If you are not employing one of the more common replacements, your teacher will tell you exactly how you are mispronouncing /oʊ/ and provide you with some discrimination drills.

---

[2]Certain words may be pronounced with either /oʊ/ or /ɔ/. In these words the vowel letters o, oa, ou, and oo combine with r. Examples include score, board, four, floor. Words of this type are found in Chapter 38. If this chapter is not assigned to you and you have occasion to use words of this nature, use whatever pronunciation is easier for you, unless there is a preference for one particular pronunciation in your area. If you have any questions about which pronunciation, if any, is the preferred one in your area, ask your instructor.

[3]A related problem is the use of /ə/ as in about for /o/ in words like yellow and potato. Some instructors consider this replacement undesirable under all speaking conditions, while others believe that the /ə/ pronunciation should be limited to informal or casual speaking circumstances. If you substitute /ə/ for /o/, your instructor will indicate the preferences in your area for /ə/ and /o/ in words of this nature.

B.   PAIRED LISTS OF WORDS

The words in the following paired lists are identical, except that the words in Column 1 contain the target, and the words in Column 2 contain one of the replacements. Complete instructions for this type of exercise are given in Chap. 5, 5-2B.

1.	**Column 1** /ou/	**Column 2** /ɔ/	2.	**Column 1** /ou/	**Column 2** /ʌ/[4]
	oat	ought		boast	bust
	woke	walk		roast	rust
	boat	bought		phone	fun
	bowl	ball		roam	rum
	coal	call		soak	suck
	coast	cost		wrote	rut
	cold	called		boat	but
	hole	hall		hole	hull
	loan	lawn		most	must
	so	saw		bone	bun
	low	law		coat	cut
				note	nut

C.   PAIRED SENTENCES

The following paired sentences are identical, except that the final word in the first sentence contains /ou/, and the final word in the second sentence contains one of the replacements. Complete instructions for this type of exercise are given in Chap. 5, 5-2C.

/ou/ – /ɔ/	/ou/ – /ʌ/[5]
1. I need the bowl.	1. Where's the roast?
I need the ball.	Where's the rust?
2. It's in the hole.	2. It's a large hole.
It's in the hall.	It's a large hull.
3. Do you want a loan?	3. I dropped the bone.
Do you want a lawn?	I dropped the bun.
4. Did you get the coal?	4. She has a small coat.
Did you get the call?	She has a small cut.
	5. He left a note.
	He left a nut.

[4] If your replacement is /o/, your instructor will carry out this drill with you by changing the /ou/ – /ʌ/ pairs to /ou/ – /o/ pairs.

[5] See footnote 4.

D. Listening for Replacements in Familiar /ou/ Words

You will hear a list of words containing /ou/. Sometimes the words will be pronounced correctly with /ou/; other times the words will be said incorrectly with your replacement. Complete instructions for this type of drill are found in Chap. 5, 5-2D.

37–3. A FEW REMINDERS ABOUT ORAL PRACTICE PROCEDURES

If this is the first practice chapter assigned to you by your instructor, you may wish to review the comments about beginning oral practice in Chap. 2, 2-4. Before you actually begin practicing each individual pronunciation drill, you may also desire to review the supplementary explanations about the exercise in Chap. 2, 2-5.

37–4. THE PRONUNCIATION OF /ou/

A. Pronouncing Isolated /ou/

In the event that you cannot pronounce /ou/ through imitation alone, your instructor will help you with the following suggestions about placement. Should placement be required, you should review the explanatory comments about back vowels in Chap. 4, 4-4F, the comments about diphthongs in Chap. 4, 4-4G, and the description of /ou/ in Figure 4 of Chapter 4.

1. The Position of the Lips

The target /ou/ is considered round, and your lips should be well rounded for both vowels. As the articulators glide from /o/ up to /u/ as in (pull), your lips gradually close and become more rounded. Note that your lips are less rounded and farther apart for /ɔ/, and that your lips are unrounded for the /ʌ/ and /ɚ/ replacements.

2. Tongue Position, Length, and Muscular Tension

Place your tongue tip near the bottoms of your lower, middle front teeth. You may or may not touch your teeth with your tongue tip. Note that your upper and lower front teeth are farther apart for /ɔ/ than for the target. Arch the back of the tongue in the direction of the soft palate, remembering that the arch is higher for the first sound /o/ than for /ɔ/. If you place your tongue too low—and open your mouth too much—you may pronounce /ɔ/ rather than the target.

The most important thing to remember about the arched tongue position for the target is its movement. The tongue moves from an initial arched position for /o/ up to the arched tongue position for /ʊ/, traveling with a smooth, continuous gliding movement. This causes your mouth to close slightly, because your lower jaw is simultaneously rising with your tongue. Watch your instructor pronounce /oʊ/ for you several times, and observe the closing movements of his lips and lower jaw. Because of the lip, tongue, and jaw movements associated with the pronunciation of /oʊ/, the target is heard as a long sound; you will pronounce the target more accurately if you prolong it. The length is especially important if your replacement is /o/, because you eliminate the diphthongal gliding movements up to /ʊ/ when you produce the single vowel. The target is also pronounced with fairly strong tensing of the tongue muscles. Tense your tongue when you pronounce the target; this will also help you acquire the required gliding movements of tongue and jaw. Remember that it is very difficult to place your tongue in the correct beginning position of the target for two reasons: (1) the difference between the tongue positions of the target and the replacements is very small, and (2) the tongue positions for /oʊ/ are not visible, the position for the /ʌ/ and /ɝ/ replacements is not visible, and the position for the /ɔ/ replacement is only partially visible.

3. *Pronouncing the Target*

Try pronouncing /oʊ/, keeping in mind the suggestions given above. Because of the difficulty you may have in placing your tongue in the proper beginning position for the target, listen intently to your instructor's pronunciation as he helps you pronounce the target. Try to feel the movements of your tongue, lips, and lower jaw while pronouncing /oʊ/. Use a mirror to observe your lips and jaw movements.

B.   PRONOUNCING /oʊ/ IN FAMILIAR WORDS

Pronounce each of the following words carefully. If you are either practicing with your instructor or listening to the exercise on tape, imitate your speech model as accurately as possible.

Beginning	Middle		End	
1. only	1. alone	11. don't	1. potato	12. window
2. old	2. spoke	12. hold	2. tomato	13. ago
3. over	3. both	13. drove	3. tomorrow	14. below
4. own	4. told	14. fold	4. pillow	15. slow
5. open	5. bold	15. float	5. piano	16. go
6. ocean	6. sold	16. roast	6. yellow	17. so
7. oats	7. bowl	17. goes	7. fellow	18. low
8. oak	8. notice	18. going	8. hollow	19. grow
9. odor	9. cold	19. scold	9. follow	20. know
10. oval	10. most	20. poker	10. shallow	21. hello
			11. shadow	22. show

C.   Pronouncing Word Pairs Containing /ou/ and a Replacement

Select some of the words from the paired lists in Section 37-2B containing /ou/ and your replacement. Read one pair of words at a time, pronouncing the word with the target first (e.g., **coal–call**). Make sure that you are saying /ou/ first and /ɔ/ second. Reverse the procedure, and pronounce the replacement word first and the target word second, making certain that you say /ɔ/ first and /ou/ second. Try to develop speed and accuracy as you do the drill. If you are either practicing with your instructor or listening to the exercise on tape, imitate your speech model as accurately as possible. If you are listening to the taped exercise, listen *only* to the drill that compares the target with your particular replacement. You will find this drill more difficult than the word list in Section 37-4B because of the closeness of target and replacement.

D.   Pronouncing /ou/ in Phrases

Pronounce each of the phrase carefully. If you mispronounce a word, say it over again several times, and then repeat the entire phrase. If you are either practicing with your instructor or listening to the drill on tape, imitate your speech model as accurately as possible.

1.   **coke** and jelly **rolls tomorrow**
2.   **snow** on the **road** in **October**
3.   **won't throw** the **stone** in the **hole**
4.   **don't vote** for **both**
5.   **told** to use **soap** on the **window**
6.   **holding both bones** for **Rose**
7.   **know** the **soldier's yellow boat**
8.   to **go** and **row slowly** where it's **shallow**

E.   Pronouncing Short Phrases Containing /ou/ and /ɔ/

This drill is similar to the exercise in Section 37-4C, except that your /ɔ/ replacement precedes the target in each phrase. Pronounce each of the phrases carefully. If you are either practicing with your instructor or listening to the exercise on tape, imitate your speech model as accurately as possible. Although these phrases are shorter than those in the preceding drill, you may find this exercise more difficult, because your replacement directly precedes /ou/ in each phrase.

/ɔ/ – /ou/

1. saw over	3. raw oats	5. straw odor
2. to draw only	4. a jaw open	

F. PRONOUNCING /ou/ IN SENTENCES

Pronounce each of the sentences carefully. If you use a replacement, say the word over again several times, and then repeat the entire sentence. If you are either practicing with your instructor or listening to the exercise on tape, imitate your speech model as accurately as possible.

1. He **hoped** that the wind hadn't **broken** the **pole holding** the **tomato** plants.
2. **Joe boasted** that he could **throw a snowball** with his eyes **closed** and hit the **hollow post.**
3. The **slowly floating snowflakes** had **coated** the **stones** with **snow.**
4. **Joan** said, "I **suppose** a **pony** likes the **odor** of **clover** and **oats.**"
5. When he **drove home** the **following October,** the **broken motorboat** was **frozen** in the lake.

G. PRONOUNCING /ou/ IN BEGINNING CONVERSATION

This exercise gives you an opportunity to begin using some of your previously learned /ou/ words in beginning conversation. Complete instructions for this type of drill are given in Chap. 5, 5-4H. Read the instructions, and adapt them to practice with /ou/.

1. "I'm **going** to _____ **tomorrow.**"
2. "The **gold piano** cost _____ dollars."
3. "They **broke** the **window** with a _____."
4. "Are **those** your _____?"
5. "Give me **most** of the _____."
6. "**Don't** you like the _____?"
7. "Please **don't scold** _____."
8. "I want a **bowl** of _____ soup."
9. "**Show** him **both** _____."
10. "I **noticed** the **bathrobe** at _____."
11. "_____ is **located** in the Pacific **Ocean.**"
12. "I like the **odor** of **roast** _____."

37-5. CONVERSATION PRACTICE

So far you have learned how to pronounce your target by reading various kinds of exercises which contain /ou/ words. Now you are ready to move into the final and most important part of your training program—learning to pronounce /oʊ/ automatically while you are talking more or less spontaneously. If this is the first practice chapter assigned to you by your instructor, you may wish to review the introductory comments on conversation practice in Chap. 2, 2-6 to 2-7.

A.   CARRYING /oʊ/ INTO SPONTANEOUS DAILY CONVERSATION

This exercise requires you to use /oʊ/ in daily conversation, starting with key words and expanding to all the /oʊ/ words in your particular vocabulary. Complete instructions for this type of drill are given in Chap. 5, 5-5A, and there are supplementary comments about the exercise in Chap. 2, 2-7A.

B.   GENERAL CLASSROOM EXERCISES IN SPEAKING

Your instructor will plan a series of classroom conversation activities, and each assignment will be discussed fully in class before you carry it out. When your instructor announces the first speaking activity, you may wish to review the introductory comments on classroom speaking in Chap. 2, 2-7B.

chapter thirty-eight

The Vowel Target
/ɔ/ (call)[1]

COMMON SPELLINGS FOR /ɔ/

The most frequent spellings are found in the words s**aw** and f**au**lt; less frequent spellings include **a**ll, th**ough**t, c**o**st, br**oa**d, and t**a**lk.

[1]It should be noted that there is widespread use of alternate acceptable pronunciations of the target with /ou/ as in post and /ɑ/ as in father. A few words of explanation at this point should help you in learning to use /ɔ/.

1. The vowel /ɑ/ is the typical pronunciation for the majority of American English speakers in the so-called "short o" words (marked diacritically with ŏ in many dictionaries). This is particularly true of "short o" before the following sounds: /p/ as in t**o**p, /b/ as in j**o**b, /t/ as in n**o**t, /d/ as in G**o**d, /k/ as in r**o**ck, and /l/ between vowels as in p**o**licy. However in certain "short o" words such as doll, golf, on, and gone, /ɔ/ as well as /ɑ/ is heard frequently.

2. The spelling **or** or **orr**—plus a vowel—is typically pronounced /ɔ/ by General American speakers, although /ɑ/ is also heard occasionally. Examples include **or**ange, f**or**est, h**orr**or.

3. The spelling **o** before the following sounds is typically pronounced /ɔ/ by General American speakers, although /ɑ/ is also heard occasionally. Examples include /g/ as in fr**o**g and /ŋ/ as in l**o**ng.

4. The spelling **wa** in certain words varies between /ɔ/ and /ɑ/ in General American speech. Examples include wash, want, water, and watch.

38–1. EAR TRAINING FOR THE /ɔ/ TARGET

A. A Few Reminders About Ear Training

The following test exercises will help you learn to recognize your /ɔ/ target. If this is the first practice chapter assigned to you by your instructor, you may wish to review the discussion about listening practice in Chap. 2, 2-B to 2-3C.

B. Recognizing /ɔ/ in Words

You will hear a list of words containing /ɔ/. After listening to each word, write *B* if you heard /ɔ/ at the beginning of the word, *M* if you heard /ɔ/ in the middle, and *E* if you heard /ɔ/ at the end of the word. The answers will be read to you at the end of the drill. This exercise is found in Appendix 1. If you have difficulty recognizing the target, you may find it worthwhile to review the test with somebody outside class.

C. Recognizing /ɔ/ in Sentences

You will listen to a series of sentences containing a number of /ɔ/ words. Each sentence will be read several times. Try to locate the /ɔ/ words in each test sentence, and write them down. The /ɔ/ words in each test sentence will be read to you at the end of the drill. The sentences appear later in the chapter in Section 38-4F. If you have difficulty recognizing the target, you may find it worthwhile to review the test with somebody outside class.

38–2. DISCRIMINATING BETWEEN /ɔ/ AND THE VARIOUS REPLACEMENTS

A. Probable Types of Replacement

The following exercises will help you learn to compare /ɔ/ with your replacement. You are probably substituting one of the following common replacements for /ɔ/: (1) /ou/ as in post, or (2) /ɑ/ as in father. Your instructor will tell you which replacement you are using. If you are not employing one of the more common replacements, your teacher will tell you exactly how you are mispronouncing /ɔ/ and provide you with some discrimination drills.

---

5. Certain words are pronounced with either /ɔ/ or /ou/ by General American speakers. In these words the vowel letters **o, oa, ou,** and **oo** combine with **r.** Examples include s**core, board, four,** and **floor.**

If the dialectal preference in your area is for either /ɑ/ or /ou/, rather than /ɔ/, in the word types listed above, your instructor will help you determine which words should be learned with /ɔ/ and which words should be pronounced with /ɑ/ or /ou/. If there is no preference in your area in these special words, use whatever pronunciation is easiest for you.

B.   PAIRED LISTS OF WORDS

The words in the following paired lists are identical, except that the words in Column 1 contain the target, and the words in Column 2 contain one of the replacements. Complete instructions for this type of exercise are given in Chap. 5, 5-2B.

1.	Column 1 /ɔ/	Column 2 /ou/	2.	Column 1 /ɔ/	Column 2 /ɑ/
	ought	oat		caught	cot
	walk	woke		pawned	pond
	bought	boat		naughty	knotty
	ball	bowl		pork	park
	call	coal		port	part
	cost	coast		score	scar
	called	cold		tore	tar
	hall	hole		born	barn
	lawn	loan		court	cart
	saw	so		four	far
	law	low		Gordon	garden
				former	farmer

C.   PAIRED SENTENCES

The following paired sentences are identical, except that the final word in the first sentence contains /ɔ/, and the final word in the second sentence contains the /ou/ replacement. Complete instructions for this type of exercise are given in Chap. 5, 5-2C.

/ɔ/ – /ou/

1. I need the ball.   3. Do you want a lawn?
   I need the bowl.   Do you want a loan?
2. It's in the hall.   4. Did you get the call?
   It's in the hole.   Did you get the coal?

D.   LISTENING FOR REPLACEMENTS IN FAMILIAR /ɔ/ WORDS

You will hear a list of words containing /ɔ/. Sometimes the words will be pronounced correctly with /ɔ/; other times the words will be said incorrectly with your replacement. Complete instructions for this type of drill are found in Chap. 5, 5-2D.

38–3.   A FEW REMINDERS ABOUT ORAL PRACTICE PROCEDURES

If this is the first practice chapter assigned to you by your instructor, you may wish to review the comments about beginning oral practice in Chap. 2, 2-4.

Before you actually begin practicing each individual pronunciation drill, you may also desire to review the supplementary explanations about the exercise in Chap. 2, 2-5.

38–4. THE PRONUNCIATION OF /ɔ/

A. PRONOUNCING ISOLATED /ɔ/

In the event that you cannot pronounce /ɔ/ through imitation alone, your instructor will help you with the following suggestions about placement. Should placement be required, you should review the explanatory comments about back vowels in Chap. 4, 4-4F, and the description of /ɔ/ in Figure 3 of Chapter 4.

1. The Position of the Lips

The target /ɔ/ is considered round. Note that your lips are more rounded and closer together for the /oʊ/ replacement, and unrounded and farther apart for the /a/ replacement. Watch your instructor pronounce /ɔ/ and your replacement several times, and observe the differences between them. If your replacement is /oʊ/, note that the lips tend to close slightly during the pronunciation of this replacement.

2. The Position of the Tongue and Muscular Tension

Place your tongue tip near the bottoms of your lower, middle front teeth. You may or may not touch your teeth with your tongue tip. Note that your jaws are farther apart for the target than for the /oʊ/ replacement. However, the jaws are opened wider for the /a/ replacement than for the target. Arch the back of the tongue in the direction of the soft palate, remembering that the arch is lower and flatter than for /oʊ/. However, the tongue arch is lower and flatter for /a/ than for /ɔ/. Actually the tongue is almost flat in the mouth for /a/. You will notice in Figure 3 of Chapter 4 that the target is positioned between /oʊ/ and /a/. If you place your tongue too high—and close your mouth too much—you may pronounce the higher-positioned /oʊ/; conversely if you place your tongue too low—and open your mouth too much—you may pronounce the lower-positioned /a/. It is very difficult to place your tongue in the correct position for the target for two reasons: (1) the difference between the tongue position of the target and the two replacements is very small, and (2) the tongue position for /ɔ/ is only partially visible, and the tongue position for /oʊ/ is not visible. However, the tongue position for /a/ is easily seen. The target is usually pronounced with little muscular tension. Keep your tongue fairly relaxed when you pronounce /ɔ/.

3. Pronouncing the Target

Try pronouncing /ɔ/, keeping in mind the suggestions given above. Because of the difficulty you may have in placing your tongue in the proper position for

/ɔ/, listen intently to your instructor's pronounciation as he helps you pronounce the target. Note how much he opens his mouth, and use a mirror to aid you with your own pronunciation.

B. PRONOUNCING /ɔ/ IN FAMILIAR WORDS

Pronounce each of the following words carefully. If you are either practicing with your instructor or listening to the exercise on tape, imitate your speech model as accurately as possible.

Beginning		Middle		End
1. all	1. across	16. toss	31. north	1. straw
2. always	2. chalk	17. along	32. morning	2. jaw
3. ought	3. fault	18. belong	33. torn	3. paw
4. autumn	4. cost	19. strong	34. orange	4. saw
5. off	5. crawl	20. song	35. forest	5. draw
6. awful	6. call	21. wrong	36. horror	6. law
7. already	7. lawn	22. long	37. four	7. raw
8. August	8. laundry	23. frog	38. floor	
9. author	9. thought	24. log	39. door	
10. also	10. halt	25. dog	40. board	
	11. caught	26. corn	41. more	
	12. crossing	27. horse	42. sport	
	13. taught	28. order	43. port	
	14. frost	29. cord	44. store	
	15. talk	30. pork	45. score	

C. PRONOUNCING WORD PAIRS CONTAINING /ɔ/ AND A REPLACEMENT

Select some of the words from the paired lists in Section 38-2B containing /ɔ/ and your replacement. Read one pair of words at a time, pronouncing the word with the target first (e.g., **ought–oat**). Make sure that you are saying /ɔ/ first and /oʊ/ second. Reverse the procedure, and pronounce the replacement word first and the target word second, making certain that you say /oʊ/ first and /ɔ/ second. Try to develop speed and accuracy as you do the drill. If you are either practicing with your instructor or listening to the exercise on tape, imitate your speech model as accurately as possible. If you are listening to the taped exercise, listen *only* to the drill that compares the target with your particular replacement. You will find this drill more difficult than the word list in Section 38-4B because of the closeness of target and replacement.

D. PRONOUNCING /ɔ/ IN PHRASES

Pronounce each of the phrases carefully. If you mispronounce a word, say it over again several times, and then repeat the entire phrase. If you are either practicing with your instructor or listening to the drill on tape, imitate your speech model as accurately as possible.

1. **orange** juice through a **straw**
2. **order** some **pork** and **corn**
3. a **dog's soft paw**
4. **bought** a **long tablecloth**

5. **saw** the **horse** in **August**
6. **walk** with a **small daughter**
7. **talk** with the **author**
8. **call often** for **salt**

E.   PRONOUNCING SHORT PHRASES CONTAINING /ɔ/ AND /ou/

This drill is similar to the exercise in Section 38-4C, except that your /ou/ replacement precedes the target in each phrase. Pronounce each of the phrases carefully. If you are either practicing with your instructor or listening to the exercise on tape, imitate your speech model as accurately as possible. Although these phrases are shorter than those in the preceding drill, you may find this exercise more difficult, because your replacement directly precedes /ɔ/ in each phrase.

/ou/ – /ɔ/

1. to show all
2. to go off
3. to blow always

4. to know autumn
5. a slow author
6. to grow already

F.   PRONOUNCING /ɔ/ IN SENTENCES

Pronounce each of the sentences carefully. If you use a replacement, say the word over again several times, and then repeat the entire sentence. If you are either practicing with your instructor or listening to the exercise on tape, imitate your speech model as accurately as possible.

1. The **officer offered** to help **Walter walk across** the **broad** street.
2. **Paul** told the **naughty** boy not to **toss** the **ball** into the **crosswalk**.
3. He **also tore** his **cloth** gloves while playing on the **long seesaw**.
4. The early **morning frost** that **fall caused all** the **lawns** to turn brown.
5. He **taught** him to fix the **four awful**-looking **faucets** in his **laundry** room.

G.   PRONOUNCING /ɔ/ IN BEGINNING CONVERSATION

This exercise gives you an opportunity to begin using some of your previously learned /ɔ/ words in beginning conversation. Complete instructions for this type of drill are given in Chap. 5, 5-4H. Read the instructions, and adapt them to practice with /ɔ/.

1. "My _____ is in the **hall** near the **wall**."
2. "Does he **always talk** about _____ ?"
3. "I want some _____ colored **chalk**."
4. "**Draw** me a picture of a _____ ."
5. "My favorite **song** is _____ ."
6. "I **almost bought** some _____ today."
7. "I **thought** I'd play with a _____ **ball**."
8. "Can you **call** about the cost of the _____ ?"
9. "Does the _____ **belong** to her?"
10. "I'm driving **north** today to _____ ."
11. "I want to **order** some _____ ."
12. "My favorite **sport** is _____ ."
13. "The **score** in the **baseball** game was _____ ."
14. "My new _____ is the **wrong** size."

38–5. CONVERSATION PRACTICE

So far you have learned how to pronounce your target by reading various kinds of exercises which contain /ɔ/ words. Now you are ready to move into the final and most important part of your training program—learning to pronounce /ɔ/ automatically while you are talking more or less spontaneously. If this is the first practice chapter assigned to you by your instructor, you may wish to review the introductory comments on conversation practice in Chap. 2, 2-6 to 2-7.

A. CARRYING /ɔ/ INTO SPONTANEOUS DAILY CONVERSATION

This exercise requires you to use /ɔ/ in daily conversation, starting with key words and expanding to all the /ɔ/ words in your particular vocabulary. Complete instructions for this type of drill are given in Chap. 5, 5-5A, and there are supplementary comments about the exercise in Chap. 2, 2-7A.

B. GENERAL CLASSROOM EXERCISES IN SPEAKING

Your instructor will plan a series of classroom conversation activities, and each assignment will be discussed fully in class before you carry it out. When your instructor announces the first speaking activity, you may wish to review the introductory comments in classroom speaking in Chap. 2, 2-7B.

chapter thirty-nine

The Vowel Target
/ɑ/ (father)¹

COMMON SPELLINGS FOR /ɑ/

The most frequent spellings are found in the words **father** and **hot**; less frequent spellings include **sergeant, heart,** and **guard.**

39–1. EAR TRAINING FOR THE /ɑ/ TARGET

A.   A FEW REMINDERS ABOUT EAR TRAINING

The following test exercises will help you learn to recognize your /ɑ/ target. If this is the first practice chapter assigned to you by your instructor, you may wish to review the discussion about listening practice in Chap. 2, 2-2B to 2-3C.

¹The target /ɑ/ tends to vary acceptably with the vowel /ɔ/ as in call in certain special word types. These variations are discussed in footnote 1 of Chapter 38. Look at them before starting this unit.

B.   Recognizing /ɑ/ in Words

You will hear a list of words containing /ɑ/. After listening to each word, write *B* if you heard /ɑ/ at the beginning of the word and *M* if you heard /ɑ/ in the middle of the word. The answers will be read to you at the end of the drill. This exercise is found in Appendix 1. If you have difficulty recognizing the target, you may find it worthwhile to review the test with somebody outside of class.

C.   Recognizing /ɑ/ in Sentences

You will listen to a series of sentences containing a number of /ɑ/ words. Each sentence will be read several times. Try to locate the /ɑ/ words in each test sentence and write them down. The /ɑ/ words in each test sentence will be read to you at the end of the drill. The sentences appear later in the chapter in Section 39-4F. If you have difficulty recognizing the target, you may find it worthwhile to review the test with somebody outside class.

39–2.   DISCRIMINATING BETWEEN /ɑ/ AND THE /ɔ/ REPLACEMENT

A.   Probable Types of Replacement

The following exercises will help you learn to compare /ɑ/ with your probable replacement of /ɔ/ as in call. This replacement typically occurs in two different situations.

1. You substitute /ɔ/ in words in which the stressed or emphasized syllables are spelled either with final **ar** or **ar** plus another consonant. Examples include **car, yard,** and **part.** If you happen to live in an "r-less" area of the United States and normally eliminate the consonant /r/ in certain instances, you are likely to employ the same substitution but will omit the /r/.[2]

2. You substitute /ɔ/ in the so-called "short o" words (marked diacritically with **ŏ** in many dictionaries). The vowel /ɑ/ is the typical pronunciation for the majority of American English speakers in "short o" words, particularly when "short o" precedes the following sounds: /p/ as in **top,** /b/ as in **job** /t/ as in **not,** /d/ as in **God,** /k/ as in rock, and /l/ between vowels as in **policy.** You are likely to substitute /ɔ/ for /ɑ/ in these words. Note that in certain "short o" words such as doll, golf, **on,** and gone /ɔ/ as well as /ɑ/ is heard frequently.

---

[2]A discussion of an "r"-less dialect is found in footnote 1 of Chapter 17.

If you are not employing the common /ɔ/ for /ɑ/ replacement, your instructor will tell you exactly how you are mispronouncing /ɑ/ and provide you with some discrimination drills.

B. PAIRED LISTS OF WORDS

The words in the following paired list are identical, except that the words in Column 1 contain the target, and the words in Column 2 contain the /ɔ/ replacement. Complete instructions for this type of exercise are given in Chap. 5, 5-2B.

Column 1 /ɑ/	Column 2 /ɔ/
cot	caught
pond	pawned
knotty	naughty
park	pork
part	port
scar	score
tar	tore
barn	born
cart	court
far	for
garden	Gordon
farmer	former

C. PAIRED SENTENCES

The following paired sentences are identical, except that the final word in the first sentence contains /ɑ/, and the final word in the second sentence contains the /ɔ/ replacement. Complete instructions for this type of exercise are given in Chap. 5, 5-2C.

/ɑ/ – /ɔ/

1. I see the park.
   I see the pork.
2. Do you have a scar?
   Do you have a score?
3. I see the star.
   I see the store.
4. Is it a cart?
   Is it a court?
5. He said it was knotty.
   He said it was naughty.

D. LISTENING FOR REPLACEMENTS IN FAMILIAR /ɑ/ WORDS

You will hear a list of words containing /ɑ/. Sometimes the words will be pronounced correctly with /ɑ/; other times the words will be said incorrectly with your replacement. Complete instructions for this type of drill are found in Chap. 5, 5-2D.

39–3. A FEW REMINDERS ABOUT ORAL PRACTICE PROCEDURES

If this is the first practice chapter assigned to you by your instructor, you may wish to review the comments about beginning oral practice in Chap. 2, 2-4. Before you actually begin practicing each individual pronunciation drill, you may also desire to review the supplementary explanations about the exercise in Chap. 2, 2-5.

39-4. THE PRONUNCIATION OF /ɑ/

A. PRONOUNCING ISOLATED /ɑ/

In the event that you cannot pronounce /ɑ/ through imitation alone, your instructor will help you with the following suggestions about placement. Should placement be required, you should review the explanatory comments about back vowels in Chap. 4, 4-4F, and the description of /ɑ/ in Figure 3 of Chapter 4.

1. The Position of the Lips

The target /ɑ/ is considered unround. Note that your lips are somewhat rounded and closer together for /ɔ/. Watch your instructor pronounce /ɑ/ and your replacement several times, and observe the differences between them.

2. The Position of the Tongue and Muscular Tension

Place your tongue tip near the floor of your mouth, under the bottoms of your lower, middle front teeth. You may or may not touch this gum area with your tongue tip. Your jaws are farther apart for /ɑ/ than for /ɔ/; in fact, your tongue is lower in your mouth for /ɑ/ than it is for any other sound, and your mouth is open wider for /ɑ/ than for any other sound. Your tongue is almost flat in your mouth with the back only slightly arched. If you place your tongue too high—and close your mouth too much—you will pronounce the higher-positioned /ɔ/. The target is pronounced with little muscular tension. Keep your tongue relaxed when you pronounce /ɑ/.

3. Pronouncing the Target

Try pronouncing /ɑ/, keeping in mind the suggestions given above. Because your mouth is open so wide for the target, you should have little difficulty in placing your tongue in the proper position. Listen intently to your instructor's pronunciation as he helps you pronounce /ɑ/. Observe how much he opens his mouth, and use a mirror to aid you with your own pronunciation.

B. Pronouncing /ɑ/ in Familiar Words

Pronounce each of the following words carefully. If you are either practicing with your instructor or listening to the exercise on tape, imitate your speech model as accurately as possible.

Beginning

1. arch
2. article
3. arm
4. arbor
5. argue
6. armor
7. Arthur
8. artist
9. art
10. army

Middle

1. large	15. bark	29. not	43. rocket
2. marble	16. barn	30. dot	44. doctor
3. march	17. car	31. lot	45. knock
4. market	18. cart	32. plot	46. Bob
5. mark	19. charge	33. follow	47. sob
6. park	20. dark	34. college	48. mob
7. part	21. far	35. dollar	49. rotten
8. party	22. farm	36. God	50. bottle
9. scar	23. farther	37. nod	51. cotton
10. smart	24. hard	38. block	52. copper
11. spark	25. jar	39. lock	53. top
12. star	26. harm	40. dock	54. crops
13. start	27. hot	41. rock	
14. apart	28. pot	42. pocket	

C. Pronouncing Word Pairs Containing /ɑ/ and the /ɔ/ Replacement

Select some of the words from the paired list in Section 39-2B containing /ɑ/ and your /ɔ/ replacement. Read one pair of words at a time, pronouncing the word with the target first (e.g., **cot–caught**). Make sure that you are saying /ɑ/ first and /ɔ/ second. Reverse the procedure, and pronounce the replacement word first and the target word second, making certain that you say /ɔ/ first and /ɑ/ second. Try to develop speed and accuracy as you do the drill. If you are either practicing with your instructor or listening to the exercise on tape, imitate your speech model as accurately as possible. You will find this drill more difficult than the word list in Section 39-4B because of the closeness of target and replacement.

D. Pronouncing /ɑ/ in Phrases

Pronounce each of the phrases carefully. If you mispronounce a word, say it over again several times, and then repeat the entire phrase. If you are either practicing with your instructor or listening to the drill on tape, imitate your speech model as accurately as possible.

1. a **large market**
2. a **harmless mob**
3. the **sparkling stars**
4. **dark tar** on the **arch**
5. a **marching army** is **starting**
6. too **far apart** on the **dock**
7. **not charge** a **dollar**
8. a **cotton pocket** for the **doctor**
9. **follow Bob** to **college**
10. too **hot** for the **farm crops**

E.   PRONOUNCING SHORT PHRASES CONTAINING /ɑ/ AND /ɔ/

This drill is similar to the exercise in Section 39-4C, except that your /ɔ/ replacement precedes the target in each phrase. Pronounce each of the phrases carefully. If you are either practicing with your instructor or listening to the exercise on tape, imitate your speech model as accurately as possible. Although these phrases are shorter than those in the preceding drill, you may find this exercise more difficult, because your replacement directly precedes /ɑ/ in each phrase.

/ɔ/ – /ɑ/

1. a straw arm	4. to draw arches	6. a law article
2. saw art there	5. a raw army	7. make a straw artist
3. a law argument		

F.   PRONOUNCING /ɑ/ IN SENTENCES

Pronounce each of the sentences carefully. If you use a replacement, say the word over again several times, and then repeat the entire sentence. If you are either practicing with your instructor or listening to the exercise on tape, imitate your speech model as accurately as possible.

1.   He bought a **marble** statue at the **party** in the **park**.
2.   He found a **large cart** filled with **rocks** in the **yard**.
3.   **Arthur parked** his **car** near the **garden**.
4.   The **carpenter charged** ten **dollars** to fix the **barn**.
5.   It wasn't **hard** to find the empty **lot** on his **block**.

G.   PRONOUNCING /ɑ/ IN BEGINNING CONVERSATION

This exercise gives you an opportunity to begin using some of your previously learned /ɑ/ words in beginning conversation. Complete instructions for this type of drill are given in Chap. 5, 5-4H. Read the instructions, and adapt them to practice with /ɑ/.

1.   "Get me some _____ at the **market**."
2.   "My new _____ is too **large**."
3.   "The dog was **barking** at the _____ ·."
4.   "Buy me a **large jar** of _____."
5.   "I bought my **car** in _____."
6.   "I need _____ **yards** of **yarn** for **art** class."
7.   "My favorite **card** game is _____."

  8. "How **far** is it to _____?"
  9. "I read the **article** in the _____."
  10. "When can you **start** fixing the _____?"
  11. "My new **lock** cost _____."
  12. "The **rocket** flew to the moon in _____."
  13. "A good **rock** group is _____."
  14. "The _____ I bought were **rotten**."
  15. "Where is the **bottle** of _____ soda?"

39–5. CONVERSATION PRACTICE

So far you have learned how to pronounce your target by reading various kinds of exercises which contain /ɑ/ words. Now you are ready to move into the final and most important part of your training program—learning to pronounce /ɑ/ automatically while you are talking more or less spontaneously. If this is the first practice chapter assigned to you by your instructor, you may wish to review the introductory comments on conversation practice in Chap. 2, 2-6 to 2-7.

A. CARRYING /ɑ/ INTO SPONTANEOUS DAILY CONVERSATION

This exercise requires you to use /ɑ/ in daily conversation, starting with key words and expanding to all the /ɑ/ words in your particular vocabulary. Complete instructions for this type of drill are given in Chap. 5, 5-5A, and there are supplementary comments about the exercise in Chap. 2, 2-7A.

B. GENERAL CLASSROOM EXERCISES IN SPEAKING

Your instructor will plan a series of classroom conversation activities, and each assignment will be discussed fully in class before you carry it out. When your instructor announces the first speaking activity, you may wish to review the introductory comments on classroom speaking in Chap. 2, 2-7B.

chapter forty

The Vowel Target
/ʌ/ (rub)

COMMON SPELLINGS FOR /ʌ/

The most frequent spellings are found in the words sh**u**t and d**o**ve; less frequent spellings include c**ou**ntry, fl**oo**d, and d**oes**.

40–1. EAR TRAINING FOR THE /ʌ/ TARGET

A. A FEW REMINDERS ABOUT EAR TRAINING

The following test exercises will help you learn to recognize your /ʌ/ target. If this is the first practice chapter assigned to you by your instructor, you may wish to review the discussion about listening practice in Chap, 2, 2-2B to 2-3C.

B. RECOGNIZING /ʌ/ IN WORDS

You will hear a list of words containing /ʌ/. After listening to each word, write *B* if you heard /ʌ/ at the beginning of the word or *M* if you heard /ʌ/ in the middle of the word. The answers will be read to you at the end of the drill. This

exercise is found in Appendix 1. If you have difficulty recognizing the target, you may find it worthwhile to review the test with somebody outside class.

C. Recognizing /ʌ/ in Sentences

You will listen to a series of sentences containing a number of /ʌ/ words. Each sentence will be read several times. Try to locate the /ʌ/ words in each test sentence, and write them down. The /ʌ/ words in each test sentence will be read to you at the end of the drill. The sentences appear later in the chapter in Section 40-4E. If you have difficulty recognizing the target, you may find it worthwhile to review the test with somebody outside class.

40–2. DISCRIMINATING BETWEEN /ʌ/ AND THE VARIOUS REPLACEMENTS

A. Probable Types of Replacement

The following exercises will help you learn to compare /ʌ/ with your replacement. You are probably substituting one of the following common replacements for /ʌ/: (1) /ɑ/ as in father, (2) /ɛ/ as in bed, (3) /ɪ/ as in bid, or (4) /ɝ/ as in bird. Your instructor will tell you which replacement you are using. If you are not employing one of the more common replacements, your teacher will tell you exactly how you are mispronouncing /ʌ/ and provide you with some discrimination drills.

B. Paired Lists of Words

The words in the following paired lists are identical, except that the words in Column 1 contain the target, and the words in Column 2 contain one of the replacements. Complete instructions for this type of exercise are given in Chap. 5, 5-2B.

1. Column 1 /ʌ/	Column 2 /ɑ/	2. Column 1 /ʌ/	Column 2 /ɛ/
color	collar	duck	deck
stuck	stock	nut	neck
duck	dock	done	den
puppy	poppy	butter	better
hug	hog	puppy	peppy
nut	knot	bus	Bess
hut	hot	money	many
luck	lock	rust	rest
shut	shot	ton	ten
rub	rob	bud	bed
wonder	wander	bug	beg
come	calm	putt	pet
cup	cop		
cut	cot		
some	psalm		

3.   Column 1 /ʌ/   Column 2 /ɪ/

rub	rib
duck	Dick
butter	bitter
won	win
love	live
rust	wrist
ton	tin
bud	bid
putt	pit
bug	big

4.   Column 1 /ʌ/   Column 2 /ɝ/

cub	curb
ton	turn
bud	bird
shut	shirt
bun	burn
fun	fern

C.   PAIRED SENTENCES

The following paired sentences are identical, except that the final word in the first sentence contains /ʌ/, and the final word in the second sentence contains one of the replacements. Complete instructions for this type of exercise are given in Chap. 5, 5-2C.

/ʌ/ – /ɑ/

1. Do you like the color?
   Do you like the collar?
2. I see the duck.
   I see the dock.
3. Look at the puppy.
   Look at the poppy.
4. It's a hard nut.
   It's a hard knot.
5. I want a cup.
   I want a cop.
6. I have a cut.
   I have a cot.

/ʌ/ – /ɛ/

1. I see the duck.
   I see the deck.
2. I dropped the nut.
   I dropped the net.
3. Do you need money?
   Do you need many?
4. I like the bud.
   I like the bed.
5. I need the rust.
   I need the rest.

/ʌ/ – /ɪ/

1. I think it's butter.
   I think it's bitter.
2. I see the rust.
   I see the wrist.
3. I got the bud.
   I got the bid.
4. It's a good putt.
   It's a good pit.

/ʌ/ – /ɝ/

1. I see the cub.
   I see the curb.
2. It's a ton.
   It's a turn.
3. It looks like a bud.
   It looks like a bird.

D.   LISTENING FOR REPLACEMENTS IN FAMILIAR /ʌ/ WORDS

You will hear a list of words containing /ʌ/. Sometimes the words will be pronounced correctly with /ʌ/; other times the words will be said incorrectly with your replacement. Complete instructions for this type of drill are found in Chap. 5, 5-2D.

40–3. A FEW REMINDERS ABOUT ORAL PRACTICE PROCEDURES

If this is the first practice chapter assigned to you by your instructor, you may wish to review the comments about beginning oral practice in Chap. 2, 2-4. Before you actually begin practicing each individual pronunciation drill, you may also desire to review the supplementary explanations about the exercise in Chap. 2, 2-5.

40–4. THE PRONUNCIATION OF /ʌ/

A. PRONOUNCING ISOLATED /ʌ/

In the event that you cannot pronounce /ʌ/ through imitation alone, your instructor will help you with the following suggestions about placement. Should placement be required, you should review the explanatory comments about central vowels in Chap. 4, 4-4F, and the description of /ʌ/ in Figure 3 of Chap. 4.

1. The Position of the Lips

The lips are unround for /ʌ/, and they are very slightly spread. The lips are unround for the /ɑ/ replacement, but they tend to be much farther apart. The lips are also unround for the /ɪ/, /ɛ/, and /ɝ/ replacements, and the lip positions for these vowels look basically like the lip position for the target.

2. The Position of the Tongue and Muscular Tension

Place your tongue tip near the bottoms of your lower, middle front teeth. You may or may not touch your teeth with your tongue tip. The middle of your tongue is very slightly arched. Note that the tongue is much lower for the /ɑ/ replacement—it is almost flat in your mouth—and your jaws are much farther apart than for /ʌ/. The jaws are approximately in the same position for the target and the /ɛ/ and /ɝ/ replacements, but the jaws tend to be closer together for the /ɪ/ replacement. If you place your tongue too low—and open your mouth too much—you may pronounce the lower-positioned /ɑ/; conversely if you place your tongue too high—and close your mouth too much—you may pronounce the higher-positioned /ɪ/. Observe also that /ɪ/ and /ɛ/ are pronounced with the tongue blade arched in the direction of the front of the hard palate, while the tongue arching for /ɝ/ is virtually identical to the arching for the target. Remember that it is very difficult to place your tongue in the correct position for the target. Although the tongue position for /ɑ/ is easily observed, the tongue positions for the other replacements range from partially visible to not visible at all. More important, the tongue position for /ʌ/ cannot be seen. The target is pronounced with little muscular tension. Keep your tongue relaxed when you pronounce /ʌ/.

3. Pronouncing the Target

Try pronouncing /ʌ/, keeping in mind the suggestions given above. Because of the difficulty you may have in placing your tongue in the proper position for /ʌ/, listen intently to your instructor's pronunciation as he helps you pronounce the target. Use a mirror if it helps you with your own pronunciation.[1]

B. Pronouncing /ʌ/ in Familiar Words

Pronounce each of the following words carefully. If you are either practicing with your instructor or listening to the exercise on tape, imitate your speech model as accurately as possible.

Beginning

1. other
2. under
3. oven
4. onion
5. uncle
6. upper

Middle

1. month
2. nothing
3. couple
4. brother
5. company
6. above
7. among
8. another
9. become
10. discover
11. come
12. shut
13. country
14. once
15. cover
16. trouble
17. wonder
18. cousin
19. touch
20. customer
21. does
22. number
23. none
24. mother
25. done
26. luck
27. double
28. love
29. hunger
30. hug
31. just
32. brush
33. blush
34. hush
35. crush
36. rush
37. mushroom
38. judge
39. ton
40. rust

C. Pronouncing Word Pairs Containing /ʌ/ and a Replacement

Select some of the words from the paired lists in Section 40-2B containing /ʌ/ and your replacement. Read one pair of words at a time, pronouncing the word with the target first (e.g., **color–collar**). Make sure that you are saying /ʌ/ first and /ɑ/ second. Reverse the procedure, and pronounce the replacement word first and the target word second, making certain that you say /ɑ/ first and /ʌ/ second. Try to develop speed and accuracy as you do the drill. If you are either practicing with your instructor or listening to the exercise on tape, imitate your speech model as accurately as possible. If you are listening to the taped exercise, listen *only* to the drill that compares the target with your particular replacement.

[1] For all practical purposes there is little difference between /ʌ/ and /ə/ as in about, when the two vowels are pronounced in isolation. In words /ʌ/ tends to be slightly more tense than /ə/, /ʌ/ is always given strong stress or emphasis while /ə/ is given weak stress, and /ʌ/ is longer in duration. The target /ə/ is discussed in Chapter 41.

You will find this drill more difficult than the word list in Section 40-4B because of the closeness of target and replacement.

D.   Pronouncing /ʌ/ in Phrases

Pronounce each of the phrases carefully. If you mispronounce a word, say it over again several times, and then repeat the entire phrase. If you are either practicing with your instructor or listening to the drill on tape, imitate your speech model as accurately as possible.

1.   **honey** and **butter** for **supper**
2.   **plums** and **onions** for **lunch**
3.   a **puppy running** in the **sun**
4.   **duck** with **mustard** and **mushrooms** for **lunch**
5.   a **bus** and a **truck** in the **tunnel**
6.   **just** too **much money** for a **haircut**
7.   **discovered** with a **rusty brush**

E.   Pronouncing /ʌ/ in Sentences

Pronounce each of the sentences carefully. If you use a replacement, say the word over again several times, and then repeat the entire sentence. If you are either practicing with your instructor or listening to the exercise on tape, imitate your speech model as accurately as possible.

1.   The **buzzing bumblebees suddenly stung** my **uncle** on his **thumb**.
2.   **One** of the **young runners** tried to **jump** over the **mud puddle** and **stumbled**.
3.   They **stuffed** the **funny**-looking **rubber rug** into the **front** of the **trunk**.
4.   She **stubbornly struggled** to **scrub** the floor and **brush up** the **dust** and **crumbs**.
5.   He bought a **dozen** pieces of **bubble gum** at the **drugstore** last **summer**.

F.   Pronouncing /ʌ/ in Beginning Conversation

This exercise gives you an opportunity to begin using some of your previously learned /ʌ/ words in beginning conversation. Complete instructions for this type of drill are given in Chap. 5, 5-4H. Read the instructions, and adapt them to practice with /ʌ/.

1.   "My new _____ is **rusty**."
2.   "When did you **discover** the _____?"
3.   "Please **brush** my _____ so I can wear it."
4.   "Did you **shut** the _____?"

5. "Does **somebody** want a **dozen** _____?"

6. "Be careful not to **touch** the hot _____."

7. "Did you see **another** _____ last **Monday**?"

8. "Will you **study** about _____ this semester?"

9. "What **color** is the _____?"

10. "Please **come** and put the _____ in the **oven**."

11. "I **wonder** if he has **enough money** for the _____."

12. "Did the **other customer** buy the _____?"

13. "Did your **younger brother** hear about the _____?"

40-5. CONVERSATION PRACTICE

So far you have learned how to pronounce your target by reading various kinds of exercises which contain /ʌ/ words. Now you are ready to move into the final and most important part of your training program—learning to pronounce /ʌ/ automatically while you are talking more or less spontaneously. If this is the first practice chapter assigned to you by your instructor, you may wish to review the introductory comments on conversation practice in Chap. 2, 2-6 to 2-7.

A. CARRYING /ʌ/ INTO SPONTANEOUS DAILY CONVERSATION

This exercise requires you to use /ʌ/ in daily conversation, starting with key words and expanding to all the /ʌ/ words in your particular vocabulary. Complete instructions for this type of drill are given in Chap. 5, 5-5A, and there are supplementary comments about the exercise in Chap. 2, 2-7A.

B. GENERAL CLASSROOM EXERCISES IN SPEAKING

Your instructor will plan a series of classroom conversation activities, and each assignment will be discussed fully in class before you carry it out. When your instructor announces the first speaking activity, you may wish to review the introductory comments on classroom speaking in Chap. 2, 2-7B.

chapter forty-one

The Vowel Target
/ə/ (about)[1,2]

COMMON SPELLINGS FOR /ə/

The target /ə/ is always pronounced with weak stress or emphasis. It may be spelled by every letter vowel in English, and by many combinations of letter symbols. Here is a partial list of the more characteristic spellings for /ə/.

1. **a** as in **a**bout
2. **e** as in **e**lephant
3. **i** as in pres**i**dent
4. **o** as in c**o**nsider

5. **u** as in circ**u**s
6. **io** as in nat**io**n
7. **eo** as in pig**eo**n

8. **ou** as in danger**ou**s
9. **iou** as in delic**iou**s
10. **ai** as in cert**ai**n

---

[1]The frequent use of /ə/ in one-syllable words is explained in Chapter 48 as part of the discussion and practice of weak stress.

[2]If you speak Eastern or Southern American English, look at the comments in footnote 1 of Chapter 43 about your regional use of /ə/ for /ɚ/ as in (paper). You may wish to use the materials in Chapter 43 for additional practice.

41–1.   EAR TRAINING FOR THE /ə/ TARGET

A.   A Few Reminders About Ear Training

The following test exercises will help you learn to recognize your /ə/ target. If this is the first practice chapter assigned to you by your instructor, you may wish to review the discussion about listening practice in Chap. 2, 2B to 2-3C.

B.   Recognizing /ə/ in Words

You will hear a list of words containing /ə/. After listening to each word, write *B* if you heard /ə/ at the beginning of the word, *M* if you heard /ə/ in the middle, and *E* if you heard /ə/ at the end of the word. The answers will be read to you at the end of the drill. This exercise is found in Appendix 1. You may find /ə/ particularly difficult to recognize, because it is typically pronounced with a rapid, somewhat indistinct quality. If you have difficulty recognizing the target, you may find it worthwhile to review the test with somebody outside class.

41–2.   DISCRIMINATING BETWEEN /ə/ AND THE VARIOUS REPLACEMENTS

A.   Probable Types of Replacement

The following exercises will help you learn to compare /ə/ with your replacement. The wide variety of spellings for /ə/ may cause you to use various weak-stressed replacements that are suggested by English spelling. More common examples include (1) /ɑ/ as in father in words like typical and agree, (2) /ou/ as in post in words like wagon and reason, and (3) /u/ as in pool in words like circus and campus. A less common possibility is the use of /ɛ/ as in bed in words like greeted, passes, jacket, bravest, and darkness.

The discrimination drills are limited to a few of the more common replacements, because of the variety of potential substitutions. Your instructor will tell you exactly how you are mispronouncing /ə/, and which exercises you are to do. He may also provide you with some additional discrimination exercises in the event that you are employing other replacements.[3]

[3] It should be remembered that in many weak-stressed syllables both /ə/ and /ɪ/ as in bid are acceptable. Examples of this variation in middle and final weak-stressed syllables include the following: telephone, passes, boasted, market, rapid, circus, visit, broken, and gallop. When words like these appear in this chapter, use whatever pronunciation is easiest for you, unless there is a preference for one particular pronunciation in your area. If you have any questions about which pronunciation, if any, is the preferred one in your area, ask your instructor. Note that /ə/ also varies with /ɪ/ and /i/ as in bead in other types of words. This variation is discussed in footnote 1 of Chapter 31.

B.   LISTENING FOR REPLACEMENTS IN
     FAMILIAR WORDS CONTAINING THE LETTER **a**

You will hear a list of words containing /ə/ in the weak-stressed syllable. In each instance the syllable is spelled with the letter **a**. Sometimes the words will be pronounced correctly with /ə/; other times the words will be said incorrectly with the /ɑ/ replacement. Complete instructions for this type of exercise are found in Chap. 5, 5-2D. This exercise is found in Appendix 1.

C.   LISTENING FOR REPLACEMENTS IN
     FAMILIAR WORDS CONTAINING THE LETTER **o**

This exercise is identical to Exercise B, except that the spelling in the weak-stressed syllable is **o**, and the incorrect pronunciation is /oʊ/.

D.   LISTENING FOR REPLACEMENTS IN
     FAMILIAR WORDS CONTAINING THE LETTER **u**

This exercise is identical to Exercise B, except that the spelling in the weak-stressed syllable is **u**, and the incorrect pronunciation is /u/.

41–3.   A FEW REMINDERS ABOUT ORAL PRACTICE PROCEDURES

If this is the first practice chapter assigned to you by your instructor, you may wish to review the comments about beginning oral practice in Chap. 2, 2-4. Before you actually begin practicing each individual pronunciation drill, you may also desire to review the supplementary explanations about the exercise in Chap. 2, 2-5.

41–4.   THE PRONUNCIATION OF /ə/

A.   PRONOUNCING ISOLATED /ə/

In the event that you cannot pronounce /ə/ through imitation alone, your instructor will help you with the following suggestions about placement. Should placement be required, you should review the explanatory comments about central vowels in Chap. 4, 4-4F, and the description of /ə/ in Figure 3 of Chapter 4.

1.   The Position of the Lips

The lips are unround for /ə/, and they are very slightly spread.

2. The Position of the Tongue and Muscular Tension

Place your tongue tip near the bottoms of your lower, middle front teeth. You may or may not touch your teeth with your tongue tip. The middle of your tongue is very slightly arched. It is very difficult to place your tongue in the correct position for the target, because you cannot see what you are doing. The target is pronounced with very little muscular tension, and you should keep your tongue relaxed when you pronounce /ə/.

3. Pronouncing the Target

Try pronouncing /ə/, keeping in mind the suggestions given above. Because of the difficulty you may have in placing your tongue in the proper position for /ə/, listen intently to your instructor's pronunciation as he helps you with the target. Use a mirror if it helps you with your own pronunciation.[4]

B. PRONOUNCING /ə/ IN FAMILIAR WORDS

Pronounce each of the following words carefully. If you are either practicing with your instructor or listening to the exercise on tape, imitate your speech model as accurately as possible.

Beginning		Middle		End
1. agree	1. greeted	13. darkness	25. lesson	1. sofa
2. about	2. invited	14. kindness	26. lemons	2. America
3. around	3. rested	15. toothless	27. campus	3. soda
4. asleep	4. passes	16. national	28. circus	4. idea
5. arrive	5. dishes	17. signal	29. nation	5. Santa
6. announce	6. inches	18. capital	30. famous	6. Sarah
7. away	7. jacket	19. typical	31. delicious	7. Africa
8. ashamed	8. blanket	20. special	32. marvelous	8. papa
9. amount	9. market	21. Christmas	33. dangerous	9. mamma
10. attack	10. bravest	22. breakfast	34. certain	
	11. fastest	23. capitol	35. courteous	
	12. nearest	24. reason		

C. SPECIAL /ə/ WORDS

Many speakers omit an /ə/ syllable in a number of commonly spoken words. Some instructors consider this omission undesirable under all speaking conditions, while others believe that omission of an /ə/ syllable should be limited

---

[4] For all practical purposes there is little difference between /ə/ and /ʌ/ as in **rub** when the two vowels are pronounced in isolation. In words /ə/ tends to be slightly less tense than /ʌ/, /ə/ is always given weak stress while /ʌ/ is always given strong stress, and /ə/ is shorter in duration. The target /ʌ/ is discussed in Chapter 40.

to informal or casual speaking circumstances. I have included a brief list of familiar /ə/ words in which I tend to omit an /ə/ under all speaking conditions. The omitted syllable is in boldface. Your instructor will indicate the preference in your area for the pronunciation of the target in these words.

Middle

1. history
2. sophomore
3. family
4. camera
5. favorable
6. grocery
7. several
8. vegetable

D. PRONOUNCING /ə/ IN SENTENCES

Pronounce each of the sentences carefully. If you use a replacement, say the word over again several times, and then repeat the entire sentence. If you are either practicing with your instructor or listening to the exercise on tape, imitate your speech model as accurately as possible.

1. The **stewardess** brought the **magazines** after a **delicious breakfast**.
2. He **started** his **special celebration** when he **arrived** on **campus**.
3. I'm **delighted** to **celebrate** my birthday by seeing the **marvelous circus**.
4. They **agreed** to buy a **blanket** and a **sofa** at the **special** sale.
5. Her **necklace** was **supposed** to be worth a **million** dollars.

E. PRONOUNCING /ə/ IN BEGINNING CONVERSATION

This exercise gives you an opportunity to begin using some of your previously learned /ə/ words in beginning conversation. Complete instructions for this type of drill are given in Chap. 5, 5-4H. Read the instructions, and adapt them to practice with /ə/.

1. "I'd like a **ticket** for _____."
2. "The town **nearest** my home is _____."
3. "I want a pound of _____ at the **market**."
4. "The **capital** of _____ is _____."
5. "I want _____ for **Christmas**."
6. "I think **Africa** is _____."
7. "The **lesson** for **tomorrow** is _____."
8. "The plane will **arrive about** _____."
9. "Do you **suppose** this is the **biggest** _____?"
10. "I think **America** is _____."

11. "I think _____ tastes **delicious**."
12. "I'm going **away** on _____."
13. "I need **about** _____ dollars."
14. "I think buying a _____ is a good **idea**."
15. "I want a can of _____ **soda**."

41–5.   CONVERSATION PRACTICE

So far you have learned to pronounce your target by reading various kinds of exercises which contain /ə/ words. Now you are ready to move into the final and most important part of your training program—learning to pronounce /ə/ automatically while you are talking more or less spontaneously. If this is the first practice chapter assigned to you by your instructor, you may wish to review the introductory comments on conversation practice in Chap. 2, 2-6 to 2-7.

A.   CARRYING /ə/ INTO SPONTANEOUS DAILY CONVERSATION

This exercise requires you to use /ə/ in daily conversation, starting with key words and expanding to all the /ə/ words in your particular vocabulary. Complete instructions for this type of drill are given in Chap. 5, 5-5A, and there are supplementary comments about the exercise in Chap. 2, 2-7A.

B.   GENERAL CLASSROOM EXERCISES IN SPEAKING

Your instructor will plan a series of classroom conversation activities, and each assignment will be discussed fully in class before you carry it out. When your instructor announces the first speaking activity, you may wish to review the introductory comments on classroom speaking in Chap. 2, 2-7B.

chapter forty-two

The Vowel Target
/ɝ/ (**bird**)¹

COMMON SPELLINGS FOR /ɝ/

The most frequent spellings are found in the words **bir**th, **chur**ch, and **ser**ve; less frequent spellings include h**ear**d, w**or**k, and j**our**ney.

¹Certain regional variations among standard American English dialects need to be mentioned in connection with the improvement of the /ɝ/ target. If you speak General American, you typically employ /ɝ/ in your dialect. If you speak either Eastern or Southern American, you typically use /ɜ/ in your dialect. English spellings are identical for both vowels so that the two sounds employ the same vocabulary. The typical replacements for the target /ɝ/ tend to parallel the typical replacements for /ɜ/. For these reasons, although I have only shown the target /ɝ/ in this chapter, you may easily adapt the comments and practice materials to /ɜ/ if that vowel happens to be your preferred pronunciation. If you have any questions about which vowel is the preferred one in your dialect, ask your instructor. It might be noted at this point that the basic difference between /ɝ/ and /ɜ/ is the degree of so-called "r"-coloring suggested by the vowels. The pronunciation of General American /ɝ/ strongly suggests a prolonged /r/ as in **r**ap. The pronunciation of /ɜ/ basically eliminates the "r"-coloring, although there is a definite similarity between the two sounds. The specific positional differences between /ɝ/ and /ɜ/ are compared in Section 42-4. If you have any questions about the pronunciation of /ɝ/ or /ɜ/ in your dialect, ask your instructor. If you speak Eastern or Southern American, note the discussion of your regional pronunciation of /ə/ as in **a**bout in place of the General American "r"-colored /ɚ/ as in pap**er** in footnote 2 of Chapter 43. Similarly, note your regional pronunciation of the related consonant /r/ in footnote 1 of Chapter 17.

42–1.   EAR TRAINING FOR THE /ɝ/ TARGET

A.   A FEW REMINDERS ABOUT EAR TRAINING

The following test exercises will help you learn to recognize your /ɝ/ target. If this is the first practice chapter assigned to you by your instructor, you may wish to review the discussion about listening practice in Chap. 2, 2-2B to 2-3C.

B.   RECOGNIZING /ɝ/ IN WORDS

You will hear a list of words containing /e/. After listening to each word, write *B* if you heard /ɝ/ at the beginning of the word, *M* if you heard /e/ in the middle, and *E* if you heard /ɝ/ at the end of the word. The answers will be read to you at the end of the drill. This exercise is found in Appendix 1. If you have difficulty recognizing the target, you may find it worthwhile to review the test with somebody outside class.

C.   RECOGNIZING /ɝ/ IN SENTENCES

You will listen to a series of sentences containing a number of /ɝ/ words. Each sentence will be read several times. Try to locate the /ɝ/ words in each test sentence, and write them down. The /ɝ/ words in each test sentence will be read to you at the end of the drill. The sentences appear later in the chapter in Section 42-4E. If you have difficulty recognizing the target, you may find it worthwhile to review the test with somebody outside class.

42–2.   DISCRIMINATING BETWEEN /ɝ/ AND THE VARIOUS REPLACEMENTS

A.   PROBABLE TYPES OF REPLACEMENT

The following exercises will help you learn to compare /ɝ/ with your replacement. Keep in mind that these replacements are also used in place of /ɜ/, with the exception of the first two replacements. You are probably substituting one of the following common replacements for /ɝ/: (1) /ɑr/ with /ɑ/ as in father and /r/ as in rap, (2) /ɔr/ with /ɔ/ as in call and /r/, (3) /ɑ/ or /ɔ/ without /r/, (4) /ʌ/ as in rub, (5) /ɔɪ/ as in boy, or (6) the substandard diphthong /ɜɪ/. Your instructor will tell you which replacement you are using. If you are not employing one of the more common replacements, your teacher will tell you exactly how you are mispronouncing /ɝ/ and provide you with some discrimination drills.

B.   PAIRED LISTS OF WORDS

The words in the following paired lists are identical, except that the words in Column 1 contain the target, and the words in Column 2 contain one of the replacements. Complete instructions for this type of exercise are given in Chap. 5, 5-2B.

1.	Column 1 /ɝ/	Column 2 /ɑr/[2]	2.	Column 1 /ɝ/	Column 2 /ɔr/[3]
	dirt	dart		burn	born
	heard	hard		perch	porch
	hurt	heart		turn	torn
	curve	carve		word	ward
	curl	Carl		firm	form
	burn	barn		shirt	short
	firm	farm		worm	warm

3.	Column 1 /ɝ/	Column 2 /ʌ/	4.	Column 1 /ɝ/	Column 2 /ɔɪ/[4]
	hurt	hut		verse	voice
	bird	bud		Earl	oil
	burn	bun		learn	loin
	turn	ton		early	oily
	shirt	shut		curl	coil
	burst	bust		furl	foil
	curd	cud			
	curt	cut			

C.   PAIRED SENTENCES

The following paired sentences are identical, except that the final word in the first sentence contains /ɝ/, and the final word in the second sentence contains one of the replacements. Complete instructions for this type of drill are given in Chap. 5, 5-2C.

/ɝ/ – /ɑr/[5]

1. I see the dirt.
   I see the dart.
2. Did it curve?
   Did it carve?
3. I have a burn.
   I have a barn.
4. He owns that firm.
   He owns that farm.

/ɝ/ – /ɔr/[6]

1. I see the perch.
   I see the porch.
2. Give him the word.
   Give him the ward.
3. That's a new firm.
   That's a new form.

[2]If your replacement is /ɑ/, your instructor will carry out this drill with you by changing the /ɝ/ – /ɑr/ pairs to /ɝ/ – /ɑ/ pairs.

[3]If your replacement is /ɔ/, your instructor will carry out this drill with you by changing the /ɝ/ – /ɔr/ pairs to /ɝ/ – /ɔ/ pairs.

[4]If your replacement is /ɝɪ/, your instructor will carry out this drill with you by changing the /ɝ/ – /ɔɪ/ pairs to /ɝ/ – /ɝɪ/ pairs.

[5]See footnote 2.

[6]See footnote 3.

/ɝ/ – /ʌ/

1. It's a turn.
   It's a ton.
2. Is it a burn?
   Is it a bun?
3. Did it burst?
   Did it bust?

/ɝ/ – /ɔɪ/[7]

1. I heard the verse.
   I heard the voice.
2. Is it early?
   Is it oily?
3. I see the curl.
   I see the coil.

D.   LISTENING FOR REPLACEMENTS IN FAMILIAR /ɝ/ WORDS

You will hear a list of words containing /ɝ/. Sometimes the words will be pronounced correctly with /ɝ/; other times the words will be said incorrectly with your replacement. Complete instructions for this type of drill are found in Chap. 5, 5-2C.

42–3. A FEW REMINDERS ABOUT ORAL PRACTICE PROCEDURES

If this is the first practice chapter assigned to you by your instructor, you may wish to review the comments about beginning oral practice in Chap. 2, 2-4. Before you actually begin practicing each individual pronunciation drill, you may also desire to review the supplementary explanations about the exercise in Chap. 2, 2-5.

42–4. THE PRONUNCIATION OF /ɝ/

A.   PRONOUNCING ISOLATED /ɝ/

In the event that you cannot pronounce /ɝ/ through imitation alone, your instructor will help you with the following suggestions about placement. Should placement be required, you should review the explanatory comments about central vowels in Chap. 4, 4-4F, and the description of /ɝ/ in Figure 3 of Chapter 4.

1.   The Position of the Lips

The lips are unround for /ɝ/, and they are very slightly spread. The lips are basically the same for the /ʌ/ and /ɝ/ replacements, they are unround and much farther apart for the /ɑ/ replacement, and the lips are round for the /ɔ/ and /ɔɪ/ replacements.

2.   The Position of the Tongue and Muscular Tension

Press the edges of your tongue against the bottoms of your upper back teeth. Now try to curl and raise your tongue tip back toward the area just behind your upper gum ridge. Be careful not to touch your gum ridge with your

[7]See footnote 4.

tongue tip. The middle of your tongue is very slightly arched. If you find that you have difficulty pronouncing /ɝ/ in this position, try an alternative one. Arch the blade of your tongue toward the front of your hard palate, and keep your tongue tip low and pointed toward the bottoms of your lower, middle front teeth. It is hard to place your tongue correctly in either position, because you cannot see what you are doing. Regardless of the position you use, the target is pronounced with a slight tensing of the tongue muscles, and it may help you to tense your tongue slightly as you say the target. Note that the tongue is lower for /ɑ/ and /ɔ/ than for the target, and the jaws are also farther apart for these replacements. The jaws are basically in the same position for /ʌ/ and the target. If you place your tongue too low—and open your mouth too much—you may pronounce the lower-positioned /ɔ/ or /ɑ/. If you glide your tongue upward from /ɔ/, you may pronounce the dipthongal replacement /ɔɪ/. If your replacement is the /ɜɪ/ diphthong, avoid the upward movement of your tongue and develop more "r"-coloring for /ɝ/.[8]

3. Pronouncing the Target

Try pronouncing /ɝ/, keeping in mind the suggestions given above. Because of the difficulty you may have in placing your tongue in the proper position for /ɝ/, listen intently to your instructor's pronunciation as he helps you pronounce the target. Use a mirror if it helps you with your own pronunciation.[9]

B. Pronouncing /ɝ/ in Familiar Words

Pronounce each of the following words carefully. If you are either practicing with your instructor or listening to the exercise on tape, imitate your speech model as accurately as possible.

Beginning		Middle		End
1. early	1. world	14. heard	26. girl	1. purr
2. earth	2. work	15. bird	27. deserve	2. stir
3. earn	3. birth	16. hurt	28. curb	3. blur
4. Earl	4. dirt	17. worse	29. verb	4. fur
5. Earnest	5. burst	18. word	30. curve	
	6. first	19. circus	31. worth	
	7. third	20. learn	32. certainly	
	8. reserve	21. turn	33. birthday	
	9. rehearse	22. serve	34. perfectly	
	10. term	23. turtle	35. Thursday	
	11. reverse	24. burned	36. church	
	12. churn	25. firmly	37. jerking	
	13. shirt			

[8] The main positional differences between /ɝ/ and /ɜ/ are as follows: (1) there is little or no contact between the edges of your tongue and the bottoms of your upper back teeth for /ɜ/, (2) there is no elevation of the front of the tongue—it is relatively low and flat in your mouth

C. Pronouncing Word Pairs Containing /ɜ/ and a Replacement

Select some of the words from the paired lists in Section 42-2B containing /ɜ/ and your replacement. Read one pair of words at a time, pronouncing the word with the target first (e.g., **hurt–hut**). Make sure that you are saying /ɜ/ first and /ʌ/ second. Reverse the procedure, and pronounce the replacement word first and the target word second, making certain that you say /ʌ/ first and /ɜ/ second. Try to develop speed and accuracy as you do the drill. If you are either practicing with your instructor or listening to the exercise on tape, imitate your speech model as accurately as possible. If you are listening to the taped exercise, listen *only* to the drill that compares the target with your particular replacement. You will find this drill more difficult than the word list in Section 42-4B because of the closeness of target and replacement.

D. Pronouncing /ɜ/ in Phrases

Pronounce each of the phrases carefully. If you mispronounce a word, say it over again several times, and then repeat the entire phrase. If you are either practicing with your instructor or listening to the drill on tape, imitate your speech model as accurately as possible.

1. a **shirt** for a **birthday** present
2. a **girl's perfumed skirt**
3. **Shirley's first** hair **curlers**
4. a **circle** of **dirt** on the **earth**
5. the **nurse's purple curtains**
6. **thirty ferns** by the **curve**
7. **certainly deserve** a **third term**
8. caught his **first Perch** with a **worm**

E. Pronouncing /ɜ/ in Sentences

Pronounce each of the sentences carefully. If you use a replacement, say the word over again several times, and then repeat the entire sentence. If you are either practicing with your instructor or listening to the exercise on tape, imitate your speech model as accurately as possible.

---

for /ə/—behind the bottoms of your lower, middle front teeth, and (3) the tongue muscles are less tense for /ə/. This combination, particularly the flattened tip and blade of your tongue, eliminates most of the characteristic "r"-coloring of /ɜ/.

[9] For all practical purposes there is little difference between /ɜ/ and /ə/, when the two vowels are pronounced in isolation. In words /ɜ/ tends to be slightly more tense than /ə/, /ɜ/ is always given strong stress or emphasis while /ə/ is always given weak stress, and /ɜ/ is longer in duration. The target /ə/ is discussed in Chapter 43.

1. They **heard** the **workers** calling in the **burning** field.
2. He was **certain** the **pearl** was **perfect** and was **worth** a lot of money.
3. **Bert** said, "Yes, **sir**! I **earn** my living raising **turkeys** and **turnips**."
4. He **firmly** planned to **return** from **Germany** on the **third Thursday** in July.
5. The **servant served** the **thirsty workmen** after their long **search**.

F. PRONOUNCING /ɝ/ IN BEGINNING CONVERSATION

This exercise gives you an opportunity to begin using some of your previously learned /ɝ/ words in beginning conversation. Complete instructions for this type of drill are given in Chap. 5, 5-4H. Read the instructions, and adapt them to practice with /ɝ/.

1. "I like to eat _____ at the **circus**."
2. "Did you **purchase** the _____ from that **clerk**?"
3. "Let's have some _____ for **dessert**."
4. "Did the _____ get **burned**?"
5. "Was the _____ **dirty**?"
6. "I want a _____ on my next **birthday**."
7. "Did you **learn** about _____ at school?"
8. "I plan to **work** next _____."
9. "My **term** paper in _____ is due next week."
10. "Our next **rehearsal** is _____."
11. "The color of my new **shirt** is _____."
12. "Our cook **burned** the _____ last night."
13. "Please **stir** the _____."

42–5. CONVERSATION PRACTICE

So far you have learned how to pronounce your target by reading various kinds of exercises which contain /ɝ/ words. Now you are ready to move into the final and most important part of your training program—learning to pronounce /ɝ/ automatically while you are talking more or less spontaneously. If this is the first practice chapter assigned to you by your instructor, you may wish to review the introductory comments on conversation practice in Chap. 2, 2-6 to 2-7.

A. CARRYING /ɝ/ INTO SPONTANEOUS DAILY CONVERSATION

This exercise requires you to use /ɝ/ in daily conversation, starting with key words and expanding to all the /ɝ/ words in your particular vocabulary.

Complete instructions for this type of drill are given in Chap. 5, 5-5A, and there are supplementary comments about the exercise in Chap. 2, 2-7A.

B.   GENERAL CLASSROOM EXERCISES IN SPEAKING

Your instructor will plan a series of classroom conversation activities, and each assignment will be discussed fully in class before you carry it out. When your instructor announces the first speaking activity, you may wish to review the introductory comments on classroom speaking in Chap. 2, 2-7B.

chapter forty-three

The Vowel Target
/ɚ/ (paper)[1,2]

COMMON SPELLINGS FOR /ɚ/

The most frequent spellings are found in the words sug**ar**, pap**er**, and col**or**; less frequent spellings include Arth**ur** and pict**ure**.

[1] The frequent use of /ɚ/ in one-syllable words is explained in Chapter 48 as part of the discussion and practice of weak stress.

[2] Certain regional variations among standard American English dialects need to be mentioned in connection with the improvement of the /ɚ/ target. If you speak General American, you typically use the "**r**"-colored /ɚ/ in your dialect, and you will use /ɚ/ in all of the practice words in this chapter. The term "**r**"-coloring is employed because the pronunciation of /ɚ/ strongly suggests a prolonged /r/ as in **r**ap. If you speak either Eastern or Southern American, you typically use /ə/ as in **a**bout in your pronunciation of the practice words in this chapter (e.g., **paper**: /peɪpə/ and **sugar**: /ʃʊgə/). If your standard dialect is either Eastern or Southern, you will not normally study the /ɚ/ target. However, /ə/ is presented as a target in Chapter 41. Your instructor may assign you the practice items containing /ɚ/ in order to give you additional practice with /ə/ if this vowel is one of your study targets. If you have any questions about the pronunciation of /ɚ/ or /ə/ in your dialect, ask your instructor. If you speak Eastern or Southern American, note the discussion of your regional pronunciation of /ɜ/ as in b**ir**d in place of the General American "**r**"-colored /ɝ/ as in b**ir**d in footnote 1 of Chapter 42. Similarly, note your regional pronunciation of the related consonant /r/ in footnote 1 of Chapter 17.

43–1. EAR TRAINING FOR THE /ɚ/ TARGET

A. A FEW REMINDERS ABOUT EAR TRAINING

The following test exercises will help you learn to recognize your /ɚ/ target. If this is the first practice chapter assigned to you by your instructor, you may wish to review the discussion about listening practice in Chap. 2, 2-2B to 2-3C.

B. RECOGNIZING /ɚ/ IN WORDS

You will hear a list of words containing /ɚ/. After listening to each word, write *M* if you heard /ɚ/ in the middle of the word or *E* if you heard /ɚ/ at the end of the word. The answers will be read to you at the end of the drill. This exercise is found in Appendix 1. If you have difficulty recognizing the target, you may find it worthwhile to review the test with somebody outside class.

43–2. DISCRIMINATING BETWEEN /ɚ/ AND THE VARIOUS REPLACEMENTS

A. PROBABLE TYPES OF REPLACEMENT

The following exercises will help you learn to compare /ɚ/ with your replacement. The target may be replaced in several different ways.

1. You may use various weak-stressed vowels that are suggested by the English spelling for /ɚ/. Examples of this type of replacement include (a) /ɑ/ as in father in words like sugar and collar, (b) /ɛ/ as in bed in words like ruler and paper, (c) /ɔ/ as in call or /ou/ as in post in words like favor and color, and (d) /u/ as in pool in words like picture and pasture.
2. You may pronounce the **r** in the spelling with a trill; for example, you pronounce a consonant /r/ as in rap with one or more strokes or taps of the tongue tip against the upper gumridge. You are most likely to use the trill when /ɚ/ comes at the end of a word.
3. You may combine the vowel replacement and the trilled /r/.

The discrimination drills are limited to a few of the more common replacements, because of the variety of potential weak-stressed vowel substitutions. Your instructor will tell you exactly how you are mispronouncing /ɚ/, and which exercises you are to do. He may also provide you with some additional discrimination exercises in the event that you are employing other replacements.

B. LISTENING FOR REPLACEMENTS IN
   FAMILIAR WORDS CONTAINING THE LETTERS **ar**

You will hear a list of words containing /ɚ/ in the weak-stressed syllable. In each instance the syllable is spelled with the letters **ar**. Sometimes the words will be pronounced correctly with /ɚ/; other times the words will be said incorrectly with the /ɑ/ replacement. Complete instructions for this type of exercise are found in Chap. 5, 5-2D. This exercise is found in Appendix 1.

C. LISTENING FOR REPLACEMENTS IN
   FAMILIAR WORDS CONTAINING THE LETTERS **er**

This exercise is identical to Exercise B, except that the spelling in the weak-stressed syllable is **er** and the incorrect pronunciation is /ɛ/.

D. LISTENING FOR REPLACEMENTS IN
   FAMILIAR WORDS CONTAINING THE LETTERS **or**

This exercise is identical to Exercise B, except that the spelling in the weak-stressed syllable is **or**, and the incorrect pronunciation is either /ɔ/ or /ou/.

E. LISTENING FOR REPLACEMENTS IN
   FAMILIAR WORDS CONTAINING THE LETTERS **ure**

This exercise is identical to Exercise B, except that the spelling in the weak-stressed syllable is **ure**, and the incorrect pronunciation is /u/.

F. LISTENING FOR A VOWEL REPLACEMENT FOLLOWED BY A TRILLED /r/

You will hear a list of words containing /ɚ/ in the weak-stressed syllable. Sometimes the words will be pronounced correctly with /ɚ/; other times the words will be said incorrectly with one of the various vowel replacements and a trilled /r/. Complete instructions for this type of exercise are found in Chap. 5, 5-2D. This exercise is found in Appendix 1.

43–3. A FEW REMINDERS ABOUT
    ORAL PRACTICE PROCEDURES

If this is the first practice chapter assigned to you by your instructor, you may wish to review the comments about beginning oral practice in Chap. 2, 2-4. Before you actually begin practicing each individual pronunciation drill, you may also desire to review the supplementary explanations about the exercise in Chap. 2, 2-5.

43–4.   THE PRONUNCIATION OF /ɚ/

A.   PRONOUNCING ISOLATED /ɚ/

In the event that you cannot pronounce /ɚ/ through imitation alone, your instructor will help you with the following suggestions about placement. Should placement be required, you should review the explanatory comments about central vowels in Chap. 4, 4-4F, and the description of /ɚ/ in Figure 3 of Chapter 4.

1.   The Position of the Lips

The lips are unround for /ɚ/, and they are very slightly spread.

2.   The Position of the Tongue and Muscular Tension

Press the edges of your tongue against the bottoms of your upper back teeth. Now try to curl and raise your tongue tip back toward the area just behind your upper gum ridge. Be careful not to touch your gum ridge with your tongue tip. If you do this, you are liable to produce a trilled /r/. The middle of your tongue is very slightly arched. If you find that you have difficulty pronouncing /ɚ/ in this position, try an alternative one. Arch the blade of your tongue toward the front of your hard palate, and keep your tongue tip low and pointed toward the bottoms of your lower, middle front teeth. It is hard to place your tongue correctly in either position, because you cannot see what you are doing. Regardless of the position you use, the target is pronunced with very little muscular tension. Keep your tongue relaxed when you pronounce /ɚ/.

3.   Pronouncing the Target

Try pronouncing /ɚ/, keeping in mind the suggestions given above. Because of the difficulty you may have in placing your tongue in the proper position for /ɚ/, listen intently to your instructor's pronunciation as he helps you pronounce the target. Use a mirror if it helps you with your own pronunciation.[3]

B.   PRONOUNCING /ɚ/ IN FAMILIAR WORDS

Pronounce each of the following words carefully. If you are either practicing with your instructor or listening to the exercise on tape, imitate your speech model as accurately as possible.

---

[3] For all practical purposes there is little difference between /ɚ/ and /ɝ/ when the two vowels are pronounced in isolation. In words /ɚ/ tends to be slightly less tense than /ɝ/, /ɚ/ is always given weak stress or emphasis while /ɝ/ is always given strong stress, and /ɚ/ is shorter in duration. The target /ɝ/ is discussed in Chapter 42.

Middle		End		
1. wonderful	1. collar	11. senator	21. measure	31. weather
2. fisherman	2. sugar	12. favor	22. leisure	32. closer
3. backward	3. dollar	13. labor	23. after	33. clover
4. featherbed	4. color	14. razor	24. bother	34. slower
5. neighborhood	5. elevator	15. pasture	25. better	35. enter
6. flowerpot	6. actor	16. picture	26. over	36. silver
7. butterfly	7. doctor	17. nature	27. winter	
8. understand	8. tailor	18. capture	28. lower	
9. evergreen	9. equator	19. adventure	29. baker	
10. gingerbread	10. editor	20. pleasure	30. clever	

C. PRONOUNCING /ɚ/ IN PHRASES

Pronounce each of the phrases carefully. If you mispronounce a word, say it over again several times, and then repeat the entire phrase. If you are either practicing with your instructor or listening to the drill on tape, imitate your speech model as accurately as possible.

1. a **picture** of the **mayor** on the **mirror**
2. a **bigger motor** for the **better messenger**
3. **deliver** the **paper** to the **doctor** by the **river**
4. **water** in the **editor's flowerpot** at **Easter**
5. **cracker** crumbs on the **senator's collar**

D. PRONOUNCING /ɚ/ IN SENTENCES

Pronounce each of the sentences carefully. If you use a replacement, say the word over again several times, and then repeat the entire sentence. If you are either practicing with your instructor or listening to the exercise on tape, imitate your speech model as accurately as possible.

1. The **clever peddler** was **leisurely** collecting old **silver** and **pictures**.
2. **Peter** was sitting in the **rocker** eating **crackers** and **butter**.
3. The **bigger tiger** was **considered** a **clever fighter**.
4. It was a **pleasure** to eat her **wonderful sugar** and **gingerbread** cookies.
5. He plans to **deliver** the **doctor's** new **mirror after dinner**.

E. PRONOUNCING /ɚ/ IN BEGINNING CONVERSATION

This exercise gives you an opportunity to begin using some of your previously learned /ɚ/ words in beginning conversation. Complete instructions for this type of drill are given in Chap. 5, 5-4H. Read the instructions, and adapt them to practice with /ɚ/.

1. "Please **deliver** the _____."

2. "I like **sugar** with _____."

3. "Did you **remember** to bring the _____?"

4. "It's **colder** in _____ than in Hawaii."

5. "I'm going to _____ **after** the **winter** is **over**."

6. "Move the _____ **closer** to me."

7. "The **color** of my new **typewriter** is _____."

8. "That's a **wonderful picture** of _____."

9. "I need a **dollar** to buy some _____."

10. "The **tailor** fixed my new _____."

11. "Please **measure** the _____."

43–5. CONVERSATION PRACTICE

So far you have learned to pronounce your target by reading various kinds of exercises which contain /ɚ/ words. Now you are ready to move into the final and most important part of your training program—learning to pronounce /ɚ/ automatically while you are talking more or less spontaneously. If this is the first practice chapter assigned to you by your instructor, you may wish to review the introductory comments on conversation practice in Chap. 2, 2-6 to 2-7.

A. CARRYING /ɚ/ INTO SPONTANEOUS DAILY CONVERSATION

This exercise requires you to use /ɚ/ in daily conversation, starting with key words and expanding to all the /ɚ/ words in your particular vocabulary. Complete instructions for this type of drill are given in Chap. 5, 5-5A, and there are supplementary comments about the exercise in Chap. 2, 2-7A.

B. GENERAL CLASSROOM EXERCISES IN SPEAKING

Your instructor will plan a series of classroom conversation activities, and each assignment will be discussed fully in class before you carry it out. When your instructor announces the first speaking activity, you may wish to review the introductory comments on classroom speaking in Chap. 2, 2-7B.

chapter forty-four

The Diphthong Target
/aɪ/ (ride)

COMMON SPELLINGS FOR /aɪ/

The most frequent spelling is found in the word ride; less frequent spellings include **lie**, **height**, **fly**, **guide**, and **dye**.

44–1. EAR TRAINING FOR THE /aɪ/ TARGET.

A. A FEW REMINDERS ABOUT EAR TRAINING

The following test exercises will help you learn to recognize your /aɪ/ target. If this is the first practice chapter assigned to you by your instructor, you may wish to review the discussion about listening practice in Chap. 2, 2-2B to 2-3C.

B. RECOGNIZING /aɪ/ IN WORDS

You will hear a list of words containing /aɪ/. After listening to each word, write *B* if you heard /aɪ/ at the beginning of the word, *M* if you heard /aɪ/ in the middle, and *E* if you heard /aɪ/ at the end of the word. The answers will be read to you at the end of the drill. This exercise is found in Appendix 1. If you have difficulty recognizing the target, you may find it worthwhile to review the test with somebody outside class.

C. RECOGNIZING /aɪ/ IN SENTENCES

You will listen to a series of sentences containing a number of /aɪ/ words. Each sentence will be read several times. Try to locate the /aɪ/ words in each test sentence, and write them down. The /aɪ/ words in each test sentence will be read to you at the end of the drill. The sentences appear later in the chapter in Section 44-4D. If you have difficulty recognizing the target, you may find it worthwhile to review the test with somebody outside class.

44–2. DISCRIMINATING BETWEEN /aɪ/ AND THE VARIOUS REPLACEMENTS

A. PROBABLE TYPES OF REPLACEMENT

The following exercises will help you learn to compare /aɪ/ with your replacement. The most common substitution for /aɪ/ is /a/, although there is some tendency to also use /ɑ/ as in father.[1] Your instructor will tell you which replacement you are using. If you are not employing one of the more common replacements, your teacher will tell you exactly how you are mispronouncing /aɪ/ and provide you with some discrimination drills.

B. PAIRED LISTS OF WORDS

The words in the following paired list are identical, except that the words in Column 1 contain the target, and the words in Column 2 contain the /ɑ/ replacement. Complete instructions for this type of exercise are given in Chap. 5, 5-2B.[2]

Column 1 /aɪ/	Column 2 /ɑ/	Column 1 /aɪ/	Column 2 /ɑ/
height	hot	like	lock
night	not	kite	cot
right	rot	type	top
guide	God	light	lot
hike	hock	dike	dock

[1]The vowel /a/ is the lowest front vowel in American English, and /a/ is typically *not* heard in General American speech as a single vowel. It is heard, however, as a single vowel in certain words in parts of Eastern New England and New York City. These words are described in footnote 1 of Chapter 34. The vowel /a/ does appear in General American as part of the diphthongs /aɪ/ and /aʊ/ as in out. The vowel /ɑ/ is the frequently heard low, back General American vowel.

[2]If your replacement is /a/, your instructor will carry out this drill with you by changing the /aɪ/ – /ɑ/ pairs to /aɪ/ – /a/ pairs.

C. Paired Sentences

The following paired sentences are identical, except that the key word in the first sentence contains /aɪ/, and the key word in the second sentence contains the /ɑ/ replacement. Complete instructions for this type of exercise are given in Chap. 5, 5-2C.

/aɪ/ – /ɑ/[3]

1. He repaired the dike.
   He repaired the dock.
2. I need a light.
   I need a lot.
3. The kite is too small.
   The cot is too small.

4. The night is dark.
   The knot is dark.
5. It's night now.
   It's not now.

D. Listening for Replacements in Familiar /aɪ/ Words

You will hear a list of words containing /aɪ/. Sometimes the words will be pronounced correctly with /aɪ/; other times the words will be said incorrectly with your replacement. Complete instructions for this type of drill are found in Chap. 5, 5-2D.

44–3. A FEW REMINDERS ABOUT
ORAL PRACTICE PROCEDURES

If this is the first practice chapter assigned to you by your instructor, you may wish to review the comments about beginning oral practice in Chap. 2, 2-4. Before you actually begin practicing each individual pronunciation drill, you may also desire to review the supplementary explanations about the exercise in Chap. 2, 2-5.

44–4. THE PRONUNCIATION OF /aɪ/

A. Pronouncing Isolated /aɪ/

In the event that you cannot pronounce /aɪ/ through imitation alone, your instructor will help you with the following suggestions about placement. Should placement be required, you should review the explanatory comments about front vowels in Chap. 4, 4-4F, the comments about diphthongs in Chap. 4, 4-4G, and the description of /aɪ/ in Figure 4 of Chapter 4.

[3]See footnote 2.

1.   The Position of the Lips

The target /aɪ/ is considered unround, and your lips are spread considerably into an unrounded position for the first vowel in the diphthong. As the articulators glide from /a/ up to /ɪ/ as in bid, your lips close steadily and become narrowed and slit-like.

2.   Tongue Position, Length, and Muscular Tension

Place your tongue tip so that it touches the bottoms of your lower, middle front teeth. The tongue is almost flat in your mouth with a very slight arching of the tongue blade. The position for the /ɑ/ replacement differs slightly in two respects: the tongue is slightly lower in the mouth, and the back of the tongue is slightly arched instead of the blade.

The most important thing to remember about the arched tongue position for the target is its movement. The tongue moves from the very low, slightly arched tongue position for /a/ up to the much higher and steeply arched tongue position for /ɪ/, traveling with a smooth continuous gliding movement. This causes your mouth to close considerably, because your lower jaw is simultaneously rising with your tongue. Watch your instructor pronounce /aɪ/ for you several times, and observe the closing movements of his lips and lower jaw. Because of the lip, tongue, and jaw movements associated with the pronunciation of /aɪ/, the target is heard as a long sound: you will pronounce the target more accurately if you prolong it. The length is especially important if your replacement is /a/, because you eliminate the diphthongal gliding movements up to /ɪ/ when you produce the single vowel. Note that some speakers produce a diphthongal replacement /ɑɪ/, by starting from the slightly lower /ɑ/ position and gliding up to /ɪ/. The target is pronounced with little muscular tension, and you should keep your tongue relaxed when you pronounce /aɪ/.

3.   Pronouncing the Target

Try pronouncing /aɪ/, keeping in mind the suggestions given above. Because your mouth is open so wide for the first sound in the target, you should have little difficulty in placing your tongue in the proper position for /a/. Listen intently to your instructor's pronunciation as he helps you pronounce the target. Try to feel the movements of your tongue, lips, and lower jaw as you glide from /a/ up to /ɪ/. Use a mirror to observe your lip, jaw, and tongue movements.

B.   PRONOUNCING /aɪ/ IN FAMILIAR WORDS

Pronounce each of the following words carefully. If you are either practicing with your instructor or listening to the exercise on tape, imitate your speech model as accurately as possible.

Beginning	Middle			End
1. eye	1. mice	11. climb	21. mind	1. sky
2. ice	2. night	12. fine	22. pipe	2. why
3. I'll	3. nine	13. fire	23. polite	3. buy
4. I've	4. write	14. tire	24. sight	4. dry
5. I'm	5. time	15. wire	25. stripe	5. rye
6. island	6. white	16. five	26. advice	6. fly
	7. beside	17. alive	27. cried	7. reply
	8. bicycle	18. alike	28. pile	8. die
	9. bite	19. fight	29. desire	9. high
	10. bright	20. life	30. tired	10. tie

C. Pronouncing /aɪ/ in Phrases

Pronounce each of the phrases carefully. If you mispronounce a word, say it over again several times, and then repeat the entire phrase. If you are either practicing with your instructor or listening to the drill on tape, imitate your speech model as accurately as possible.

1. **bright sunshine** through the **fine pines**
2. drinking **iced** coffee **while ironing white** shirts
3. **desire** to **light** a **bright fire** at **night**
4. too **tired** to **decide** about **climbing** the **hillside**
5. the **right time** to **buy** a **pipe**

D. Pronouncing /aɪ/ in Sentences

Pronounce each of the sentences carefully. If you use a replacement, say the word over again several times, and then repeat the entire sentence. If you are either practicing with your instructor or listening to the exercise on tape, imitate your speech model as accurately as possible.

1. **I'll buy** some **ice** cream and **rice** for dinner **tonight**.
2. A **supply** of **ripe pineapples** will **arrive** in **five** to **nine** days.
3. Please **dry** your **eyes** and stop **crying** about **Mike's knife**.
4. A **pile** of **wire** was **lying beside** the **child's bike**.
5. The **bride** was both **delighted** and **excited** about winning the **prize**.

E. Pronouncing /aɪ/ in Beginning Conversation

This exercise gives you an opportunity to begin using some of your previously learned /aɪ/ words in beginning conversation. Complete instructions for this type of drill are given in Chap. 5, 5-4H. Read the instructions, and adapt them to practice with /aɪ/.

1. "I like _____ **pie**."
2. "Please **write** a letter to _____."
3. "Is your new _____ the **right size**?"
4. "Did he **find** the _____?"
5. "**I'm driving** to _____ in **July**."
6. "I live _____ **miles** from here."
7. "Where did you **hide** the _____?"
8. "**Why** did you **lie** about the _____?"
9. "**I've** never **liked fried** _____."
10. "**I applied** for a job at _____."
11. "Does the **highway sign** have a picture of a _____ on it?"
12. "The **flight might arrive** in _____ minutes."
13. "My **tie** has **bright** _____ **stripes** on it."

44–5. CONVERSATION PRACTICE

So far you have learned how to pronounce your target by reading various kinds of exercises which contain /aɪ/ words. Now you are ready to move into the final and most important part of your training program—learning to pronounce /aɪ/ automatically while you are talking more or less spontaneously. If this is the first practice chapter assigned to you by your instructor, you may wish to review the introductory comments on conversation practice in Chap. 2, 2-6, to 2-7.

A. CARRYING /aɪ/ INTO SPONTANEOUS DAILY CONVERSATION

This exercise requires you to use /aɪ/ in daily conversation, starting with key words and expanding to all the /aɪ/ words in your particular vocabulary. Complete instructions for this type of drill are given in Chap. 5, 5-5A, and there are supplementary comments about this exercise in Chap. 2, 2-7A.

B. GENERAL CLASSROOM EXERCISES IN SPEAKING

Your instructor will plan a series of classroom conversation activities, and each assignment will be discussed fully in class before you carry it out. When your instructor announces the first speaking activity, you may wish to review the introductory comments on classroom speaking in Chap. 2, 2-7B.

chapter forty-five

The Diphthong Target
/aʊ/ (**out**)

COMMON SPELLINGS FOR /aʊ/

The most frequent spellings are found in the words **out** and **cow**; a less frequent spelling is found in the word **bough**.

45–1. EAR TRAINING FOR THE /aʊ/ TARGET

A. A FEW REMINDERS ABOUT EAR TRAINING

The following test exercises will help you learn to recognize your /aʊ/ target. If this is the first practice chapter assigned to you by your instructor, you may wish to review the discussion about listening practice in Chap. 2, 2-2B to 2-3C.

B. RECOGNIZING /aʊ/ IN WORDS

You will hear a list of words containing /aʊ/. After listening to each word, write *B* if you heard /aʊ/ at the beginning of the word, *M* if you heard /aʊ/ in the middle, and *E* if you heard /aʊ/ at the end of the word. The answers will be read to you at the end of the drill. This exercise is found in Appendix 1. If you have difficulty recognizing the target, you may find it worthwhile to review the test with somebody outside class.

C.   RECOGNIZING /aʊ/ IN SENTENCES

You will listen to a series of sentences containing a number of /aʊ/ words. Each sentence will be read several times. Try to locate the /aʊ/ words in each test sentence, and write them down. The /aʊ/ words in each test sentence will be read to you at the end of the drill. The sentences appear later in the chapter in Section 45-4D. If you have difficulty recognizing the target, you may find it worthwhile to review the test with somebody outside class.

45–2.   DISCRIMINATING BETWEEN /aʊ/ AND THE /aeʊ/ REPLACEMENT

A.   PROBABLE TYPES OF REPLACEMENT

The following exercises will help you learn to compare /aʊ/ with your probable replacement of the diphthong /aeʊ/.[1] This substitution tends to vary in two additional ways: (1) you may pronounce an overly prolonged and tense /aeʊ/ diphthong, or (2) you may nasalize the tense, prolonged /aeʊ/ replacement. Your instructor will tell you which replacement you are using. If you are not employing one of the more common /aeʊ/ replacements, your teacher will tell you exactly how you are mispronouncing /aʊ/ and provide you with some discrimination drills.

B.   LISTENING FOR REPLACEMENTS IN FAMILIAR /aʊ/ WORDS

You will hear a list of words containing /aʊ/. Sometimes the words will be pronounced correctly with /aʊ/; other times the words will be said incorrectly with your replacement. Complete instructions for this type of drill are found in Chap. 5, 5-2D.

45–3.   A FEW REMINDERS ABOUT ORAL PRACTICE PROCEDURES

If this is the first practice chapter assigned to you by your instructor, you may wish to review the comments about beginning oral practice in Chap. 2, 2-4.

---

[1] This substandard diphthong is composed of the vowel /ae/ as in bad and the vowel /ʊ/ as in pull.

Before you actually begin practicing each individual pronunciation drill, you may also desire to review the supplementary explanations about the exercise in Chap. 2, 2-5.

45–4.   THE PRONUNCIATION OF /aʊ/

A.   PRONOUNCING ISOLATED /aʊ/

In the event that you cannot pronounce /aʊ/ through imitation alone, your instructor will help you with the following suggestions about placement. Should placement be required, you should review the explanatory comments about front vowels in Chap. 4, 4-4F, the comments about diphthongs in Chap. 4, 4-4G, and the description of /aʊ/ in Figure 4 of Chapter 4.

1.   The Position of the Lips

Your lips are spread considerably into an unrounded position for the first vowel in the diphthong. As the articulators glide from /a/ up and back to /ʊ/, your lips close steadily and become well rounded.

2.   Tongue Position, Length, and Muscular Tension

Place your tongue tip so that it touches the bottoms of your lower, middle front teeth. The tongue is almost flat in your mouth with a very slight tensing of the tongue blade. It is important to remember that the tongue position for /a/ is lower than the tongue position for /ae/, and if you place your tongue too high—and close your mouth too much—you will start your pronunciation with /ae/ and most likely end up using the diphthong /aeʊ/.[2]

The most important thing to remember about the arched tongue position for the target is its movement. The tongue moves from the very low, slightly arched tongue position for /a/ up and back to the much higher and steeply arched tongue position for the back vowel /ʊ/. The tongue travels with a smooth continuous gliding movement. This causes your mouth to close considerably, because your lower jaw is simultaneously rising with your tongue. Watch your instructor pronounce /aʊ/ for you several times, and observe the closing movements of his lips and lower jaw. Because of the lip, tongue, and jaw movements associated with the pronunciation of /aʊ/, the target is heard as a long sound: you will pronounce the target more accurately if you prolong it. However, if your replacement is an overly prolonged /aeʊ/, be careful not to produce an overly lengthened /aʊ/. The target is pronounced with little muscular tension, and you should keep your tongue relaxed when you pronounce /aʊ/.

[2]See footnote 1 of Chapter 44 regarding the pronunciation of /a/ as a single vowel in General American speech.

3. Pronouncing the Target

Try pronouncing /aʊ/, keeping in mind the suggestions given above. Because your mouth is open so wide for the first sound in the target, you should have little difficulty in placing your tongue in the proper position for /a/. Listen intently to your instructor's pronunciation as he helps you pronounce the target. Try to feel the movements of your tongue, lips, and lower jaw as you glide from /a/ up and back to /ʊ/. Use a mirror to observe your lip, jaw, and tongue movements.

B. PRONOUNCING /aʊ/ IN FAMILIAR WORDS

Pronounce each of the following words carefully. If you are either practicing with your instructor or listening to the exercise on tape, imitate your speech model as accurately as possible.

Beginning	Middle		End
1. out	1. around	11. growl	1. plow
2. owl	2. brown	12. power	2. allow
3. hour	3. house	13. drown	3. now
4. ouch	4. downtown	14. county	4. how
	5. found	15. couch	5. cow
	6. sour	16. loud	
	7. shower	17. frown	
	8. flower	18. ground	
	9. towel	19. shout	
	10. foul	20. mouth	

C. PRONOUNCING /aʊ/ IN PHRASES

Pronounce each of the phrases carefully. If you mispronounce a word, say it over again several times, and then repeat the entire phrase. If you are either practicing with your instructor or listening to the drill on tape, imitate your speech model as accurately as possible.

1. not a **sound** from the **county crowd**
2. a **pound** of **sour** pickles **around** the **house**
3. **found flour** on the **brown couch**
4. a **loudly howling cow**
5. a **mound** of dirt by the **towel**
6. a **bouncing** ball **outside** the **foul** line

D. PRONOUNCING /aʊ/ IN SENTENCES

Pronounce each of the sentences carefully. If you use a replacement, say the word over again several times, and then repeat the entire sentence. If you are either practicing with your instructor or listening to the exercise on tape, imitate your speech model as accurately as possible.

1. The boy **scout's towel** got wet in the **shower.**
2. He went **trout** fishing **down south.**
3. The **mouse** was squeaking **loudly** under the **house.**
4. The **owl** kept hooting **hour** after **hour.**
5. The **powerful** dog kept **growling loudly** on the **downtown** street.

E. PRONOUNCING /aʊ/ IN BEGINNING CONVERSATION

This exercise gives you an opportunity to begin using some of your previously learned /aʊ/ words in beginning conversation. Complete instructions for this type of drill are given in Chap. 5, 5-4H. Read the instructions, and adapt them to practice with /aʊ/.

1. "The _____ spoiled and became **sour.**"
2. "**How** many _____ do you want?"
3. "My favorite **flower** is the _____."
4. "My **towel** is colored _____."
5. "Let's walk **around** the _____."
6. "I'm **proud** to live in _____."
7. "He **found** the _____ on the **ground.**"
8. "I need _____ **pounds** of **flour.**"
9. "Are you **allowed** to stay **out** until _____?"
10. "I'll meet you **downtown** in _____ **hours.**"

45-5. CONVERSATION PRACTICE

So far you have learned how to pronounce your target by reading various kinds of exercises which contain /aʊ/ words. Now you are ready to move into the final and most important part of your training program—learning to pronounce /aʊ/ automatically while you are talking more or less spontaneously. If this is the first practice chapter assigned to you by your instructor, you may wish to review the introductory comments on conversation practice in Chap. 2, 2-6 to 2-7.

A.   Carrying /aʊ/ into Spontaneous Daily Conversation

This exercise requires you to use /aʊ/ in daily conversation, starting with key words and expanding to all the /aʊ/ words in your particular vocabulary. Complete instructions for this type of drill are given in Chap. 5, 5-5A, and there are supplementary comments about this exercise in Chap. 2, 2-7A.

B.   General Classroom Exercises in Speaking

Your instructor will plan a series of classroom conversation activities, and each assignment will be discussed fully in class before you carry it out. When your instructor announces the first speaking activity, you may wish to review the introductory comments on classroom speaking in Chap. 2, 2-7B.

chapter forty-six

The Diphthong Target
/ɔɪ/ (**boy**)

COMMON SPELLINGS FOR /ɔɪ/

The most frequent spellings are found in the words **oi**l and b**oy**; a less frequent spelling is found in the word l**aw**yer.

46–1. EAR TRAINING FOR THE /ɔɪ/ TARGET

A. A FEW REMINDERS ABOUT EAR TRAINING

The following test exercises will help you learn to recognize your /ɔɪ/ target. If this is the first practice chapter assigned to you by your instructor, you may wish to review the discussion about listening practice in Chap. 2, 2-2B to 2-3C.

B. RECOGNIZING /ɔɪ/ IN WORDS

You will hear a list of words containing /ɔɪ/. After listening to each word, write *B* if you heard /ɔɪ/ at the beginning of the word, *M* if you heard /ɔɪ/ in the middle, and *E* if you heard /ɔɪ/ at the end of the word. The answers will be read

to you at the end of the drill. This exercise is found in Appendix 1. If you have difficulty recognizing the target, you may find it worthwhile to review the test with somebody outside class.

C.   RECOGNIZING /ɔɪ/ IN SENTENCES

You will listen to a series of sentences containing a number of /ɔɪ/ words. Each sentence will be read several times. Try to locate the /ɔɪ/ words in each test sentence, and write them down. The /ɔɪ/ words in each test sentence will be read to you at the end of the drill. The sentences appear later in the chapter in Section 46-4D. If you have difficulty recognizing the target, you may find it worthwhile to review the test with somebody outside class.

46–2.   DISCRIMINATING BETWEEN /ɔɪ/ AND THE VARIOUS REPLACEMENTS

A.   PROBABLE TYPES OF REPLACEMENT

The following exercises will help you learn to compare /ɔɪ/ with your replacement. You are probably substituting one of the following common replacements for /ɔɪ/: (1) /ɔ/ as in call, (2) /ɝ/ as in bird, or (3) the substandard diphthong /ɜɪ/.[1] Your instructor will tell you which replacement you are using. If you are not employing one of the more common replacements, your teacher will tell you exactly how you are mispronouncing /ɔɪ/ and provide you with some discrimination drills.

B.   PAIRED LISTS OF WORDS

The words in the following paired lists are identical, except that the words in Column 1 contain the target, and the words in Column 2 contain one of the replacements. Complete instructions for this type of exercise are given in Chap. 5, 5-2B.

1.	Column 1 /ɔɪ/	Column 2 /ɔ/	2.	Column 2 /ɔɪ/	Column 2 /ɝ/[2]
	boil	ball		voice	verse
	oil	all		oil	Earl
	broil	brawl		loin	learn
	soil	Saul		oily	early
	toil	tall		coil	curl
	foil	fall		foil	furl
	joys	jaws			

[1] This substandard diphthong is composed of the Eastern and Southern American /ɜ/ as in bird and /ɪ/ as in bid. The differences between /ɜ/ and /ɝ/ are discussed in footnotes 1 and 8 of Chapter 42.

[2] If your replacement is /ɜɪ/, your instructor will carry out this drill with you by changing the /ɔɪ/ – /ɝ/ pairs to /ɔɪ/ – /ɜɪ/ pairs.

C. PAIRED SENTENCES

Then following paired sentences are identical, except that the key word in the first sentence contains /ɔɪ/, and the key word in the second sentence contains one of the replacements. Complete instructions for this type of drill are given in Chap. 5, 5-2C.

$$/ɔɪ/ - /ɔ/$$

1. Is it a boil?
   Is it a ball?
2. They were broiling.
   They were brawling.
3. His joys were small.
   His jaws were small.

$$/ɔɪ/ - /ɝ/ [3]$$

1. I heard the voice.
   I heard the verse.
2. Is it oily?
   Is it early?
3. I see the coil.
   I see the curl.

D. LISTENING FOR REPLACEMENTS IN FAMILIAR /ɔɪ/ WORDS

You will hear a list of word containing /ɔɪ/. Sometimes the words will be pronounced correctly with /ɔɪ/; other times the words will be said incorrectly with your replacement. Complete instructions for this type of drill are found in Chap. 5, 5-2D.

46–3. A FEW REMINDERS ABOUT ORAL PRACTICE PROCEDURES

If this is the first practice chapter assigned to you by your instructor, you may wish to review the comments about beginning oral practice in Chap. 2, 2-4. Before you actually begin practicing each individual pronunciation drill, you may also desire to review the supplementary explanations about the exercise in Chap. 2, 2-5.

46–4. THE PRONUNCIATION OF /ɔɪ/

A. PRONOUNCING ISOLATED /ɔɪ/

In the event that you cannot pronounce /ɔɪ/ through imitation alone, your instructor will help you with the following suggestions about placement. Should placement be required, you should review the explanatory comments about back vowels in Chap. 4, 4-4F, the comments about diphthongs in Chap. 4, 4-4G, and the description of /ɔɪ/ in Figure 4 of Chapter 4.

[3]See footnote 2.

1. The Position of the Lips

Your lips are opened considerably into a somewhat rounded position for the first vowel in the diphthong. As the articulators glide from /ɔ/ up and forward to /ɪ/, your lips close steadily and become narrowed and slit-like. The lips are unrounded for the /ɝ/ and /ɜɪ/ replacements; if you begin your pronunciation with unrounded, slightly spread lips, you are liable to pronounce one of these replacements.

2. Tongue Position, Length, and Muscular Tension

Place your tongue tip near the bottoms of your lower, middle front teeth. You may or may not touch your teeth with your tongue tip. Arch the back of the tongue moderately in the direction of the soft palate.

The most important thing to remember about the arched tongue position for the target is its movement. The tongue moves from the low, moderately arched tongue position for /ɔ/ up and forward to the much higher and steeply arched tongue position for the front vowel /ɪ/. The tongue travels with a smooth continuous gliding movement. This causes your mouth to close considerably, because your lower jaw is simultaneously rising with your tongue. Watch your instructor pronounce /ɔɪ/ for you several times, and observe the closing movements of his lips and lower jaw. Because of the lip, tongue, and jaw movements associated with the pronunciation of /ɔɪ/, the target is heard as a long sound: you will pronounce the target more accurately if you prolong it. The length is especially important if your replacement is /ɔ/, because you eliminate the diphthongal gliding movements up to /ɪ/ when you produce the single vowel. The target is usually pronounced with little muscular tension, and you should keep your tongue relaxed when you pronounce /ɔɪ/.

3. Pronouncing the Target

Try pronouncing /ɔɪ/, keeping in mind the suggestions given above. Because the tongue position for the first sound in the target is only partially visible, you may have difficulty placing your tongue in the proper position for /ɔ/. Listen intently to your instructor's pronunciation as he helps you pronounce the target. Try to feel the movements of your tongue, lips, and lower jaw as you glide from /ɔ/ up and forward to /ɪ/. Use a mirror to observe your lip and jaw movements.

B. PRONOUNCING /ɔɪ/ IN FAMILIAR WORDS

Pronounce each of the following words carefully. If you are either practicing with your instructor or listening to the exercise on tape, imitate your speech model as accurately as possible.

Beginning		Middle		End
1. oil	1. boil	8. choice	15. Detroit	1. boy
2. oily	2. coin	9. joint	16. lawyer	2. destroy
3. ointment	3. spoil	10. broil	17. coil	3. enjoy
4. oyster	4. join	11. avoid	18. poise	4. joy
	5. noise	12. sirloin	19. rejoice	5. toy
	6. point	13. appoint	20. foil	6. annoy
	7. voice	14. soil	21. Joyce	

C. PRONOUNCING /ɔɪ/ IN PHRASES

Pronounce each of the phrases carefully. If you mispronounce a word, say it over again several times, and then repeat the entire phrase. If you are either practicing with your instructor or listening to the drill on tape, imitate your speech model as accurately as possible.

1. a **boiled oyster** dinner
2. **pointing** to the **poised lawyer**
3. **avoiding** the **appointment**
4. **coiling** the **spoiled** rope
5. **joining** the **noisy** party
6. **rejoice** about the **ointment**

D. PRONOUNCING /ɔɪ/ IN SENTENCES

Pronounce each of the sentences carefully. If you use a replacement, say the word over again several times, and then repeat the entire sentence. If you are either practicing with your instructor or listening to the exercise on tape, imitate your speech model as accurately as possible.

1. The **oil**-soaked **toys** were **destroyed**.
2. The **boy's voice** was filled with **joy**.
3. My first **choice** was an old **coin**.
4. I **enjoy** eating a **broiled sirloin** steak.
5. The **royal** couple was **annoyed** by the **noise**.

E. PRONOUNCING /ɔɪ/ IN BEGINNING CONVERSATION

This exercise gives you an opportunity to begin using some of your previously learned /ɔɪ/ words in beginning conversation. Complete instructions for this type of drill are given in Chap. 5, 5-4H. Read the instructions, and adapt them to practice with /ɔɪ/.

1. "Did you **boil** the _____?"
2. "I need **oil** for my _____."
3. "I **enjoyed** my trip to _____."

4. "_____ has a **noisy voice**."

5. "Did you buy **Joyce** a new _____?"

6. "The _____ was **spoiled**."

7. "Was your _____ **annoyed**?"

8. "I'm **joining** the _____ club."

9. "Wrap the aluminum **foil** around the _____."

10. "Stop **pointing** at the _____."

46–5. CONVERSATION PRACTICE

So far you have learned how to pronounce your target by reading various kinds of exercises which contain /ɔɪ/ words. Now you are ready to move into the final and most important part of your training program—learning to pronounce /ɔɪ/ automatically while you are talking more or less spontaneously. If this is the first practice chapter assigned to you by your instructor, you may wish to review the introductory comments on conversation practice in Chap. 2, 2-6 to 2-7.

A.   CARRYING /ɔɪ/ INTO SPONTANEOUS DAILY CONVERSATION

This exercise requires you to use /ɔɪ/ in daily conversation, starting with key words and expanding to all the /ɔɪ/ words in your particular vocabulary. Complete instructions for this type of drill are given in Chap. 5, 5-5A, and there are supplementary comments about this exercise in Chap. 2, 2-7A.

B.   GENERAL CLASSROOM EXERCISES IN SPEAKING

Your instructor will plan a series of classroom conversation activities, and each assignment will be discussed fully in class before you carry it out. When your instructor announces the first speaking activity, you may wish to review the introductory comments on classroom speaking in Chap. 2, 2-7B.

part IV

THE USE OF
STRESS
AND
INTONATION

INTRODUCTION

Languages have distinctive patterns of rhythm and melody in addition to distinctive types of vowels, diphthongs, and consonants. Learning to pronounce American English often means that you have to learn how to use English stress and melody as well as learn how to pronounce various English sounds. If you are having difficulty using stress and intonation, your instructor will ask you to read over the explanatory materials and carry out the drills in the following chapters.

chapter forty-seven

The Use of Strong Stress

47-1. INTRODUCTION

Some writers define *stress* as the relative loudness or amount of vocal intensity that is given to a particular syllable.[1,2] Other writers relate changes in stress to variations in intensity, duration, and pitch.[3,4,5] I agree with the latter writers and believe that changes in stress are related to the combined effects of intensity, duration, and pitch. However, I have long felt that the time element—the duration or length of the stressed syllable—offers the student the best avenue to developing acceptable English stress patterns. This belief is based on classroom observations which have indicated that faulty stress patterns improve most rapidly when the student concentrates primarily on increasing vowel, diphthong, and consonant duration. An experiment by Fry offers evidence to substantiate this observation. Fry explored the influence of certain cues in perceiving stress.

[1] C. M. Wise, *Applied Phonetics* (Englewood Cliffs, N.J.: Prentice-Hall, Inc., 1957), p .13.
[2] C. F. Hockett, *A Course in Modern Linguistics* (New York: The Macmillan Company, 1958), p. 47.
[3] A. J. Bronstein, *The Pronunciation of American English* (New York: Appleton-Century-Crofts, 1960), p. 247.
[4] G. Fairbanks, *Voice and Articulation Drillbook* (New York: Harper & Row, Publishers, 1960), p. 159.
[5] P. Delattre, *The General Phonetic Characteristics of Language* (Final Report, Language Development Program, U.S. Office of Education, Contract SAE-8366, 1962), pp. 221 and 375.

He found that duration and intensity are both used by the speaker in evaluating stress, but that duration was more effective in helping a speaker decide how much stress he had used. In this study, vowel sounds accounted for the major differences in duration and intensity.[6]

47–2. UNDERSTANDING STRESS IN SINGLE WORDS

A. STRESS AND THE SYLLABLE

The place to begin our discussion of the English stress system is with the syllable, because all syllables are spoken with greater or lesser degrees of stress. Every English syllable normally contains one of the following: (1) a vowel alone, (2) a diphthong alone, or (3) a combination of a vowel or a diphthong and one or more consonants. The vowel is considered the strongest sound within the syllable, and it is often called the center or heart of the syllable. Consonants either precede or follow the vowel center. Examples of syllables include /θi/ and /iθ/, with /θ/ as in **th**ought and /i/ as in **bea**d. Certain consonants may become a syllable by themselves by replacing a vowel. These consonants are called syllabic consonants, and they are discussed in Chapters 16 and 22. Thus the number of spoken vowels, diphthongs, and syllabic consonants within a word tells us how many syllables the word contains, and the number of syllables within the word determines the number of stresses that will be heard.

B. LEVELS OF STRESS

Although linguists have indicated that American English utilizes four levels of stress, dictionaries have traditionally employed a three-level system of stress.[7] Although I believe that a four-stress system is theoretically more accurate, I have chosen to use a three-stress system for two reasons: (1) classroom experiences with both systems indicate that a three-stress system is easier for a student to learn, especially if the student is a nonnative speaker of English; and (2) students in speech improvement classes frequently rely on dictionaries—particularly nonnative speakers of English—and the explanatory and practice materials for a three-stress system relate very practically to most current American dictionaries. The stresses in the three-stress system include (1) primary, or most prominent /´/; (2) secondary, or less prominent /ˋ/; and (3) weak, or little prominence /˘/. Thus this system operates on two strong stresses and one weak stress. Syllables containing weak stress are commonly referred to as *unstressed syllables*, and the vowels are commonly called *unstressed vowels*. It should be remembered that the term "unstress" *does not* mean a complete lack of stress.

[6]D. B. Fry, "Duration and Intensity as Physical Correlates of Linguistic Stress," *The Journal of the Acoustical Society of America*, XXVII (1955), 765–768.
[7]G. L. Trager and H. L. Smith, Jr., *An Outline of English Structure, Studies in Linguistics, Occasional Papers, No. 3* (Norman, Okla.: Battenburg Press, 1951), pp. 35–39.

C. MARKING STRESS

You have probably noticed that the marking system used in this chapter differs from the system usually employed in most current dictionaries. Most dictionaries indicate strong stress by placing the stress mark *after* the stressed syllable. They use a short, heavy, diagonal line to show primary stress and a short, lighter, diagonal line to show secondary stress, e.g., **sand′ wich′**. Unstressed syllables are unmarked in dictionaries. In this chapter primary and secondary stress marks are placed directly *over* the syllable receiving prominence, using diagonal lines of equal weight, e.g., **móving, sáilbòat**. Unstressed syllables are normally unmarked.

D. LOCATING THE STRESSED SYLLABLE IN POLYSYLLABIC WORDS

We already know that all English syllables are uttered on one of three levels of stress, and we are now ready to examine the ways in which these stresses may be distributed—or may pattern themselves—in individual words. This distribution or patterning is sometimes referred to as *word stress* or *mechanical stress*.

When words of one syllable are pronounced alone, they are always spoken with primary stress, e.g., **áim, áll**, and **cáve**. Words of two or more syllables—polysyllabic words—are spoken in accordance with established stress patterns which are based on current usage. The source for a given stress pattern in a polysyllabic word is always found in a current dictionary. Every polysyllabic word must contain at least one primary stress, but the remaining syllables may be composed of varying combinations of secondary and weak stresses. Thus many words may contain stress patterns that are made up of all three levels of stress. Some of the more common polysyllabic stress patterns are illustrated below for you. Note that the location of the primary stress varies considerably.

1. Primary–Weak Stress Pattern: **néither, swímming**
2. Weak–Primary Stress Pattern: **remáin, alóng**
3. Weak–Primary–Weak Stress Pattern: **appéaring, Septémber**
4. Primary–Weak–Weak Stress Pattern: **yésterday, président**
5. Secondary–Weak–Primary Stress Pattern: **Hàllowéen, màthemátics**
6. Primary–Secondary Stress Pattern: **dóorbèll, páintbòx**
7. Primary–Primary Stress Pattern: **wéll-knówn, hómemáde**

A few additional comments are necessary about the compounds given in 6 and 7.[8] The primary–primary stress pattern shown in 7 is not actually a sequence

[8] Note that a compound is made up of two or more separate parts of speech—that is, nouns, verbs, adjectives, and so on. A compound has a distinctive meaning and use within a sentence.

of two identical primary stresses. Repeat the words wéll–knówn and hómemáde several times. Listen carefully, and you will notice that in each compound you are making the second word slightly longer and louder than the first word. You are also beginning the second word on a higher pitch. If you cannot hear these differences, ask your instructor to demonstrate them for you. Although the differences are small in these words, you must be able to demonstrate these changes in stress when pronouncing primary–primary words.

As you can see from the examples given above, the stress patterns found in compounds tend to vary. In addition to the *primary–secondary* sequence in a word like dóorbèll, and the *primary–primary* sequence in a word like wéll-knówn, some compounds have a *primary–weak* combination as in sálesmăn and wórkmăn. Certain other word sequences may or may not function as compounds, depending upon the intended meaning of the speaker. This is especially true of compound nouns which may become adjective–noun sequences. The change from compound nouns to adjective–noun sequences also brings about a change in meaning. Let us look at the words bláckbìrd and bláck bírd. When we are talking about a particular species of bird, the word combination functions as a compound with a primary–secondary stress pattern, e.g., bláckbìrd. When we are referring to some bird that happens to be black or is just dark, the word black functions as a modifier of the noun bird and we employ a primary–primary pattern, e.g., bláck bírd. Other contrastive examples include such pairs as gréenhòuse and gréen hóuse, and dárkròom and dárk róom. Although the meaningful differences between all of these pairs are indicated clearly by the spelling, these word combinations depend upon stress for their meaning in oral usage. You must be able to demonstrate these changes in stress when you are talking.

A similar type of change in stress occurs in sequences that do not function as compounds. These combinations are also normally pronounced with primary–primary stress patterns, but these sequences may also be said with primary–secondary stress patterns. The particular stress pattern used depends upon such factors as situation and emotional mood. When you tell a friend that you will have lunch with him on Máy fírst, you are simply telling him that the selected date is the first day in the month of May. However, if there has been some discussion about whether you are meeting on May first or June first, you would probably use a primary–secondary stress pattern and say Máy fìrst in order to avoid any confusion about a possible meeting in June. In another example you may become involved in a discussion about a néw shírt. The person you are talking to insists that the shirt in question is not new but old. After a while you become very angry and emphasize your point by using the word new very forcefully. Your stress pattern changes and you talk about a néw shìrt: e.g., "It was a néw shìrt!"

Most words are pronounced with a single acceptable pattern of stress, but certain words have more than one acceptable pattern, with variation in the location of the primary and secondary stress, e.g., cígarètte and cìgarétte, and

mágazìne and **màgazíne**. Still other words alter their stress patterns and meaning in accordance with their usage in a sentence. When words like **conduct** and **rebel** are used as nouns, the primary stress falls on the first syllable, e.g., **cóndùct** and **rébĕl**. When these words are used as verbs, the primary stress falls on the second syllable, e.g., **cŏndúct** and **rĕbél**. Note that there are certain secondary differences in pronunciation between these two types of stress patterns.

47–3.   TYPES OF FAULTY STRESS IN POLYSYLLABIC WORDS

We are concerned primarily with two basic types of incorrect stress: (1) problems which are caused by a misplaced primary or secondary stress, and (2) problems which are caused by poorly developed stress pattern contrasts. Each of these problems is discussed separately. Your instructor will tell you which type of replacement stress problem you are using. If you are not employing one of these basic types of incorrect stress, your instructor will tell you exactly how you are using English stress incorrectly.

47–4.   PROBLEMS STEMMING FROM POORLY LOCATED STRESSES IN POLYSYLLABIC WORDS

Your instructor may tell you that occasionally you mispronounce a poly-syllabic word by placing your primary or secondary stress on the wrong syllable. This does not normally mean that you have a severe stress problem. When your instructor tells you that you have stressed a word incorrectly, he will write the word out in phonetic symbols and include the correct stress marks. Then he will demonstrate the correct stress pattern for you by saying the word several times. You may wish to keep a complete list of all of these incorrectly stressed words in a small notebook so that you can review them frequently until you are automat-ically pronouncing them with the proper stress patterns. On some occasions you will hear or see a word outide class that you cannot pronounce, because you are uncertain about the correct stress pattern. When that occurs, look up the word in a standard American dictionary, and write the word down in your notebook, using phonetic symbols and the correct stress marks. Check your use of stress with your instructor when you get to class, and then memorize the correct pronunciation.

Some of the more frequently found problems involve stress difficulties with compound expressions. You may pronounce a compound taking primary–secondary stress with a secondary–primary stress pattern—e.g., **pìneápple** becomes **pìneápple**, or **cámping spòt** becomes **càmping spót**. You may also pronounce a compound taking a primary–primary stress pattern with a primary–secondary stress pattern—e.g., **hárd-bóiled** becomes **hárd bòiled**. Additional problems may develop with compound nouns which may become adjective–noun sequences. The meaning clearly requires primary–secondary stress, but you may use a primary–primary stress pattern. Thus **White Hòuse** may be pronounced as **whíte hóuse**, and **gréenhòuse** may be heard as **gréen hóuse**. You may also use the reverse of this type of error.

47–5. RHYTHM PROBLEMS STEMMING FROM POOR STRONG STRESS CONTRASTS IN POLYSYLLABIC WORDS

The severest types of stress problems relate to rhythm and come about because of poorly developed contrastive stress patterns. This lack of proper contrast or variation among the various degrees of stress present in your oral English is the element of stress that is most likely to create communication problems for you. Let us first look at the use of contrastive stress in words.

A. THE USE OF CONTRASTIVE STRESS PATTERNS IN WORDS

The English stress system is fundamentally based on variable sequences of strongly and weakly stressed syllables. Your ability to employ acceptable English stress patterns depends upon your skill in making a distinction among the various degrees of stress that are present in your speech. The strong stresses, and particularly primary stress, are especially important. Your stresses must stand in sharp contrast to each other when you speak. You must clearly indicate the length, volume, and pitch differences between the primary stress in a polysyllabic word and the weakly stressed syllable or syllables within the same word. These same oral distinctions must be made between other stress combinations, e.g., primary–secondary, secondary–weak–primary, and so on.

If your attempts at contrastive stressing are unsuccessful, your deficient use of stress will call unfavorable attention to your rhythm. Students typically employ two kinds of poor rhythm. The most common type occurs when you weaken the syllable or syllables containing strong stress, and thus impart a rapid, jerky quality to the pronunciation of the polysyllabic word. This occurs, mainly, because you are pronouncing the strongly stressed syllable with approximately the same brief period of duration and the same weak degree of loudness that is normally given to the weakly stressed syllable. If your instructor tells you that you use rapid, choppy rhythm, pay particular attention to the *length* differences between strong and weak stress. It is essential that you learn to use sufficient duration on the syllable or syllables receiving primary stress.

A second common type of poor rhythm occurs when you make the weak-stressed syllable or syllables too long. This imparts a slow, even quality to the pronunciation of the polysyllabic word. This occurs, primarily, because you are pronouncing all the syllables with too much length and loudness. You are using secondary, or even primary stress, on the weak-stressed syllables. If your instructor tells you that you are using slow, even rhythm, pay particular attention to the length differences between strong and weak stress. However, in this instance it is essential that you learn to shorten the syllable or syllables receiving weak stress. Further discussion of this type of problem is found in Chapter 48 along with additional practice exercises.

Both types of inadequate stressing lead to monotonous, uninteresting speech. The rapid, choppy style of rhythm may also lead to unintelligibility on the part of the speaker.

47–6. EAR TRAINING PRACTICE FOR STRONG STRESS CONTRASTS IN POLYSYLLABIC WORDS

A. A Few Reminders About Ear Training

If this is the first practice chapter assigned to you by your instructor, you may wish to review the discussion about listening practice in Chap. 2, 2-2B to 2-3C, before you begin your ear training practice for stress in polysyllabic words. Adapt the comments to your study of stress.

B. Recognizing Primary Stress in Simple Syllables

You will listen to a series of paired syllables containing a primary stress and a weak stress. After listening to each pair of syllables, write *1* if you heard primary stress on the first syllable and *2* if you heard primary stress on the second syllable. The answers will be read to you at the end of the drill. This exercise is found in Appendix 1. If you have difficulty recognizing primary stress, you may find it worthwhile to review the test with somebody outside class.

C. Recognizing Primary Stress in Polysyllabic Words

You will listen to a series of polysyllabic words containing one primary stress and one or more weak-stressed syllables. After listening to each word, indicate which syllable contained primary stress; that is, write *1* if it was the first syllable, *2* if it was the second syllable, and so on. The answers will be read to you at the end of the drill. This exercise is found in Appendix 1. If you have difficulty recognizing primary stress, you may find it worthwhile to review the test with somebody outside class.

D. Recognizing Primary Stress in Polysyllabic Words Also Containing Secondary Stress

You will listen to a series of polysyllabic words containing either primary–primary stress or primary–secondary stress. Sometimes there will also be syllables containing weak stress. After listening to each sequence of words, write *1* if you heard a primary–primary stress pattern and *2* if you heard a primary–secondary stress pattern. The answers will be read to you at the end of the drill. This exercise is found in Appendix 1. If you have difficulty recognizing the difference between the two types of stress patterns, you may find it worthwhile to review the test with somebody outside class.

47–7. PRACTICE EXERCISES FOR STRONG STRESS CONTRASTS IN POLYSYLLABIC WORDS

A. A FEW REMINDERS ABOUT ORAL PRACTICE PROCEDURES

If this is the first practice chapter assigned to you by your instructor, you may wish to review the comments about beginning oral practice in Chap. 2, 2-4, and the comments about oral practice procedures in Chap. 2, 2-5. Adapt the comments to your study of polysyllabic word stress.

One final word on developing adequate duration in order to alter a rapid, staccato rhythm pattern. Although this important feature of stress is most easily acquired by prolonging strongly stressed vowels and diphthongs, the durational aspect of stress is frequently reinforced by lengthening certain consonants. In particular, prolong the following consonants, especially when they come at the end of a stressed syllable or at the end of a word: /m/ as in **me**, /n/ as in **not**, /ŋ/ as in goi**ng**, /l/ as in **lap**, /r/ as in **rap**, and /v/ as in **vine**.

The drills for stress contrasts in polysyllabic words are arranged according to the more common patterns of stress, because you need to develop an awareness of specific stress patterns. This form of systematic drill will help you learn to pronounce and remember each of the more frequently occurring stress patterns of English. When you become skilled at contrasting syllables within individual words, you will be ready to handle stress patterns as they develop in groups of words.

B. PRONOUNCING WORDS OF ONE SYLLABLE

Sometimes a student finds it extremely difficult to use strong stress—especially primary stress. No matter how hard he tries to imitate his instructor's use of strong stress, the student always pronounces the syllable with a rapid, jerky quality. If you are one of these persons, your instructor will ask you to practice stressing the following one-syllable words in order to develop more accurate use of primary stress. Stress each of the following words carefully, paying particular attention to your use of length. If you are either practicing with your instructor or listening to the words on tape, imitate your speech model as accurately as possible.

1. áim	7. mán	13. háy	19. óne	25. twó
2. áll	8. fíne	14. híll	20. crów	26. díme
3. Ánn	9. fún	15. hów	21. hám	27. dóll
4. wáy	10. gún	16. bée	22. gréen	28. cómb
5. béll	11. cáve	17. bóne	23. báll	29. drúm
6. blów	12. cóol	18. blúe	24. cóal	30. níne

C. PRONOUNCING PRIMARY–WEAK STRESS PATTERNS

Stress each of the following words carefully, and concentrate on prolonging the first syllable. If you are either practicing with your instructor or listening to the words on tape, imitate your speech model as accurately as possible.

1. mórning	6. pláyful	11. séeing	16. mónkey	21. séven
2. móving	7. sáying	12. slówly	17. péncil	22. nýlon
3. néighbors	8. ríder	13. swímming	18. ísland	23. cándy
4. néither	9. róasting	14. prómise	19. mángo	24. Súnday
5. pássing	10. góing	15. Mónday	20. gúava	25. cráyon

D. PRONOUNCING WEAK–PRIMARY STRESS PATTERNS

Stress each of the following words carefully, and concentrate on prolonging the second syllable. If you are either practicing with your instructor or listening to the words on tape, imitate your speech model as accurately as possible.

1. remáin	6. arríve	11. expláin	16. guitár	21. ballóon
2. alárm	7. prepáre	12. alóne	17. cemént	22. corrál
3. retúrn	8. replý	13. alóng	18. cartóon	23. perfúme
4. becóme	9. surpríse	14. agrée	19. cigár	24. abóve
5. allów	10. todáy	15. garáge	20. paráde	25. belów

E. PRONOUNCING WEAK–PRIMARY–WEAK STRESS PATTERNS

Stress each of the following words carefully, and concentrate on prolonging the second syllable. If you are either practicing with your instructor or listening to the words on tape, imitate your speech model as accurately as possible.

1. admítted	8. collécting	15. enórmous	22. tomáto	29. Atlántic
2. advénture	9. compláining	16. detéctive	23. potáto	30. Pacífic
3. alárming	10. commánding	17. eléctric	24. vanílla	31. Septémber
4. annóuncing	11. delícious	18. torpédo	25. eléven	32. Octóber
5. becóming	12. depártment	19. volcáno	26. mosquíto	33. políceman
6. appéaring	13. destróying	20. umbrélla	27. Novémber	
7. begínning	14. enjóying	21. equátor	28. Decémber	

F. PRONOUNCING PRIMARY–WEAK–WEAK STRESS PATTERNS

Stress each of the following words carefully, and concentrate on prolonging the first syllable. If you are either practicing with your instructor or listening to the words on tape, imitate your speech model as accurately as possible.

1. áccident	7. cárefully	13. mánaging	19. pássenger	25. ámbulance
2. ánimal	8. dángerous	14. sílently	20. médicine	26. áudience
3. béautiful	9. cústomer	15. tímidly	21. Wáshington	27. bícycle
4. bóthering	10. éagerly	16. élephant	22. président	28. Cánada
5. méssenger	11. éxcellent	17. físherman	23. sýmphony	29. cárpenter
6. yésterday	12. húngrily	18. stéwardess	24. órchestra	30. góvernor

G. PRONOUNCING SECONDARY–WEAK–PRIMARY STRESS PATTERNS

Stress each of the following words carefully, and concentrate on prolonging the first and third syllables. Make sure that the third syllable is longer than the first syllable. If you are either practicing with your instructor or listening to the words on tape, imitate your speech model as accurately as possible.

1. àfternóon	3. dìsagrée	5. ùnderstánd	7. ènginéer
2. dìsappéar	4. ìntrodúce	6. Hàllowéen	8. lèmonáde

H. PRONOUNCING PRIMARY–SECONDARY STRESS PATTERNS

Stress each of the following words carefully, and concentrate on prolonging both syllables. Make sure the first syllable is longer than the second syllable.

1. áirfìeld	7. rówbòat	13. séacòast	19. básebàll
2. bédròom	8. páintbòx	14. múshròom	20. fóotbàll
3. snówbàll	9. dáybrèak	15. bédsprèad	21. sándbòx
4. dóorbèll	10. bíllbòard	16. páintbrùsh	22. sándwìch
5. blúejày	11. páncàke	17. yárdstìck	23. súnsèt
6. sáilbòat	12. stáircàse	18. hótdòg	24. Whíte Hòuse

I. PRONOUNCING PRIMARY–SECONDARY STRESS PATTERNS PLUS ONE OR MORE WEAK-STRESSED SYLLABLES

Stress each of the following words carefully, and concentrate on prolonging the primary and secondary stresses. Make sure that the primary stress is longer than the secondary stress.

1. rócket shìp	3. Chrístmas trèe	5. hámbùrger	7. píneàpple
2. mílk bòttle	4. péncil shàrpener	6. swímming pòol	8. básketbàll

J.   PRONOUNCING PRIMARY–PRIMARY STRESS PATTERNS

Stress each of the following words carefully, and concentrate on prolonging both syllables. Make sure that the second syllable is longer than the first syllable.

1. íced téa	6. ský-blúe	11. Jóhn Wóng	16. límeáde
2. gréen líght	7. hárd-bóiled	12. néw cár	17. fríed égg
3. réd líght	8. hómemáde	13. brówn shóes	18. gréen gráss
4. néw shírt	9. flát désk	14. blúe shírt	19. hót téa
5. Máy fírst	10. wéll-dóne	15. Tímes Squáre	20. hígh súrf

K.   PRONOUNCING PRIMARY–PRIMARY STRESS PATTERNS PLUS ONE OR MORE WEAK-STRESSED SYLLABLES

Stress each of the following words carefully, and concentrate on prolonging the two primary stresses. Make sure that the second primary stress is longer than the first primary stress.

1. Bíg Dípper	4. gréen ríbbon	7. United Státes	10. hót cóffee
2. róund táble	5. órange sóda	8. Julý Fóurth	11. cóld wéather
3. yéllow bóok	6. schóol líbrary	9. poláris míssile	12. Chrístmas vacátion

47–8.   UNDERSTANDING STRESS IN GROUPS OF WORDS

A.   THE THOUGHT GROUP

So far the discussion and practice of contrastive stress patterns has been limited to isolated polysyllabic words, compounds, and other two-word sequences. Now we are ready to examine stress in word groups.

Although the single word response is part of our total oral communication system, we normally communicate with others through groups of words, which are commonly referred to as *thought groups* or *phrases*. These spoken language segments may be thought of as the oral counterparts of written structural units, such as the clause and the sentence. Sentences may be short, simple structural units composed of a few words, or they may be longer, more complex units that are divided into clauses. Sentences and parts of sentences are separated from each other by such punctuation marks as commas, semicolons, and periods.

Sentences may be said to become thought groups when you read them aloud. Thus thought groups, too, may vary in size and complexity. You may communicate your thoughts in a short, simple group of words, or you may employ a longer, more complex word group. Thought groups are also punctuated. While talking, you tend to separate thought groups from each other by using clearly distinguishable pauses of varying lengths. The way you elect to break up your stream of speech is a highly individualistic matter, although it is useful to remember that structurally related words are not usually separated by pauses. There is no such thing as a recipe for effective grouping, because grouping is determined by the particular meaning you wish to convey to your listener. You decide to stop after a certain group of words, because you believe that this grouping will enable you to express an idea most clearly to your listener. However, although there is no recipe for effective grouping, there are certain guide lines you must remember for more effective communication. If your thought groups are consistently too long—and consequently there are few pauses in your speech—it may become difficult for your listener to remember all your ideas. You are throwing too many ideas at him without giving him a chance to digest your thoughts briefly during your pauses. You may also disrupt communication by using thought groups which are consistently too short. These short thought groups—and the frequent pauses that accompany them—may interrupt your flow of ideas so badly that your listener has difficulty understanding you. There is no continuity to the flow of ideas when your word groups are consistently either too long or too short. Both types of ineffective grouping contribute to monotony, and the use of frequent pauses—especially if they are short—may also contribute to a rapid, choppy style of rhythm.

Finally, it is important to remember that a change in grouping may drastically alter meaning. A lack of cooperation is apparent in the following two sentences, but the source of the negative attitude is different in each sentence.

1. The teacher / says the P.T.A. / is uncooperative.
2. The teacher says / the P.T.A. is uncooperative.

B.   THE USE OF CONTRASTIVE STRESS PATTERNS IN THOUGHT GROUPS

We have seen that polysyllabic words are pronounced according to established stress patterns and that in most instances usage allows for only one acceptable pattern of stress. The stress patterns of thought groups tend to be considerably less restrictive, and as a result we find a great deal of variety in the stressing of word groups. This contrastive variety is related to a speaker's intended meaning and is frequently referred to as *meaningful stress*. Every thought group characteristically contains one or more primary stresses. However, there is a tendency toward the use of only one primary stress per group. Theoretically any word or words within a thought group may be given primary stress, because eventually some speaker's intended meaning will call for the particular stress pattern. Observe how the sequence of strong and weak stresses may vary in accordance with the question asked by the listener. The questions are asked in a normal conversational style.

1.	What did you find?	I fòund a gréen pèncil.
2.	Did you find a red pencil?	I fòund a gréen pèncil.
3.	Did you find a green pencil or did you buy one?	I fóund a grèen pèncil.'
4.	Who found a green pencil?	Í fòund a grèen pèncil.

The first thing to notice is that in each example the primary stress occurs on a different word because the *meaning* of each response is slightly different. The meaning expressed in each particular response—and the location of the primary stress—is determined by the specific information requested in the question. Once again oral communication depends upon your ability to use clearly shown stress contrasts. Obviously certain words may be expected to take primary stress more frequently than other words. You would anticipate that words such as **found**, **green**, and **pencil** would receive primary stress much more typically than words like **I** and **a**. Your expectation would be correct. Generally speaking, English nouns, verbs, adjectives, adverbs, interrogatives, and demonstratives are assigned the primary and secondary stress values in thought groups. This is natural, because these words carry meaning in English—they are the meat-and-potato words of the language and represent the backbone of any effective oral communication. Such words are frequently referred to as *content* words. On the other hand, our less meaningful words are usually assigned weak-stressed values in thought groups. These words are commonly referred to as *function* words and include the articles, prepositions, personal pronouns, conjunctions, and auxiliary verb forms. Their role as carriers of strong stress is discussed in Chapter 48.

Another thing to notice is the continuing relationship between strong and weak stress in the polysyllabic word. The first syllable in the word **pencil** always remains stronger than the second syllable. It does not make any difference whether the polysyllabic word is pronounced alone or in a thought group. The only thing that changes is that the degree of strong meaningful stress may vary from primary to secondary when contrasted to the rest of the words in the thought group. Note also that the only time the speaker uses the typical primary –primary stress pattern of the isolated **green pencil** is in the first example. This occurs because the responses are given with normal, straightforward conversational speech. When speech becomes more forceful or emotional, the speaker tends to use primary stress on more words in the thought group. If you answer the last question with a great deal of exasperation, you might talk slowly and very emphatically, showing the forcefulness by giving primary stress to all of the words except the article **a**; for example, Í fóund a gréen péncil.

C.   THE TIMING SYSTEM OF ENGLISH RHYTHM

We have seen that the contrastive stress pattern of a thought group characteristically contains at least one primary stress and varying groups of lesser stressed syllables. The primary stress feature of this pattern tends to repeat itself when a speaker expresses himself through a series of thought groups. The primary stresses are more important rhythmically than the total number of syllables present in a thought group, and for this reason English rhythm is said to be *stress timed*. The chief distinguishing feature of stress-timed rhythm is that the primary stresses tend to recur at fairly regular intervals. This means that a speaker, if he is employing a reasonable steady rate of speech, takes about the same amount of time to get from the primary stress of one thought group to the primary stress of the following thought group. The interval of time between primary stresses is consistent, regardless of the number of intervening syllables of weaker stress. When only one or two syllables occur between primary stresses, the speaker tends to slow down slightly; when numerous syllables occur between primaries, the speaker tends to increase his rate. The more syllables a speaker uses between his primary stresses, the more rapidly he tends to say the syllables. Weak-stressed vowels particularly are crushed and blurred. Conversely, the fewer syllables a speaker inserts between primary stresses, the more slowly he pronounces the syllables.

This characteristic repetition of primary stresses is frequently illustrated in English poetry, which relies heavily on stress timing. The reiteration of strong stress is clearly demonstrated in the contrastive stress patterns of the following two lines of matching verse from Matthew Arnold's poem, "The Forsaken Merman."

Dówn, / dówn / dówn /
Dówn / to the dépths / of the séa. /

The first line contains three syllables and three primary stresses; the second line contains seven syllables and three primary stresses. The amount of time required to read each line is identical, since the determining factor is the *equal* number of primary stresses in each line. The second line is made to match the first one, because the reader increases his rate of speaking as he pronounces the weaker-stressed syllables before the second and third primary stresses.

The same fundamental repetitive feature is demonstrated in the contrastive patterns of the following prose samples. The total number of syllables per group is indicated beneath each phrase.

1. He had a stéak, / some ríce, / and that was áll./
         4   2   4
2. He sàt in the stàdium with a blánket, / a píllow, / and a jùg of cóffee./
          11   3   6

The fairly regular repetition is most easily heard when you read aloud the first sample, where the thought groups contain only one primary stress in each group. The speaker employs a series of simple weak–primary contrasts. The three weak syllables preceding the primary stress in the first and last groups are spoken more rapidly than the single weak stress in the second group. Note how the weak-stressed vowels are weakened and obscured, especially in the first and third thought groups. Compare these weak-stressed syllables to the long, heavy primary stresses at the end of the thought groups. Stress timing also appears when you read the second example, although the added strong stresses tend to slow down the rate of speaking and makes it more difficult to hear the regular primary repetition.

47–9. RHYTHM PROBLEMS STEMMING FROM POOR STRONG-STRESS CONTRASTS IN THOUGHT GROUPS

Review the comments in Section 47-5 regarding the use of contrastive stress patterns in polysyllabic words. Although a great deal more variation is permissible in stressing thought groups, the same basic skills are required. You must carry your ability to distinguish among the three degrees of stress from polysyllabic words to thought groups. Contrastive stressing is much more difficult in thought groups, because the word groups are longer and more complex. Note particularly the comments on rapid choppy rhythm. You will find that it becomes progressively more difficult to develop acceptable stress patterns as you approach conversational rhythm.

47–10. EAR TRAINING FOR STRONG STRESS CONTRASTS IN THOUGHT GROUPS

A. Recognizing Strong Stresses in Simple Sentences

You will listen to a series of sentences containing two or more words with strong stress. Each sentence will be read several times. After listening to each sentence, write down the word or words given primary stress and the word or words given secondary stress. The answers will be read to you at the end of the drill. This exercise is found in Appendix 1. If you have difficulty recognizing strong stress, you may find it worthwhile to review the test with somebody outside class. Ask them to vary the sentences by changing the location of the primary stresses.

47–11. PRACTICE EXERCISES FOR STRONG STRESS CONTRASTS IN THOUGHT GROUPS

A. Pronouncing Stress Patterns in Simple Sentences

Read each of the following sentences carefully, trying to develop well-stressed thought groups. Indicate clearly the differences among the various levels of stress, paying particular attention to prolonging the syllable or syllables carrying primary stress. If you are either practicing with your instructor or listening to the sentences on tape, imitate your speech model as accurately as possible.

1. I àte a gréen mángo.
2. She lòst her ríbbon in the schóol yàrd.
3. My bírthday is Máy fírst.
4. He is lèaving schòol at ónce.
5. Jàck is a wéll-beháved bóy.
6. The árrow flèw into the wíndow.
7. He had some frèsh éggs for brèakfast.
8. He bòught a jár of jàm.

B.   PRONOUNCING STRESS PATTERNS IN BEGINNING CONVERSATION

This exercise gives you an opportunity to begin using contrastive stress patterns in thought groups that are in conversational form. Each set of exercises employs a starter pattern which contains a specific combination of stresses. Each set of exercises also employs several groups of completion words which contain a specific stress pattern. Complete the first starter pattern by substituting one of the completion words from Group A in the blank. Continue practicing the pattern until you have tried all the completion items in that particular group. Practice the starter pattern with all the remaining word groups in the same manner, and then continue the exercise with the next starter pattern. Try to develop well-stressed thought groups. Indicate clearly the differences among the various levels of stress, paying particular attention to prolonging the syllable or syllables carrying primary stress. When you are satisfied that you are reading the patterns conversationally with acceptable stress patterns, you are ready to practice with somebody else. During class your instructor may ask you to practice the exercise with him, or he may ask you to do the patterns with another student. Outside class you may wish to practice with a friend or somebody at home.

Choose a pattern, and ask your helper to begin saying the completion words from one of the word groups. Each time your partner says a word, you repeat the pattern, completing it with the word selected from your list. You may wish to have your partner mix up the completion words by using items with different stress patterns. Pretend that you are actually talking to somebody. Look directly at your helper's face, listen for the completion word, and then complete the statement or ask the question as realistically as possible. The drill should move along smoothly and rapidly in the manner of good conversation. Keep checking to make certain that you are using well-stressed thought groups. The exercise may be expanded by asking your helper to think of additional words—

containing the same stress patterns—which may be used to complete the patterns.

1. The following starter pattern contains a sequence of two weak-stressed syllables.

    "It's a _____."

    Group A—one–syllable completion words: bóy, gírl, pén, dóg, cát, stár, drúm, bée, nóse, píg, béar, góat,ców, báll, fárm, hórse, cár, péar, dísh, bóne.

    Group B—primary–weak completion words: mángo, báby, cráyon, cóver, dríver, síster, bróther, fáther, móther, gíant, póny, méadow, wágon, túrtle, búilding, quéstion, dínner, néighbor.

    Group C—weak–primary completion words: cigár, ballóon, paráde, surpríse, guitár, garáge, cartóon, giráffe, dessért, hotél, belíef, repórt, replý.

    Group D—primary–weak–weak completion words: messenger, président, sýmphony, cústomer, bícycle, cárpenter, góvernor, mánager, físherman, pássenger, stéwardess.

    Group E—weak–primary–weak completion words: depártment, detéctive, volcáno, torpédo, tomáto, potáto, mosquíto.

    Group F—primary–secondary completion words: hótdòg, frúitcàke, schóol yàrd, básebàll, fóotbàll, gólf bàll, snówbàll, bédròom, sáilbòat, grápefrùit, páncàke, múshròom, bíllbòard, súnsèt, sándwìch, dóorbèll.

    Group G—primary–primary completion words: bláck bírd, bláck béar, blúe pén, gréen hóuse, fríed égg, gréen líght, néw cár, flát désk, límeáde. The following words contain some weak-stressed syllables: réd swéater, róund táble, brówn ríbbon, schóol líbrary, Chrístmas vacátion, yéllow bóok.

2. Redo the preceding exercises by using the various completion words in starter patterns containing sequences of three weak-stressed syllables. Use only those completion words that make sense with the starter patterns.

    a. "I have a _____."

    b. "It was a _____."

    c. "Is it a _____?"

    d. "Was it a _____?"

3. The following starter patterns all contain a word with primary stress. Select one of the patterns, and redo the preceding exercises. Use only those completion items that make sense with the starter pattern. Vary the exercise by practicing different starter patterns.

    a. "It ísn't a _____."

    b. "It wásn't a _____."

    c. "I háven't a _____."

    d. "I dón't have a _____."

    e. "The téacher has a _____."

    f. "Gíve me the _____."

47–12.   CONVERSATION PRACTICE

So far you have learned how to use strong stress by reading various kinds of exercises for strong stress contrasts. Now you are ready to move into the final and most important part of your training program—learning how to use strong stress contrasts automatically while you are talking more or less spontaneously. It this is the first practice chapter assigned to you by your instructor, you may wish to review the introductory comments on conversation practice in Chap. 2, 2-6 to 2-7.

A.   GENERAL CLASSROOM EXERCISES IN SPEAKING

Your instructor will plan a series of classroom conversation activities, and each assignment will be discussed fully in class before you carry it out. When your instructor announces the first speaking activity, you may wish to review the introductory comments on classroom speaking in Chap. 2, 2-7B.

chapter forty-eight

The Use of
Weak Stress

48–1. INTRODUCTION

In the previous chapter we concentrated on developing the strong stress features of the English stress system. You learned to sharpen your stress contrasts by prolonging strongly stressed English syllables, especially those syllables receiving primary stress. We also noted that some speakers needed to shorten weak-stressed syllables in order to avoid slow, even, or level rhythm. This chapter is devoted to further discussion of this type of problem. We are particularly interested in the weak-stressed pronunciation of certain frequently occurring one-syllable words, and observing the effect of these unstressed words on contrastive stress patterns in thought groups.

48–2. UNDERSTANDING WEAK STRESS

A. UNSTRESSED FORMS. [1]

We learned in the previous chapter that certain less meaningful words are usually pronounced with weak stress in thought groups. Such words are referred

---

[1] Because so many symbols are used in this chapter, you may wish to review the symbols listed in Figure 1 of Chapter 4.

to as "function words," and include the articles, prepositions, personal pronouns, conjunctions, and auxiliary verb forms. Actually these one-syllable words appear in English with two acceptable pronunciations: (1) a stressed pronunciation, (2) a weak-stressed pronunciation, which is sometimes referred to as an *unstressed form* or *weak form*. Typically these words are uttered with their weak-stressed pronunciation, but function words may be given primary stress because of special circumstances dictated by the speaker's intended meaning. When these one-syllable words are given primary stress, they are pronounced with various English vowels. When they are given weak stress, the stressed vowel is most frequently replaced by the typically indistinct, rapid /ə/. The stressed vowel is less frequently replaced by /ɚ/ or by a weak-stressed /ɪ/. (If you have not studied the pronunciation of these vowels, you may wish to look at the comments made about them in Chapters 31, 41, and 43.) Actually any English vowel may be given weak stress, although some of these pronunciations are quite rare.[2] My dialect frequently includes weak-stressed /ʊ/ rather than /ə/ in words like **should, would,** and **could**; weak-stressed /i/ rather than weak-stressed /ɪ/ in words like **me, we,** and **be**; and weak-stressed /ae/ rather than /ə/ in words like **that** and **as**.

An example of the replacement of the stressed vowel by /ə/ is found in the preposition **of**. When this word is stressed, it is pronounced /av/ with the vowel /a/; when it is given weak stress, the word is pronounced /əv/ with the vowel /ə/. An example of the replacement of the stressed vowel by a weak-stressed /ɪ/ is found in the pronoun **she**. When this word is stressed, it is pronounced /ʃi/ with the vowel /i/; when it is given weak stress, it is pronounced /ʃɪ/ with weak-stressed /ɪ/. An example of the replacement of the stressed vowel by /ɚ/ is found in the auxiliary verb **are**. When this word is stressed, it is pronounced /ar/ with the vowel /a/; when it is given weak stress, the word is pronounced /ɚ/ with the vowel /ɚ/. An additional type of change is seen in words like **him** and **his**. In each instance the change from strong-stressed /ɪ/ to weak-stressed /ɪ/ is accompanied by the omission of the consonant /h/. Thus /hɪm/ and /hɪz/ become /ɪm/ and /ɪz/. A list of commonly used one-syllable words having unstressed forms is found in Figure 1. Study this list carefully. Your instructor will demonstrate the various stressed and unstressed pronunciations for you.

B.   RHYTHM PROBLEMS STEMMING FROM POOR USE OF WEAK STRESS IN THOUGHT GROUPS

Students who use weak stress inadequately in thought groups typically tend to use the stressed pronunciations of the unstressed forms found in Figure

[2]H. A. Gleason, Jr., *An Introduction to Descriptive Linguistics*, rev. ed. (New York: Holt, Rinehart and Winston, Inc., 1961), p. 323.

1. Using primary stress, or even secondary stress, on these words gives their speech a slow, even, monotonous quality, because they are pronouncing these one-syllable words with too much length and volume. The use of weak stress in these monosyllables is an essential part of an acceptable contrastive English stress pattern. Your ability to pronounce weakly all the weak-stressed vowels and diphthongs in a thought group is just as important as your skill in prolonging the strong stresses in the group. It is imperative that you shorten and obscure weak-stressed syllables—primarily by employing less length on these syllables. Proper use of weak stress contributes to the rhythmical recurrence of the long primary stresses, helps you place your weak stresses in sharp contrast with your strong stresses, and thus aids you in establishing an accurately contrasted stress pattern.[3]

FIGURE 1

Commonly Used Unstressed Forms

Word	Stressed Pronunciation	Weak-Stressed Pronunciation
a	/eɪ/	/ə/
am	/aem/	/əm/
an	/aen/	/ən/
and	/aend/	/ən/ (before a consonant)
		/ənd/ (before a vowel)
		/n̩/ (when preceded by /t/ or /d/)
are	/ɑr/	/ɚ/
as	/aez/	/əz/
at	/aet/	/ət/
be	/bi/	/bɪ/
but	/bʌt/	/bət/
can	/kaen/	/kən/
could	/kʊd/	/kəd/
do	/du/	/də/ (before a consonant)
		/dʊ/ (before a vowel)
for	/fɔr/	/fɚ/
from	/frɑm/	/frəm/
had	/haed/	/həd/ or /əd/[4]
has	/haez/	/həz/ or /əz/[4]
have	/haev/	/həv/ or /əv/[4]
he	/hi/	/hɪ/ or /ɪ/[4]

[3] If you had difficulty using weak stress in polysyllabic words, you may wish to review the practice materials containing weak-stressed syllables in the preceding chapter before proceeding to the practice exercises for weak stress in thought groups.
[4] When words like **had, have, he, her, him,** and **his** occur as the first word in a sentence, alone, or the first word after a pause, /h/ is never dropped.

Word	Stressed Pronunciation	Weak-Stressed Pronunciation
her	/hɝ/	/hɚ/ or /ɚ/[4]
him	/hɪm/	/ɪm/[4]
his	/hɪz/	/ɪz/[4]
me	/mi/	/mɪ/
of	/ɑv/	/əv/
or	/ɔr/	/ɚ/
shall	/ʃael/	/ʃəl/
she	/ʃi/	/ʃɪ/
should	/ʃʊd/	/ʃəd/
some	/sʌm/	/səm/
than	/ðaen/	/ðən/
that	/ðaet/	/ðət/
the	/ði/	/ðə/ (before a consonant)
		/ðɪ/ (before a vowel)
them	/ðɛm/	/ðəm/
their	/ðɛr/	/ðɚ/
to	/tu/	/tə/ (before a consonant)
		/tʊ/ (before a vowel)
was	/wɑz/	/wəz/
we	/wi/	/wɪ/
were	/wɝ/	/wɚ/
would	/wʊd/	/wəd/
you	/ju/	/jə/ (before a consonant)
		/jʊ/ (before a vowel)
your	/jʊr/	/jɚ/

48–3. PRACTICE EXERCISES FOR WEAK STRESS CONTRASTS IN THOUGHT GROUPS

A. Pronouncing Unstressed Forms Containing /ə/ in Simple Sentences

Read each of the following sentences carefully, trying to develop well-stressed thought groups. Indicate clearly the differences among the various levels of stress, paying particular attention to shortening the unstressed forms. The unstressed forms containing /ə/ are in italics, and words containing primary stress are marked. If you are either practicing with your instructor or listening to the sentences on tape, imitate your speech model as accurately as possible. If you have difficulty pronouncing /ə/, your instructor will probably ask you to study the pronunciation of /ə/ in Chapter 43.

1. It's *a* bóok.
2. Where is *the* bóok?
3. Bill *can* gó.
4. *Was* Jóhn thére?
5. *The* boy *was* húngry.
6. Who came *from the* béach?
7. He *has a* bóok.
8. Does Bob *have the* rábbit?
9. Béth came *to* get *an* ápple.
10. Who gáve it *to them*?
11. Joe *and* Tom *can* cóme.
12. Did Álice go *as* soon *as* póssible?
13. They *have an* órange.
14. They walked *to the* cár.
15. Did they find it *at the* stóre?
16. Did *you* see *that* they áte?
17. *Could* Alice *have a* dóg?
18. They went ín *and* óut.
19. I *shall* léave now.
20. Peter *has* góne.

21. They called *at* nóon.
22. I need *some* cáke.
23. They left here *at* éight.
24. *Would* they cóme?
25. He found *a* púppy.
26. Let's go *to* Tóm's house.
27. I want fíve *of them*.
28. I wish I *could* swím.
29. *Would you* like *some* cándy?
30. Peter *can* gó, *but* Mary cán't.
31. I wísh *that* I *could* táke *them*.
32. Jóe *and* I *should* take *them* hóme.
33. *The* bread *and* cáke came *from the* bákery.
34. *Can you* take *the* canóe *to the* láke?
35. I *have* óne *but* Tom *has* thrée.
36. Í *would* like *to* cut *and* wrap *the* méat.
37. He stood *as* I éntered.
38. My bróther is afraid *of* dógs *but* Í'm not.
39. *The* tráin *should* arrive very sóon.
40. He *was* gone in *a* mínute.

B. PRONOUNCING UNSTRESSED FORMS CONTAINING /ɚ/ IN SIMPLE SENTENCES

Follow the directions in Exercise A when you do this drill. Note that the unstressed forms containing /ɚ/ are shown in italics, but that other unstressed forms are not. If you have difficulty pronouncing /ɚ/, your instructor will probably ask you to study the pronunciation of /ɚ/ in Chapter 43.

1. It's this *or* thát.
2. Is it *for* hím?
3. Gíve it to *her*.
4. Do you have *their* bóoks?
5. These *are* míne.
6. They *were* thére.
7. Is that *your* cár?
8. Do you want péas *or* béans?
9. The letter was *for* Jóhn.
10. I have *their* new blánket.
11. We gáve it to *her* last níght.
12. Where *are* you góing?
13. I didn't think they *were* réady.
14. I have *your* lúnch.

15. He'll be here on Súnday *or* Mónday.
16. I'll come *for* it at nóon.
17. They went to the stóre with *her*.
18. I ate *their* cándy.
19. I'm sure these *are* míne.
20. *Were* they cóming?
21. Is that *your* schóol?
22. The shoes *are* réady.
23. Give it to *your* móther.
24. I thought the ápples *were* rípe.
25. They took *her* to the gáme.
26. They wanted *their* íce cream.
27. Was the call *for* yóu *or for* mé?

C. PRONOUNCING UNSTRESSED FORMS
CONTAINING /ɪ/ IN SIMPLE SENTENCES

Follow the directions in Exercise A when you do this drill. Note that the unstressed forms containing /ɪ/ are shown in italics, but that other unstressed forms are not. This exercise also includes weak forms that are pronounced by omitting the initial /h/. If you have difficulty pronouncing /ɪ/, your instructor will probably ask you to study the pronunciation of /ɪ/ in Chapter 31.

1. Show *me* this afternóon.
2. Can you táke *me* to the móvies?
3. Did *he* fínd *him*?
4. I seè *him* over thére.
5. Will *he be* right óver?
6. Try to *be* on tíme.
7. Will Jack *be* thére?
8. Is *she* níce?
9. Did you say *she* can't cóme?
10. Are *we* leaving nów?
11. Can *we* go to *his* hóuse?
12. When can *we* gó?
13. Is *this his* móther?
14. That's *his* bóok.
15. Gíve it to *him*.
16. *The* egg is bróken.
17. *The* orange is rótten.
18. If Dad wants *me* láter, I'll *be* at hóme.

D. PRONOUNCING A MIXED LIST OF
UNSTRESSED FORMS IN SIMPLE SENTENCES

Follow the directions in Exercise A when you do this drill. Note that all the unstressed forms are indicated by the use of italics.

1. I saw John *as he* léft.
2. I smell *an* órange.
3. I *was* hére.
4. I *can* gó.
5. I *could* gó.
6. I *have a* cár.
7. *She has an* ápple.
8. I came *at* tén.
9. I need *the* lámp.
10. I want *the* órange.
11. I went *to the* stóre.
12. I gáve it *to them*.
13. I *shall* éat.
14. I see *the* knife *and* fórk.
15. I like bread *and* bútter.
16. I like salt *and* pépper.
17. I saw *the* shoes *that* Máry bought.
18. I came *from* Hawáii.
19. I want twó *of* those.
20. I saw *you* swímming.
21. I saw *your* dóg.
22. I thought *you were* thére.
23. *We were* hére.
24. I hope they *are* cóming.
25. I want *some* íce cream *for* dessért.
26. I want *a* pen *or* pencil *at* ónce.
27. I want *some* cáke *and* cóffee.
28. I saw it in *her* désk.
29. I found *their* báll.
30. I know *your* fáther.
31. I thought *you were* síck.
32. I think they *are* wínning.
33. I bought this *for* móther.
34. I need thís *or* thát.
35. I want *her* to gó.
36. I *have their* bóok.
37. I think *he* lóst.
38. Will they *be* láte?
39. Will they gíve it *to me*?
40. Do *you* want *the* súgar?
41. Will *you do* it nów?
42. I *would* líke it.
43. I want *some* ríce.
44. Hé went *but* Í didn't.
45. I see *his* móther.
46. I sée *him*.

48–4. CONVERSATION PRACTICE

So far you have learned how to use weak stress by reading various kinds of exercises for weak–stress contrasts. Now you are ready to move into the final and most important part of your training program—learning how to use weak–stress contrasts automatically while you are talking more or less spontaneously. Supplement your general classroom practice activities in speaking through the following exercise on the use of stress patterns in spontaneous daily conversation.

A. CARRYING CONTRASTIVE STRESS PATTERNS
INTO SPONTANEOUS DAILY CONVERSATION
THROUGH COMMON EXPRESSIONS

All of us use very short expressions as part of our daily conversation. Such conversational fragments—with suggested primary stresses—include:

1. "Hí! How áre you?"
2. "What tíme is it?"
3. "Let's have some cóffee."
4. "I need a bréak."
5. "What's your next cláss?"
6. "Got a cígarette?"
7. "See you láter."

Write down from five to ten expressions that you use in your daily conversation. Read them aloud several times, and decide what kind of stress pattern you normally use when saying each expression. Make sure that you know which word, or words, contain primary stress. Practice each expression until you are certain that you are saying it with a well-contrasted stress pattern. Then keep track of how effectively you stress each thought group during your daily conversation.

chapter forty-nine

Intonation

49–1. INTRODUCTION

This chapter is concerned primarily with changes in pitch. Pitch is familiar to all of us when it is used as a musical term to establish the key of an instrument or a singer's voice, or when it is employed to described the habitual highness or lowness of a person's vocal quality. We recognize that voices are characterized by differences in pitch; for example, childrens' voices and the voices of adult females are usually higher than the voices of adult males.

Our main concern in this chapter is not with the habitual pitch of an individual's voice. Instead, we are interested in certain basic linguistic levels of pitch, and the way in which these levels pattern or interact with each other during speech. We are especially interested in the following points: (1) the basic levels of pitch that characteristically appear in American English, and (2) the more common intonation contours formed by the contrastive interaction of these levels.

49–2. THE LINGUISTIC LEVELS OF PITCH

Linguists recognize the presence of four linguistic levels of pitch in American English: *low* or /1/, *mid* or /2/, *high* or /3/, and *extra high* or /4/.[1] These levels are shown graphically in Figure 1.

FIGURE   1

The Levels of Pitch

                                               Extra High or /4/

                             High or /3/

               Mid or /2/

Low or /1/

1. *Pitch Level* /1/. This level is the lowest level. It is approximately *2* or *3* notes below pitch level /2/.
2. *Pitch Level* /2/. This level represents the speaker's habitual pitch level. This level is relatively common and serves as a basis for comparison for the other three levels.
3. *Pitch Level* /3/. This level is approximately *2* or *3* notes higher than pitch level /2/.
4. *Pitch Level* /4/. This last level is approximately *2* or *3* notes higher than pitch level /3/. At times it may go even higher. This level is heard much less frequently than the others.

It should be noted that while these various pitch levels are found in the speech of all native speakers, the actual levels are not absolute but tend to vary from speaker to speaker. This variation is easily heard when you compare pitch level /1/ of male and female speakers. Level /1/ of the average adult male speaker is quite different from level /1/ of the average adult female speaker. Your instructor will ask several male and female students in your class to say the following sentence: "I want a hotdog." Pitch level /1/ typically occurs at the end of simple factual statements, and **dog** will be spoken on pitch level /1/ by both male and female speakers. Listen to the difference in pitch between male and female voices on **dog**. The male voices will be distinctly lower than the female voices on pitch level /1/.

Furthermore, an individual may vary his own set of pitch levels from time to time in accordance with a particular situation. Under emotional stress the speaker may use a higher pitch level /1/, /2/, /3/, or /4/, and establish a somewhat different set of pitches.

---

[1]H. A. Gleason, Jr., *An Introduction to Descriptive Linguistics*, rev. ed. (New York: Holt, Rinehart and Winston, Inc., 1961,) pp. 46–47.

49–3. CONTRASTING THE FOUR BASIC PITCH LEVELS TO FORM INTONATION CONTOURS

A. THE BASIC PITCH LEVELS AND MEANING

The four pitch levels are not meaningful by themselves. They signal meaning only when they contrast with each other and form intonation contours. The dialogue in the following hypothetical situation furnishes us with a good example of how pitch levels are combined in different ways to form meaningful intonation contours.

Mrs. Jones walks over to the fruit counter at her local supermarket and asks the clerk if he has any good peaches. The clerk points to some peaches on the counter and says: "We just received this shipment this morning. These are fresh." The second part of his reply indicates to Mrs. Jones that the peaches are fresh, because this is the word order usually employed by the speaker who is stating a simple fact. In this instance, the meaning of the words has been reinforced by the speaker's use of an intonation contour that is commonly associated with factual English statements. This intensification has been signaled specifically by pitch movements that start from level /2/, move up to level /3/ at the beginning of **fresh**, and then drop to level /1/ through the middle of **fresh**:

$$
\begin{array}{l}
^{3}\!\!\ulcorner\text{frèsh.''} \\
_{2}\underline{\text{''These are}}\!\!\rfloor \\
\qquad\qquad _{1}\llcorner
\end{array}
$$

Now suppose that our imaginary Mrs. Jones is a careful shopper, and she decides to check some of the peaches before buying any. She picks up two or three pieces of fruit and notices that the underside of each peach is soft and rotten. She turns to the clerk and says:

$$
\begin{array}{l}
\qquad\qquad ^{4}\!\!\ulcorner\quad \urcorner \\
_{2}\underline{\text{''These are}}\!\!\rfloor\ \text{frésh!''}
\end{array}
$$

Despite the identical structure the words no longer carry the meaning originally established by the clerk. Mrs. Jones's reaction to the fruit has caused her to superimpose a completely different shade of meaning upon the fundamental meaning of the sentence. She has altered the contour of pitches on **fresh** by exhibiting a sharp upward movement from level /2/ to level /4/. This has highlighted **fresh** with special emphasis and turned the factual statement into a query of disbelief and amazement. Mrs. Jones is really saying: "Come on, you must be kidding me. This fruit is anything but fresh." The meaningful difference between the two utterances lies in the different melodic contours used by the two speakers.

B. The Location of the High Pitch

You may have noticed that thus far the location of the high pitch has coincided with the syllable receiving primary stress. The pitch of the syllable carrying primary stress usually differs from the pitch of the preceding and following syllables. The change in pitch level is usually to a higher level, although on occasion it may be to a lower level. This close relationship between English stress and English intonation is demonstrated easily by repeating the basic sentences we used in Chap. 47, 47-8B to demonstrate meaningful stress. Observe how the high pitch consistently coincides with the syllable or syllables receiving primary stress (if you have not studied the materials on strong stress, your instructor will explain the relationship between English stress and melody):

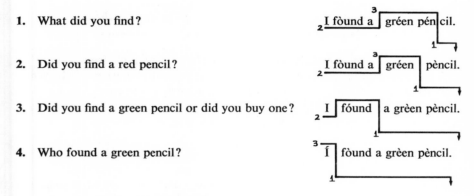

1. What did you find?

2. Did you find a red pencil?

3. Did you find a green pencil or did you buy one?

4. Who found a green pencil?

C. The Use of a Pitch Level
over a Long Sequence of Syllables

Frequently the speaker's pitch level will appear to be the same over long sequences of syllables. This continuing pitch will often occur at level /2/:

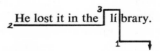

When this sentence is verbalized, all the syllables preceding the first syllable in **library** are uttered on pitch level /2/. The first important melody change does not come until the speaker raises his voice between **the** and **library** and utters the first syllable of **library** at pitch level /3/. The second important change comes as the speaker drops to level /1/ before saying the second syllable. The fact that the speaker's pitch level remains constant until he reaches the first syllable of **library** does not mean that this entire word sequence is said on a monopitch at level /2/. The portion of the sentence preceding the initial syllable of **library** is actually spoken over a range of shorter pitches. These brief rising-and-falling inflectional changes do not affect the speaker's meaning, but nevertheless they are important aspects of the speaker's total melodic pattern. These less noticeable fluctuations contribute to the melodic variations that typify English speech. Without these movements our intonation, and consequently our speech, would appear stilted, artificial, and monotonous.

D.   THE SHIFT AND THE GLIDE

You have probably noticed that there are two basic types of inflectional movement. When you inflect between the syllables of a word, or between words, you *shift* or *step* up or down:

There is a brief moment of silence as you shift in each example from level /3/ to level /1/. This slight break is most obvious when you shift between words. When you inflect through the syllable of a word you *glide* up or down:

Thus, in this instance, you slide your voice with continuous sound through the vowel or diphthong as you glide from level /3/ to level /1/.

49–4.   COMMON INTONATION CONTOURS

American English pitch contours are extremely variable and complex. Our hypothetical Mrs. Jones has already demonstrated how a speaker's particular attitude may alter the meaning of words. A multitude of other fine shades of meaning may be superimposed upon the dictionary denotation of words, depending upon such factors as the speaker's mood, his immediate situation, and the particular meaning he wishes to convey. In each case the slightly different connotation is transmitted largely by the speaker's choice of intonation contours. Good speakers effectively combine both intonation and stress in order to produce meaningfully spoken thought groups. Although there exists a wide variety of potential contours, the more common melody patterns of American English have been identified for us by such linguists as Pike,[2] and Trager and Smith.[3] The intonation contours illustrated in the following sections are considered to be the more frequently employed melody patterns of American English.

A. MID–HIGH–LOW /2 3 1 ↓/ OR HIGH–LOW /3 1 ↓/
FALLING INTONATION

The /2 3 1 ↓/ and its slightly different /3 1 ↓/ variation constitute the commonest intonation contours in English. The /2 3 1 ↓/ contour is typically found at the end of simple factual statements, at the end of commands, and at the end of questions beginning with interrogatives:

$$_2\underline{\text{These are}}\ ^3\text{fresh.}_1\!\downarrow \qquad _2\underline{\text{I need a}}\ ^3\text{ride.}_1\!\downarrow$$

$$_2\underline{\text{He lost it in the}}\ ^3\text{car.}_1\!\downarrow$$

When the contour is /2 3 1 ↓/, the voice is given a general mid–high–low direction. The speaker begins on level /2/, moves up to level /3/, and then drops to level /1/. The falling arrow, /↓/, emphasizes that the speaker's pitch continues to drop as his voice fades away at the end of the thought group.

The contour does not necessarily have to occur at the end of the statement. We have seen already in Section 49-3B that the high pitch usually coincides with the syllable receiving primary stress. The rise to level /3/ and the subsequent drop to /1/ may appear at varying points within the thought group, depending upon the intended meaning of the speaker:

$$_2\underline{\text{I found a}}\ ^3|\text{green}|\,_1\text{pencil.}\!\downarrow \qquad _2\underline{\text{I}}\ ^3|\text{found}|\,_1\text{a green pencil.}\!\downarrow$$

The /2 3 1 ↓/ contour may also be used to separate two closely related ideas and to attach strong importance to the second thought. The emphasis is increased by the use of a long pause following the first intonation contour:

$$_2\underline{\text{I}}\ ^3|\text{told}|\,_1\text{you,}\ _2\underline{\text{we're}}\ ^3|\text{through!}_1\!\downarrow$$

[2]K. L. Pike, *The Intonation of American English* (Ann Arbor, Mich.: University of Michigan Press, 1946).
[3]G. L. Trager and H. L. Smith, *An Outline of English Structure* (Norman, Okla.: Battenburg Press, 1951).

The /2 3 1 ↓/ contour is also typically heard with questions that start with an interrogative. These questions might be termed information questions, because they require more than a simple affirmative or negative response:

Finally, the /2 3 1 ↓/ contour is frequently employed when we issue commands:

In a /3 1 ↓/ or high–low contour, the speaker commences talking on level /3/ and drops immediately to level /1/:

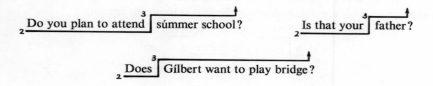

Note that the use of /3 1 ↓/ intonation on the preceding statements makes the thought groups more emphatic.

The /3 1 ↓/ contour is also employed with single-word responses:

Are you married? ³Yes.   Were you late to school? ³No.

B.   MID–HIGH /2 3 ↑/ RISING INTONATION

The mid–high /2 3 ↑/ contour is most frequently heard with questions that may be answered with a simple "yes" or "no" response:

₂Do you plan to attend ³sùmmer school?   Is that your ³father?

₂Does ³Gílbert want to play bridge?

The voice is given a mid–high direction by moving from level /2/ up to level /3/. The significant change is the speaker's rise to level /3/. The rising arrow, /↑/, emphasizes that the speaker's pitch continues to rise slightly as his voice fades away at the end of the thought group. When there are several syllables preceding the upward movement from /2/ to /3/, the voice tends to continue rising throughout the contour. This tendency is most obvious in the third example where the initial upward movement comes early in the thought group. Note that *primary stress* is normally used on the *first word* that the speaker utters at pitch level /3/.

The /2 3 ↑/ contour is also heard in certain instances in questions commencing with interrogatives. Observe the following example: Jack is talking to his friend Bob on the telephone; during the conversation Jack inquires about a baseball score and uses a /2 3 1 ↓/ contour, as he asks:

$$\text{Who won the } \boxed{\text{game?}}$$

The connection is poor and Jack does not hear Bob's reply. He repeats his question but alters his intonation to a /2 3 ↑/ pattern:

$$\text{Who won the game?}$$

The switch in intonation tells Bob that Jack did not hear him the first time and that Jack wants the information repeated.

The /2 3 ↑/ contour is commonly utilized when the speaker is enumerating a series of items connected by **and**. All the enumerated items preceding **and** are said with rising /2 3 ↑/ intonation; the final item in the series is given a /2 3 1 ↓/ falling contour:

$$\text{I visited } \boxed{\text{Maine, Ver}}\text{mont, and New } \boxed{\text{Hamp}}\text{shire.}$$

$$\text{We bought } \boxed{\text{grapes, or}}\text{anges, lem}\boxed{\text{ons, and}}\text{peach}\boxed{\text{es.}}$$

Note that the syllable carrying primary stress in **oranges** and **lemons** is low rather than high in order to allow the speaker to make the transition to the higher pitch level.

When a series of items is connected by **and** in a question form, the /2 3 ↑/ contour is used on all of the items in the series:

$$\text{Did you buy some to}\boxed{\text{matoes, rice, and cof}}\text{fee?}$$

The /2 3 ↑/ contour is also used in a series that offers a choice when the various choices are connected by **or**. Everything prior to the final choice takes the /2 3 ↑/ contour, while the final choice takes a /2 3 1 ↓/ contour:

You have a choice of jello, cake, or pie.

Did they suggest you take Japanese, Italian, or French?

The same contour is frequently heard when the speaker is concerned with only two choices:

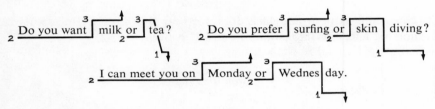

Do you want milk or tea?   Do you prefer surfing or skin diving?

I can meet you on Monday or Wednesday.

C.   MID–HIGH–MID /2 3 2 →/ OR HIGH–MID /3 2 →/ SUSTAINED INTONATION

The mid–high–mid /2 3 2 →/ contour is typically heard at the end of a thought group that is closely related by meaning to the following thought group.

If you're at the store, please buy some dog food.

I'll give you a test, but not until Friday.

The voice is given a general mid–high–mid direction as the speaker begins on level /2/, moves up to level /3/, and then returns to level /2/. The horizontal arrow, /→/, emphasizes that the speaker's pitch remains level or sustained as his voice fades away at the end of the thought group.

The /2 3 2 →/ contour may be heard as part of a single thought group that contains more than one primary stress. This type of thought group ends with a /2 3 1 ↓/ contour:

The flight is due at noon.

The /3 2 →/ or high–mid contour may also be heard as part of a single thought group that contains more than one primary stress:

D. THE USE OF PITCH LEVEL /4/

Pitch level /4/ is heard much less frequently than the other linguistic levels, and it is associated with the expression of emotional feelings such as anger, surprise, or fear. The speaker employs this pitch level to indicate the greater emphasis associated with his emotional reaction. We have already seen one example of this level in Mrs. Jones's sharp reaction to the fresh fruit with a /2 4 ↑/ or mid–extra-high rising contour. The following situation is another example of a /2 4 ↑/ contour. A neighbor becomes ill very suddenly and is rushed to the hospital. When learning about the emergency trip, you might well exclaim:

A /2 4 1 ↓/ or mid–extra-high–low falling contour is also possible. An angry child who does not want to go to bed might very well emphatically state:

49–5. INTONATION PROBLEMS STEMMING FROM POORLY USED COMMON INTONATION CONTOURS

A number of potential replacement contours are possible, but the most predictable intonation problems are described briefly in the following sections.

A. THE /2 3 1 ↓/ INTONATION CONTOUR

Some speakers find it difficult to lower their voices sufficiently on thought groups requiring a /2 3 1 ↓/ or a /3 1 ↓/ contour. They normally replace this type of intonation with a /2 3 2 →/ or /3 2 →/ contour. Consistent use of this type of intonation pattern gives the speaker's conversation an incomplete or unfinished quality. Your instructor will illustrate this usage for you, if you have difficulty employing the /2 3 1 ↓/ or /3 1 ↓/ contour.

³
₂ Please buy me some ⌐eggs.
₂

³
₂They didn't ⌐have it.
₂

Note that some speakers may vary the pitch of the final syllable or syllables and end their thought group with a slight rise or drop in intonation. The incomplete quality is still present. Sometimes the listener expects more information, not realizing that the speaker is through talking. This occurs because level /2/ does not normally signal completion to the listener; it does not carry the finality of the "I'm through now" signal of level /1/.

B.   THE /2 3 ↑/ INTONATION CONTOUR

Some speakers find it difficult to use the /2 3 ↑/ contour on questions requiring a simple "yes" or "no" response. They typically employ a replacement contour which is best described as a /2 3 2 3 ↑/ circumflex contour. This pattern begins with a movement from level /2/ to level /3/. At level /3/ the pitch abruptly plunges downward, and it continues its fall until it reaches the vicinity of level /2/. At this point the voice rapidly reverses itself and rises back toward level /3/. The contour fades away someplace in the vicinity of level /3/. The movement just described tends to give this contour a definite lilt. There is no real problem with occasional use of this circumflex contour, but the speaker who uses it with frequency tends to develop a singsong quality in his speech. Your instructor will illustrate this usage for you, if you have difficulty using the /2 3 ↑/ contour.

₂ Did he tell her?   ₂ Are you going?   ₂ Did he write?

C.   THE /2 3 2 →/ INTONATION CONTOUR

Some speakers use the /2 3 2 3 ↑/ circumflex contour as a replacement for the /2 3 2 →/ pattern. Frequent use of this replacement for the /2 3 2 →/ contour adds to the singsong quality mentioned in Section 49-5B.

₂ If you don't come, I'm going home.

49–6.   PRACTICE EXERCISES FOR INTONATION

A.   A FEW REMINDERS ABOUT PRACTICE PROCEDURES

If this is the first practice chapter assigned to you by your instructor, you may wish to review the comments about beginning oral practice in Chap. 2, 2-4 and the comments about oral practice procedures in Chap. 2, 2-5A and 2-5B. Adapt the comments to your study of intonation.

49–7. USING THE /2 3 1 ↓/ OR /3 1 ↓/ INTONATION CONTOUR

A. USING THE /2 3 1 ↓/ OR /3 1 ↓/ CONTOUR IN A NONSENSE SYLLABLE

Sometimes a student finds it extremely difficult to use the /2 3 1 ↓/ or /3 1 ↓/ contour. No matter how hard he tries to imitate his instructor's use of the intonation contour, the student's intonation always resembles his replacement. If you are one of these persons, your instructor will ask you to practice using the contour in the following nonsense syllables and words. If you are either practicing with your instructor or listening to the syllables on tape, imitate your speech model as accurately as possible.

B. USING THE /2 3 1 ↓/ OR /3 1 ↓/ CONTOUR IN STATEMENTS

Read each of the following sentences carefully, trying to develop accurate intonation in the thought groups. Pay particular attention to using level /3/ and primary stress on the appropriate word, and to dropping your pitch accurately to level /1/ where indicated. Remember that primary stress will usually coincide with the high pitch in each thought group. You may wish to review the comments in Section 49-3C regarding the use of monopitch. If you are either practicing with your instructor or listening to the sentences on tape, imitate your speech model as accurately as possible.

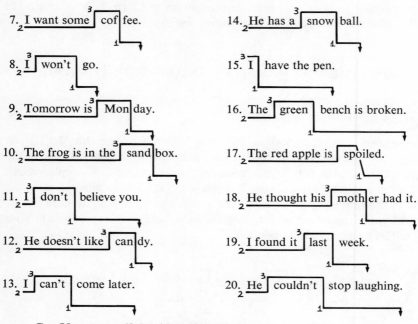

7. ₂I want some ³cof fee.

8. ₂I³ won't go.

9. ₂Tomorrow is ³Mon day.

10. ₂The frog is in the ³sand box.

11. ₂I³ don't believe you.

12. ₂He doesn't like ³can dy.

13. ₂I³ can't come later.

14. ₂He has a ³snow ball.

15. ₂I³ have the pen.

16. ₂The ³green bench is broken.

17. ₂The red apple is spoiled.

18. ₂He thought his ³moth er had it.

19. ₂I found it ³last week.

20. ₂He ³couldn't stop laughing.

C. USING THE /2 3 1 ↓/ OR /3 1 ↓/ CONTOUR IN QUESTIONS

Follow the directions in Exercise B when you do this drill.

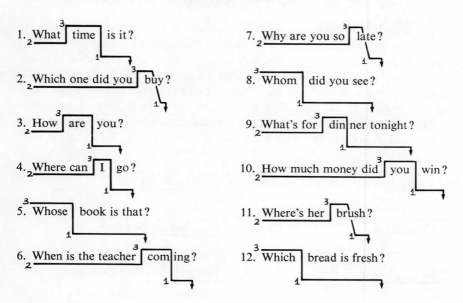

1. ₂What ³time is it?

2. ₂Which one did you ³buy?

3. ₂How ³are you?

4. ₂Where can ³I go?

5. ³Whose book is that?

6. When is the teacher ³com ing?

7. ₂Why are you so ³late?

8. ³Whom did you see?

9. ₂What's for ³din ner tonight?

10. ₂How much money did ³you win?

11. ₂Where's her ³brush?

12. ³Which bread is fresh?

D.   USING THE /2 3 1 ↓/ OR /3 1 ↓/ CONTOUR IN COMMANDS

Follow the directions in Exercise B when you do this drill.

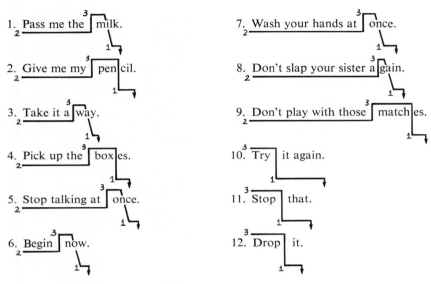

1. Pass me the milk.

2. Give me my pencil.

3. Take it away.

4. Pick up the boxes.

5. Stop talking at once.

6. Begin now.

7. Wash your hands at once.

8. Don't slap your sister again.

9. Don't play with those matches.

10. Try it again.

11. Stop that.

12. Drop it.

E.   ANSWERING QUESTIONS USING THE /2 3 1 ↓/ OR /3 1 ↓/ CONTOUR

Your instructor or another student will ask you a series of questions about one of the following basic statements. You are to answer each question using a /2 3 1 ↓/ or /3 1 ↓/ contour, whichever is appropriate. Pay particular attention to using level /3/ and primary stress on the appropriate word in your response.

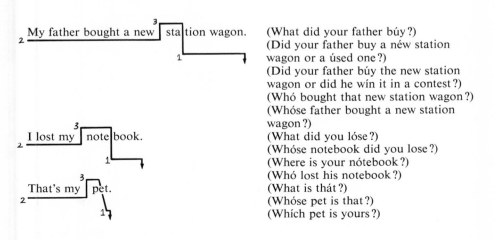

My father bought a new station wagon.

I lost my notebook.

That's my pet.

(What did your father búy?)
(Did your father buy a néw station wagon or a úsed one?)
(Did your father búy the new station wagon or did he wín it in a contest?)
(Whó bought that new station wagon?)
(Whóse father bought a new station wagon?)
(What did you lóse?)
(Whóse notebook did you lose?)
(Where is your nótebook?)
(Whó lost his notebook?)
(What is thát?)
(Whóse pet is that?)
(Whích pet is yours?)

49–8.   USING THE /2 3 ↑/ INTONATION CONTOUR

A.   USING THE /2 3 ↑/ CONTOUR IN QUESTIONS

Read each of the following sentences carefully, trying to develop accurate intonation in the thought groups. Pay particular attention to your rise in pitch from level /2/ to level /3/, making sure that you are using primary stress appropriately. Remember that primary stress is normally used on the first word in the thought group that is said at level /3/. Once you have inflected up to pitch level /3/, be sure to keep your voice there throughout the rest of the thought group. You may wish to review the comments in Section 49-3C regarding the use of monopitch. If you are either practicing with your instructor or listening to the sentences on tape, imitate your speech model as accurately as possible.

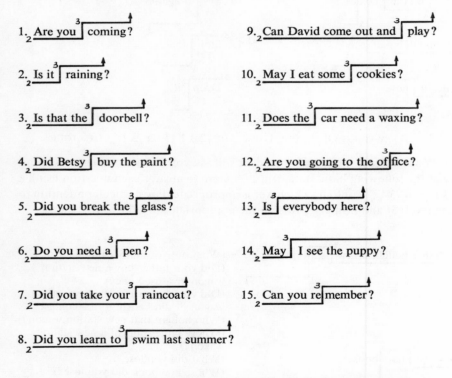

1. Are you coming?

2. Is it raining?

3. Is that the doorbell?

4. Did Betsy buy the paint?

5. Did you break the glass?

6. Do you need a pen?

7. Did you take your raincoat?

8. Did you learn to swim last summer?

9. Can David come out and play?

10. May I eat some cookies?

11. Does the car need a waxing?

12. Are you going to the office?

13. Is everybody here?

14. May I see the puppy?

15. Can you remember?

B.   USING THE /2 3 ↑/ CONTOUR IN A SERIES CONNECTED BY **and**

Read each of the following sentences carefully, trying to develop accurate intonation in the thought groups. Pay particular attention to your upward inflections from level /2/ to level /3/, and to your final drop to level /1/. Remember that primary stress will usually coincide with the high pitch in each thought group. You may wish to review the comments in Section 49-3C regarding the use of monopitch. If you are either practicing with your instructor or listening to the sentences on tape, imitate your speech model as accurately as possible.

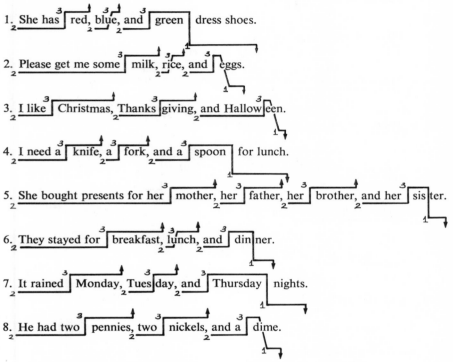

1. She has red, blue, and green dress shoes.

2. Please get me some milk, rice, and eggs.

3. I like Christmas, Thanksgiving, and Halloween.

4. I need a knife, a fork, and a spoon for lunch.

5. She bought presents for her mother, her father, her brother, and her sister.

6. They stayed for breakfast, lunch, and dinner.

7. It rained Monday, Tuesday, and Thursday nights.

8. He had two pennies, two nickels, and a dime.

C. USING THE /2 3 ↑/ CONTOUR IN A SERIES
   WHEN THE CHOICES ARE CONNECTED BY **or**

Follow the directions in Exercise B when you do this drill.

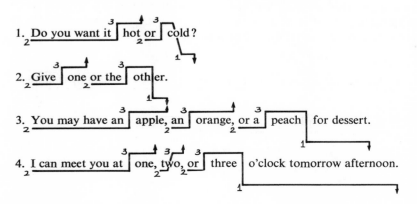

1. Do you want it hot or cold?

2. Give one or the other.

3. You may have an apple, an orange, or a peach for dessert.

4. I can meet you at one, two, or three o'clock tomorrow afternoon.

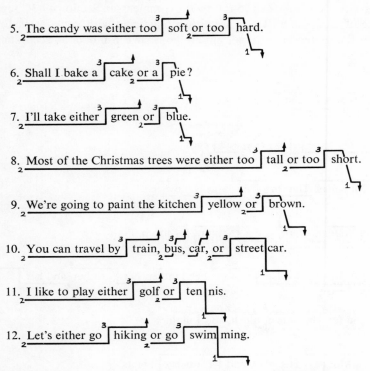

5. The candy was either too soft or too hard.

6. Shall I bake a cake or a pie?

7. I'll take either green or blue.

8. Most of the Christmas trees were either too tall or too short.

9. We're going to paint the kitchen yellow or brown.

10. You can travel by train, bus, car, or street car.

11. I like to play either golf or tennis.

12. Let's either go hiking or go swimming.

49–9. USING THE /2 3 2 →/ INTONATION CONTOUR

A. USING THE /2 3 2 →/ CONTOUR

Read each of the following sentences carefully, trying to develop accurate intonation in the thought groups. Pay particular attention to using level /3/ and primary stress on the appropriate word, and to dropping your pitch accurately to level /2/ where indicated. Remember that primary stress will usually coincide with the high pitch in each thought group. You may wish to review the comments in Section 49-3C regarding the use of monopitch. If you are either practicing with your instructor or listening to the sentences on tape, imitate your speech model as accurately as possible.

1. Autumn came early that year, and the trees were bare by October.

2. Ann has a bad cold, so she can't come today.

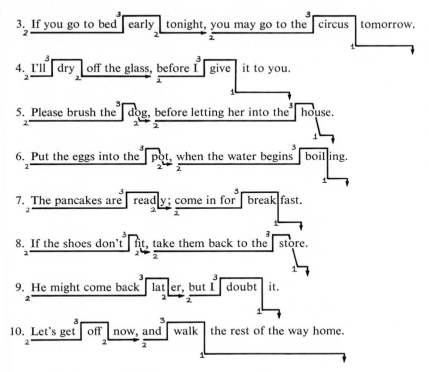

3. If you go to bed early tonight, you may go to the circus tomorrow.

4. I'll dry off the glass, before I give it to you.

5. Please brush the dog, before letting her into the house.

6. Put the eggs into the pot, when the water begins boiling.

7. The pancakes are ready; come in for breakfast.

8. If the shoes don't fit, take them back to the store.

9. He might come back later, but I doubt it.

10. Let's get off now, and walk the rest of the way home.

49–10. USING INTONATION CONTOURS IN BEGINNING CONVERSATION

This exercise gives you an opportunity to begin using intonation contours in thought groups that are in conversational form. Each set of drills utilizes one or more intonation contours in a variety of different starter patterns. Complete the patterns that are listed in each group of exercises by finding from five to ten words that you can substitute meaningfully in the blanks for each pattern. If some of your previous practice has been in pronunciation, you may wish to use some of your former target words in this exercise. Write the words on a sheet of paper, and begin practicing the / 2 3 1 ↓/ contour in Section 49-10A. Practice the first starter pattern with each of your completion words, placing primary stress and high pitch on the completion word. Do this with each of the starter patterns in *A*, and then continue the drill with the next contour and starter patterns. When you are satisfied that you are using the contours and patterns accurately and conversationally, you are ready to practice with somebody else. During class your instructor may ask you to practice the exercise with him, or he may ask you to do it with another student. Outside class you may wish to practice with a friend or somebody at home.

Choose a pattern, and ask your helper to begin saying the completion words. Each time your partner says a word, you repeat the pattern, using the appropriate intonation contour or contours with the completion word. Note that in C and D your helper will use more than one word for each pattern. Pretend that you are actually talking to somebody. Look directly at your helper's face, listen for the completion word, and then ask the question or complete the statement as realistically as possible. The drill should move along smoothly and rapidly in the manner of good conversation. Keep checking to make certain that you are using accurate intonation contours. The exercise may be expanded by asking your helper to think of additional words which may be used to complete the patterns. You may also wish to vary, where feasible, the location of the high pitch and primary stress.

A.   PRACTICING THE /2 3 1 ↓/ CONTOUR

1. "I see the _____."
2. "Give me the _____."
3. "Please pick up the _____."
4. "I'm going to visit the _____."
5. "I have a _____."
6. "How many _____ do you have?"
7. "Which _____ is yours?"

B.   PRACTICING THE /2 3 ↑/ CONTOUR

1. "Do you like _____?"
2. "Can I buy a _____?"
3. "Did you get me some _____?"
4. "Will you give me the _____?"
5. "Is that your _____?"

C.   PRACTICING THE /2 3 ↑/ CONTOUR
IN A SERIES FOLLOWED BY A FINAL /2 3 1 ↓/ CONTOUR

1. "I bought some _____, _____, and _____."
2. "My three favorite desserts are _____, _____, and _____."
3. "My favorite subjects are _____, _____, and _____."

4. "My best friends are _____, _____, and

_____."

5. "My favorite games are _____, _____, and

_____."

D. **PRACTICING THE /2 3 ↑/ CONTOUR
   IN A CHOICE SITUATION
   FOLLOWED BY A FINAL /2 3 1 ↓/ CONTOUR**

1. "Is your favorite color _____ or _____?"

2. "You may have either _____ or _____ for
breakfast."

3. "You may have a choice of _____ or _____ for
lunch today."

4. "You may watch either _____ or _____ on
television."

5. "You may have either _____ or _____ ice cream."

6. "Please buy me some _____ or _____ at the
market."

E. **PRACTICING THE /2 3 2 →/ CONTOUR
   FOLLOWED BY A FINAL /2 3 1 ↓/ CONTOUR**

1. "May I have a dime, so I can buy some _____?"

2. "Vacation starts next week, and I expect to _____."

3. "The recess bell just rang, and I'm going to _____."

4. "Christmas is coming soon, and I'm planning to buy mother a

_____."

49–11. CONVERSATION PRACTICE

So far you have learned how to use intonation by reading various kinds of exercises for melody. Now you are ready to move into the final and most important part of your training program—learning how to use typical English intonation contours automatically while you are talking more or less spontaneously. If this is the first practice chapter assigned to you by your instructor, you may wish to review the introductory comments on conversation practice in Chap. 2, 2-6 to 2-7.

A.   GENERAL CLASSROOM EXERCISES IN SPEAKING

Your instructor will plan a series of classroom conversation activities, and each assignment will be discussed fully in class before you carry it out. When your instructor announces the first speaking activity, you may wish to review the introductory comments on classroom speaking in Chap. 2, 2-7B.

appendix one

Ear Training Exercises

THE RECOGNITION OF PRONUNCIATION TARGETS IN WORDS

Review the instructions for the listening test in the appropriate chapter with your student. Read the words to him, making sure that his book is closed and that he is not watching your mouth for visual clues. You may wish to alter the order of target words. Most of the ear training drills may be carried out in the preceding manner. In a few instances special instructions are given for a particular exercise.

Chapter 5, 5–1B—Recognizing /θ/ in Words

1. thumb	4. birthday	7. third	10. bathroom	13. cloth
2. mouth	5. bath	8. nothing	11. both	14. thick
3. thorn	6. path	9. think	12. everything	15. anything

Chapter 6, 6–1B—Recognizing /ð/ in Words

1. brother	5. their	9. then	13. than	17. leather
2. other	6. bathe	10. weather	14. these	18. they
3. that	7. though	11. bothering	15. lathe	19. teethe
4. breathe	8. rather	12. smooth	16. either	20. bother

Chapter 7, 7–1B—Recognizing /f/ in Words

1. fixing	5. half	9. handkerchief	13. sniff	17. food
2. found	6. forever	10. laughing	14. himself	18. cornfield
3. difference	7. affair	11. surface	15. rough	19. knife
4. office	8. folding	12. fun	16. February	20. suffer

Chapter 8, 8–1B—Recognizing /v/ in Words

1. alive	5. silver	9. receiver	13. serve	17. covering
2. clover	6. starving	10. deliver	14. violin	18. give
3. very	7. various	11. voice	15. elevator	19. valley
4. gave	8. have	12. television	16. heaven	20. visiting

Chapter 9, 9–1B—Recognizing /s/ in Words

1. goose	5. introduce	9. dancing	13. sailboat	17. handsome
2. goodness	6. sour	10. consider	14. necklace	18. hillside
3. sell	7. increase	11. unless	15. ceiling	19. chase
4. silently	8. messenger	12. disagree	16. sea	20. century

Chapter 10, 10–1B—Recognizing /z/ in Words

1. zebra	5. zoo	9. cries	13. ponies	17. using
2. does	6. pigs	10. husband	14. visiting	18. zipper
3. dozen	7. zip code	11. whose	15. music	19. noise
4. bees	8. pleasant	12. zone	16. drums	20. desire

Chapter 11, 11–1B—Recognizing /ʃ/ in Words

1. ashes	5. sharp	9. flashing	13. delicious	17. national
2. shone	6. show	10. shoe	14. push	18. English
3. wash	7. crushing	11. fisherman	15. finish	19. share
4. ashamed	8. bush	12. shade	16. Chicago	20. dish

Chapter 12, 12–1B—Recognizing /ʒ/ in Words

1. measure	4. rouge	7. television	10. invasion	13. Asia
2. pleasure	5. usual	8. collision	11. leisure	14. garage
3. treasure	6. unusual	9. measuring	12. message	15. usually

Chapter 13, 13–1B—Recognizing /h/ in Words

1. behind	4. overhead	7. hungrier	10. unhappy
2. handsome	5. hurrying	8. heavily	11. harmless
3. perhaps	6. beehive	9. sawhorse	12. downhill

Chapter 14, 14–1B—Recognizing /tʃ/ in Words

1. adventure	5. chance	9. inch	13. coach	17. chilly
2. beaches	6. cheat	10. matching	14. branching	18. butcher
3. bench	7. witch	11. French	15. hitch	19. bunch
4. chase	8. pitcher	12. children	16. charge	20. patching

Chapter 15, 15–1B—Recognizing /dʒ/ in Words

1. vegetable	5. package	9. joke	13. gentleman	17. bridge
2. joy	6. enjoying	10. jacket	14. magic	18. stranger
3. language	7. passenger	11. hedge	15. cabbage	19. cage
4. jewel	8. manage	12. imagining	16. jumping	20. January

Chapter 16, 16–1B—Recognizing /l/ in Words

1. allowed	5. heel	9. lost	13. hillside	17. light
2. letter	6. smell	10. licking	14. leader	18. fully
3. along	7. laughing	11. mile	15. especially	19. tailor
4. language	8. belonged	12. lettuce	16. call	20. lucky

Chapter 16, 16–1D—Recognizing Dark /l/ in Words

Review the instructions for this drill. You may wish to complicate the exercise by asking the student to indicate if he heard dark /l/ at the beginning, in the middle, or at the end of the word.

1. lose	5. loan	9. fool	13. hall	17. believe
2. loose	6. look	10. call	14. shell	18. telephone
3. loop	7. law	11. mill	15. gulf	19. million
4. low	8. full	12. feel	16. salt	20. fully

Chapter 16, 16–1E—Recognizing Syllabic /l̩/ in Words

1. battle	5. kettle	9. cradle	13. riddle	17. saddle
2. cattle	6. little	10. handle	14. model	18. paddle
3. gentle	7. rattle	11. middle	15. middle	
4. gentleman	8. petal	12. needle	16. pedal	

Chapter 17, 17–1B—Recognizing /r/ in Words

1. rest	5. cherry	9. receive	13. errand	17. refuse
2. tomorrow	6. raincoat	10. remain	14. cigar	18. berry
3. story	7. pear	11. around	15. radio	19. tomorrow
4. beer	8. eraser	12. racing	16. direction	20 sure

Chapter 18, 18–1B—Recognizing /j/ in Words

1. yesterday	5. opinion	9. yardstick	13. senior	17. yeast
2. youngest	6. yawning	10. younger	14. year	18. canyon
3. barnyard	7. companion	11. beyond	15. union	19. beyond
4. onion	8. yet	12. yacht	16. behavior	20. yonder

Chapter 19, 19–1B—Recognizing /w/ in Words

1. otherwise	5. anyway	9. Wednesday	13. workman
2. waitress	6. Washington	10. Halloween	14. between
3. sandwich	7. underwater	11. wonderful	15. wandering
4. sidewalk	8. wagonload	12. highway	16. awakening

Chapter 20, 20–1B—Recognizing /ʍ/ in Words

1. what
2. wheat
3. anywhere
4. when
5. whether
6. whispering
7. nowhere
8. whine
9. bobwhite
10. while
11. everywhere
12. which
13. wherever
14. white
15. whistling
16. somewhere

Chapter 21, 21–1B—Recognizing /m/ in Words

1. aim
2. became
3. shoemaker
4. Mike
5. promise
6. scream
7. mystery
8. bottom
9. steam
10. room
11. meadow
12. same
13. coming
14. became
15. most
16. lime

Chapter 22, 22–1B—Recognizing /n/ in Words

1. again
2. frown
3. narrow
4. sunny
5. new
6. grown
7. never
8. cannot
9. clean
10. nice
11. north
12. began
13. dinner
14. between
15. nose
16. ten
17. honey
18. neat
19. drawn
20. funny

Chapter 22, 22–1D—Recognizing Syllabic /n̩/

1. button
2. cotton
3. couldn't
4. kitten
5. mitten
6. hidden
7. wouldn't
8. written
9. certain
10. shouldn't
11. sudden
12. didn't
13. bitten
14. gotten
15. garden
16. needn't

Chapter 23, 23–1B—Recognizing /ŋ/ in the Suffix -ing in Words

1. waiting
2. walking
3. tickling
4. biting
5. building
6. aching
7. according
8. rushing
9. paddling
10. looking
11. losing
12. lowering
13. raising
14. racing
15. pushing

Chapter 24, 24–1B—Recognizing /p/ in Words

1. appear
2. part
3. sleep
4. stopper
5. pass
6. pine
7. put
8. ripe
9. point
10. bumper
11. pen
12. repeat
13. stopping
14. tulip
15. pound
16. pillow
17. leaping
18. tip
19. stupid
20. peace

Chapter 24, 24–1D—Recognizing /p/ in Words
When the Target Is Said with a Strong Puff of Air

1. appear
2. part
3. pass
4. pillow
5. peace
6. pine
7. put
8. apart
9. point
10. report
11. pen
12. repeat
13. pound
14. suppose
15. pan

Chapter 25, 25–1B—Recognizing /b/ in Words

1. back	5. grab	9. club	13. backward	17. busy
2. bank	6. horseback	10. rainbow	14. cub	18. robe
3. about	7. motorboat	11. basement	15. doorbell	19. nobody
4. stubborn	8. ball	12. maybe	16. storybook	20. obey

Chapter 26, 26–1B—Recognizing /t/ in Words

1. winter	5. chocolate	9. telephone	13. lighting	17. telegram
2. take	6. toward	10. laughed	14. teaching	18. daytime
3. lifting	7. beautiful	11. tomorrow	15. fighting	19. tar
4. put	8. carpenter	12. slight	16. wheat	20. pretend

Chapter 26, 26–1D—Recognizing /t/ in Words
When the Target Is Said with a Strong Puff of Air

1. take	5. television	9. tone	13. tire	17. telegram
2. toward	6. telephone	10. tip	14. toe	18. daytime
3. attend	7. attention	11. teaching	15. return	19. tar
4. attach	8. attack	12. retake	16. retain	20. pretend

Chapter 26, 26–1E—Recognizing /t/ in Words
When the Target Is Said Without a Strong Puff of Air

1. better	5. cutting	9. matter	13. battle	17. twenty
2. bitter	6. getting	10. pretty	14. little	18. seventy
3. butter	7. notice	11. lighter	15. bottle	19. sweater
4. Betty	8. later	12. hotter	16. kettle	20. invited

Chapter 26, 26–1F—Recognizing /t/ in Words
in Which the Target Is Typically Omitted

1. twenty	5. costly	9. almost	13. correct	17. lift
2. center	6. softly	10. against	14. expect	18. tastes
3. plenty	7. mostly	11. biggest	15. act	19. pastes
4. printed	8. swiftly	12. rest	16. left	20. rests

Chapter 27, 27–1B—Recognizing /d/ in Words

1. add	5. hiding	9. odd	13. duck	17. Monday
2. dare	6. dime	10. radio	14. sand	18. disappear
3. model	7. nod	11. held	15. dream	19. overhead
4. made	8. ready	12. greedy	16. bolder	20. window

Chapter 27, 27–1D—Recognizing /d/ in Words
in Which the Target Is Typically Omitted

1. shoulder	4. children	7. laundry	10. told	13. behind
2. colder	5. hundred	8. standing	11. hold	14. round
3. bolder	6. wondering	9. window	12. sold	15. blind

Chapter 28, 28–1B—Recognizing /k/ in Words
When the Replacement Is Caused by Poor Contact

1. keep	5. account	9. candy	13. cup
2. require	6. picking	10. copper	14. cook
3. lake	7. packing	11. became	15. raccoon
4. kiss	8. luck	12. working	16. cover

Chapter 28, 28–1C—Recognizing /k/ When
the Target Is Said with a Strong Puff of Air

1. couple	5. kill	9. because	13. mechanic	17. company
2. cowboy	6. camp	10. kind	14. kid	18. cold
3. color	7. became	11. raccoon	15. kiss	19. cousin
4. require	8. cord	12. corner	16. account	20. candy

Chapter 28, 28–1D—Recognizing /k/ When
the Target Is Omitted in Certain Final Consonant Clusters

1. desk	4. risk	7. risks	10. risked
2. ask	5. masks	8. tasks	11. masked
3. task	6. tusks	9. asked	

Chapter 29, 29–1B—Recognizing /g/ in Words

1. gave	5. wig	9. gone	13. tiger	17. begin
2. rug	6. game	10. language	14. hug	18. geese
3. gun	7. eagerly	11. foggy	15. snug	19. egg
4. again	8. bargain	12. guest	16. gallop	20. nightgown

Chapter 30, 30–1B—Recognizing /i/ in Words

1. seacoast	5. freeze	9. green	13. either	17. east
2. agree	6. tea	10. bumblebee	14. three	18. free
3. Easter	7. eaten	11. scene	15. weaker	19. peach
4. even	8. agreed	12. degree	16. between	20. equal

Chapter 31, 31–1B—Recognizing /ɪ/ in Words

1. little	5. sister	9. if	13. will	17. middle
2. big	6. illness	10. isn't	14. filled	18. kitchen
3. into	7. quit	11. sting	15. minute	19. silver
4. instant	8. swing	12. ink	16. interested	20. interview

Chapter 32, 32–1B—Recognizing /eɪ/ in Words

1. May	5. obey	9. showcase	13. today	17. agent
2. able	6. train	10. blue jay	14. playground	18. stage
3. ashamed	7. pray	11. eight	15. age	19. highway
4. awakening	8. ate	12. straightened	16. grain	20. acorn

Chapter 33, 33–1B—Recognizing /ɛ/ in Words

1. Ellen
2. election
3. remembered
4. anyway

5. attempt
6. elephant
7. celebrate
8. elevator

9. nonsense
10. November
11. umbrella
12. messenger

13. everybody
14. footsteps
15. empty
16. ever

17. better
18. lettuce
19. pleasantly
20. regulate

Chapter 34, 34–1B—Recognizing /ae/ in Words

1. add
2. understand
3. magic
4. dandelion

5. ask
6. character
7. ashes
8. candle

9. attic
10. branch
11. slap
12. Valentine

13. accident
14. handsome
15. angry
16. apple

17. Halloween
18. sandwiches
19. answer
20. phonograph

Chapter 35, 35–1B—Recognizing /u/ in Words

1. teaspoon
2. gluing
3. school

4. too
5. smoothly
6. scooping

7. fooling
8. produce
9. who

10. afternoon
11. movement
12. zoo

13. truly
14. grapefruit
15. throughout

Chapter 37, 37–1B—Recognizing /oʊ/ in Words

1. telephone
2. clothesline
3. below
4. goldfish

5. ocean
6. whole
7. woke
8. open

9. glow
10. grown-up
11. toasted
12. snowshoes

13. only
14. though
15. ago
16. moment

17. over
18. homemade
19. flow
20. zip code

Chapter 38, 38–1B—Recognizing /ɔ/ in Words

1. all
2. across
3. tall
4. law

5. daughter
6. frosting
7. cautious
8. always

9. soft
10. paw
11. strawberry
12. author

13. crossing
14. draw
15. ought
16. claws

17. belong
18. fawn
19. offering
20. raw

Chapter 39, 39–1B—Recognizing /ɑ/ in Words

1. large
2. scarlet
3. far
4. argument

5. carpenter
6. car
7. arch
8. artery

9. garden
10. darting
11. hot

12. not
13. cotton
14. pocket

15. dollar
16. arbor
17. Argentina

Chapter 40, 40–1B—Recognizing /ʌ/ in Words

1. something
2. oven
3. mushroom
4. under

5. government
6. onion
7. wondered
8. uncle

9. youngest
10. suppertime
11. bumblebee
12. other

13. drugstore
14. monkey
15. husband
16. sundown

17. buttoned
18. tumbled
19. jumping
20. upper

Chapter 41, 41–1B—Recognizing /ə/ in Words

1. alive	5. telephone	9. along	13. alike	17. goodness
2. control	6. pocket	10. idea	14. Sarah	18. arrived
3. aloud	7. attend	11. foxes	15. lighted	19. tonight
4. Santa	8. disappear	12. famous	16. papa	20. mamma

Chapter 41, 41–2B—Listening for
Replacements in Words Containing the Letter a

Review the instructions for the listening test with the student. Read the words and mix up your use of /ə/ and /ɑ/. The difficulty of the test may be increased by reading the items more rapidly. The test may be varied by saying the same word over several times, using /ə/ and /ɑ/ pronunciations.

1. alike	5. several	9. appear	12. Africa	15. Christmas
2. agree	6. afraid	10. Texas	13. typical	16. Santa
3. signal	7. special	11. national	14. breakfast	17. capital
4. sofa	8. idea			

Chapter 41, 41–2C—Listening for
Replacements in Words Containing the Letter o

Follow the instructions in the preceding exercise, but use /ə/ and /oʊ/.

1. season	3. reasons	5. gallop	7. lessons	9. pilot
2. contain	4. command	6. control	8. lemons	10. capitol

Chapter 41, 41–2D—Listening for
Replacements in Words Containing the Letter u

Follow the instructions in the preceding exercises, but use /ə/ and /u/.

1. suppose   2. succeed   3. supply   4. support   5. circus   6. campus

Chapter 42, 42–1B—Recognizing /ɝ/ in Words

1. bird	5. perfectly	9. Thursday	13. blur	17. occur
2. church	6. terminal	10. stir	14. Earnest	18. blackbird
3. early	7. earn	11. turned	15. alert	19. searching
4. fur	8. certainly	12. workman	16. servant	20. courteous

Chapter 43, 43–1B—Recognizing /ɚ/ in Words

1. entering	5. doctor	9. picture	13. hammer	16. discover
2. baker	6. another	10. evergreen	14. favor	17. featherbed
3. laughter	7. dollar	11. number	15. wonderful	18. backward
4. butterfly	8. neighborhood	12. fisherman		

Chapter 43, 43–2B—Listening for
Replacements in Words Containing the Letters ar

Review the instructions for the listening test with the student. Read the words, and mix up your use of /ɚ/ and /ɑ/. The difficulty of the test may be increased by reading the items more rapidly. The test may be varied by saying the same word over again several times, using /ɚ/ and /ɑ/ pronunciations.

1. collar
2. sugar
3. backward
4. dollar
5. forward
6. steward
7. cougar

Chapter 43, 43–2C—Listening for
Replacements in Words Containing the Letters er

Follow the instructions in the preceding exercise, but use /ɚ/ and /ɛ/.

1. after
2. better
3. bigger
4. center
5. closer
6. finger
7. louder
8. quicker
9. power
10. water

Chapter 43, 43–2D—Listening for
Replacements in Words Containing the Letters or

Follow the instructions in the preceding exercises, but use /ɚ/ and /ɔ/ or /oʊ/.

1. sailor
2. color
3. doctor
4. effort
5. actor
6. tailor

Chapter 43, 43–2E—Listening for
Replacements in Words Containing the Letters ure

Follow the instructions in the preceding exercises, but use /ɚ/ and /u/.

1. picture
2. nature
3. pasture
4. juncture
5. rapture
6. capture

Chapter 43, 43–2F—Listening for
a Vowel Replacement Followed by a Trilled /r/

Select some of the test words from the preceding exercises for Chapter 43. Vary your pronunciation with /ɚ/ and a probable vowel replacement plus trilled /r/. If necessary, use only the trilled /r/.

Chapter 44, 44–1B—Recognizing /aɪ/ in Words

1. island
2. ride
3. try
4. might
5. reply
6. admire
7. outside
8. ice
9. fireplace
10. apply
11. acquire
12. ice cream
13. buy
14. climbing
15. dye
16. eye

Chapter 45, 45–1B—Recognizing /aʊ/ in Words

1. clown	4. amount	7. proud	10. allow	13. outside
2. out	5. bough	8. account	11. plow	14. sundown
3. cow	6. owl	9. hour	12. loudest	15. ouch

Chapter 46, 46–1B—Recognizing /ɔɪ/ in Words

1. boiling	4. destroy	7. point	10. enjoying	13. join
2. oil	5. ointment	8. toy	11. oyster	14. oiling
3. spoiled	6. Detroit	9. boy	12. soiled	15. voice

THE RECOGNITION OF STRESS

Chapter 47, 47–6B—Recognizing Primary Stress in Simple Syllables

1. lá	la	3. lu	lú	5. ló	lo	7. lú	le	9. lu	lá
2. la	lá	4. lé	le	6. la	lé	8. ló	la	10. le	lú

Chapter 47, 47–6C—Recognizing Primary Stress in Polysyllabic Words

1. chíldren	5. torpédo	9. sýmphony	13. excíting	17. góvernment
2. sándwich	6. básement	10. foréver	14. accépt	18. sýmpathy
3. garáge	7. afráid	11. grúnting	15. sóldier	19. impátient
4. víolet	8. enórmous	12. gálloping	16. umbrélla	20. machíne

Chapter 47, 47–6D—Recognizing Primary Stress
in Polysyllabic Words Also Containing Secondary Stress

1. bláckbìrd	6. gréenhòuse	11. dárk róom	16. Chrístmas trèe
2. gréen hóuse	7. réd bóok	12. Jóhn Smíth	17. swìmming pòol
3. blúe béll	8. Rédbòok	13. dárkròom	18. poláris míssile
4. Whíte Hòuse	9. stréet càr	14. spécial delívery	19. péncil shàrpener
5. bláck bírd	10. frúit càke	15. více-président	20. rócket shìp

Chapter 47, 47–10A—Recognizing Strong Stresses in Simple Sentences

1. I'll sèe you at lúnch.
2. Gìve it to the téacher.
3. Did he sày nó?
4. We néed it at ónce.
5. Pául isn't còming.
6. I líke the nèw instrúctor.
7. Can you màke some ápplesàuce?
8. The ténnis còurts are búsy.
9. I sàid gíve me the móney.
10. Péter's fàther is làte.

appendix two

Test Sentences
for Articulation

1. /θ/   I think Arthur is coming to my birthday party on Thursday at three.
2. /ð/   Neither their father nor their mother were bothered with the weather.
3. /f/   Her nephew offered to fix the fan himself if Fay telephoned the factory.
4. /v/   David was invited to spend five days of his vacation, camping at the cove near the valley.
5. /s/   The second excited nurse suddenly discovered that the medicine was harmless.
6. /z/   He didn't realize that his fingers and his nose were almost frozen by the freezing weather.
7. /ʃ/   The shower had passed, the air was fresh, and the sun was shining over the ocean at the seashore.
8. /ʒ/   As usual he had a collision with the garage door.
9. /h/   She hopped halfway down the hill to the schoolhouse by the highway.

10. /tʃ/   Which teacher gave the child another chance to answer the question about the ranch?

11. /dʒ/   Jill gave some juicy oranges, some gingerbread, and a jar of cabbage to George.

12. /l/   Paul was allowed a late snack of cold milk and a full slice of delicious lime pie.

13. /l̩/   The little petals fell onto the rattle in the baby's cradle.

14. /r/   He ate a pear and rice cereal with very sweet raisins and cream at breakfast.

15. /j/   Did you eat a few yellow onions yesterday?

16. /w/   The wild wind was always chasing the swamp weeds through the open doorway.

17. /ʌ/   What kind of wheat did they see everywhere?

18. /m/   He came home at suppertime for a steamed clam dinner.

19. /n/   My nice neighbor is eating alone again in the fancy dining room.

20. /n̩/   The kitten wouldn't have bitten him, if he hadn't teased it.

21. /ŋ/   Mother shook her finger in anger, because the boys kept laughing, singing, and playing.

22. /p/   Peter was supposed to take some cold potato soup, rice pudding, and a piece of pie to the picnic.

23. /b/   Bob decided to have a boiled crab dinner at a nearby beach in October.

24. /t/   They told him it was better to return the rest of his tickets to the city office at once.

25. /d/   They had some wonderful roast duck, with cold homemade pudding, for dinner last Monday.

26. /k/   They drank some coffee, and asked for a snack in the kitchen while packing the candy.

27. /g/   The big dog stopped growling, and gaily began wagging his grey tail.

28. /i/   The three speakers at each meeting said the Peace Corps needed eager workers.

29. /ɪ/   Jim isn't interested in walking home, since he lives over this hill.

30. /eɪ/   Jay explained that he may spend his April vacation raking hay and picking grapes at his favorite farm.

31. /ɛ/   The smell of breakfast was getting everybody hungry at the hotel.

32. /ae/   Sam was asked to wrap up some apples and bananas with the crackers and jam.

33. /u/   Whose shoe did Susan find in the schoolroom this afternoon?

34. /ʊ/   The woman stood up and put on the wonderful looking woolen hood.

35. /ou/   He hoped that the wind hadn't broken the old pole that was holding the yellow tomato plants.

36.	/ɔ/	He saw the officer offer to help her walk across the broad street yesterday morning.
37.	/ɑ/	Arthur parked his hot car near the empty lot on his block.
38.	/ʌ/	She baked a duck in the oven with onions, mustard, and crushed mushrooms.
39.	/ə/	They agreed to buy a blanket and a sofa at the special sale at the campus store.
40.	/ɝ/	Earl said, "Yes, sir! I earn my living selling pearls, and this perfect pearl is worth a lot of money."
41.	/ɚ/	It was a pleasure for the doctor to eat the wonderful sugar and gingerbread cookies.
42.	/aɪ/	I wish you'd dry your eyes and stop crying about Mike's ice cream.
43.	/aʊ/	The shower lasted an hour, and the boy scout's towel got wet.
44.	/ɔɪ/	I enjoy eating a broiled sirloin steak with boiled potatoes.

Evaluation Form

NAME _____   DATE _____

I. PRONUNCIATION TARGETS[1]

1.	/θ/	_____	**11.**	/dʒ/	_____
2.	/ð/	_____	**12.**	/l/	_____
3.	/f/	_____	**13.**	/l̩/	_____
4.	/v/	_____	**14.**	/r/	_____
5.	/s/	_____	**15.**	/j/	_____
6.	/z/	_____	**16.**	/w/	_____
7.	/ʃ/	_____	**17.**	/ʌ/	_____
8.	/ʒ/	_____	**18.**	/m/	_____
9.	/h/	_____	**19.**	/n/	_____
10.	/tʃ/	_____	**20.**	/ŋ/	_____

[1]Suggested code based on *Chapter 3*.
Substitution: diagonal line e.g., ___ / ___
Distortion: **dst.**
Omission: circled sound – ◯ **init., mdl., fnl.**
Addition: **ad. – init., fnl.**

21.	/ŋ/	_____	**33.**	/u/ _____
22.	/p/	_____	**34.**	/ʊ/ _____
23.	/b/	_____	**35.**	/oʊ/ _____
24.	/t/	_____	**36.**	/ɔ/ _____
25.	/d/	_____	**37.**	/ɑ/ _____
26.	/k/	_____	**38.**	/ʌ/ _____
27.	/g/	_____	**39.**	/ə/ _____
28.	/i/	_____	**40.**	/ɝ/ _____
29.	/ɪ/	_____	**41.**	/ɚ/ _____
30.	/eɪ/	_____	**42.**	/aɪ/ _____
31.	/ɛ/	_____	**43.**	/aʊ/ _____
32.	/ae/	_____	**44.**	/ɔɪ/ _____

II. STRESS

Place a check next to the category that best describes the student's problem in using stress. Use the additional space for needed comments.

_____ A. *Poorly Located Stress in Polysyllabic Words.*

_____ B. *Rapid, Choppy Rhythmic Quality:* uses weak stress for primary stress.

_____ C. *Slow, Even Rhythmic Quality:* uses strong stress for weak stress in polysyllabic words.

_____ D. *Slow, Even Rhythmic Quality:* uses strong stress for weak stress in unstressed forms.

_____ E.   *Other Stress Problems.*

III.   INTONATION

Place a check next to the category that best describes the student's problem in using intonation. Use the additional space for needed comments.

_____ A.   */2 3 2 →/ or /3 2 →/ for /2 3 1 ↓/ or /3 1 ↓/.*

_____ B.   */2 3 2 3 ↑/ (circumflex) for /2 3 ↑/.*

_____ C.   */2 3 2 3 ↑/ (circumflex) for /2 3 2 →/.*

_____ D.   *Other Intonation Problems.*

IV.   CLARITY

Place a check next to the category that best describes the reason for the student's lack of clarity. Use the additional space for needed comments.

_____ A.   *Mispronunciation.*

_____ B. *Extremely Rapid and Choppy Rhythm.*

_____ C. *Inadequate Projection.*

_____ D. *Slurred or Slushy Pronunciation.*

_____ E. *Clenched or Tight Jaw.*

appendix three b

Evaluation Form

NAME _____   DATE _____

I. PRONUNCIATION TARGETS[1]

1. /θ/	_____	**13.** /l̩/	_____
2. /ð/	_____	**14.** /r/	_____
3. /f/	_____	**15.** /j/	_____
4. /v/	_____	**16.** /w/	_____
5. /s/	_____	**17.** /ʍ/	_____
6. /z/	_____	**18.** /m/	_____
7. /ʃ/	_____	**19.** /n/	_____
8. /ʒ/	_____	**20.** /n̩/	_____
9. /h/	_____	**21.** /ŋ/	_____
10. /tʃ/	_____	**22.** /p/	_____
11. /dʒ/	_____	**23.** /b/	_____
12. /l/	_____	**24.** /t/	_____

[1]Suggested code based on *Chapter 3*.
  Substitution: diagonal line, e.g., ___ / ___
  Distortion: **dst.**
  Omission: circled sound – ◯ **init., mdl., fnl.**
  Addition: **ad. – init., fnl.**

25.	/d/	_____	**35.**	/ou/	_____
26.	/k/	_____	**36.**	/ɔ/	_____
27.	/g/	_____	**37.**	/a/	_____
28.	/i/	_____	**38.**	/ʌ/	_____
29.	/ɪ/	_____	**39.**	/ə/	_____
30.	/eɪ/	_____	**40.**	/ɝ/	_____
31.	/ɛ/	_____	**41.**	/ɚ/	_____
32.	/ae/	_____	**42.**	/aɪ/	_____
33.	/u/	_____	**43.**	/au/	_____
34.	/ʊ/	_____	**44.**	/ɔɪ/	_____

II. STRESS

Place a check next to the category that best describes the student's problem in using stress. Use the additional space for needed comments.

_____A. *Poorly Located Stress in Polysyllabic Words.*

_____B. *Rapid, Choppy Rhythmic Quality:* uses weak stress for primary stress.

_____C. *Slow, Even Rhythmic Quality:* uses strong stress for weak stress in polysyllabic words.

_____D. *Slow, Even Rhythmic Quality:* uses strong stress for weak stress in unstressed forms.

_____E. *Other Stress Problems.*

III.   INTONATION

Place a check next to the category that best describes the student's problem in using intonation. Use the additional space for needed comments.

_____A.   /2 3 2 →/ or /3 2 →/ for /2 3 1 ↓/ or /3 1 ↓/.

_____B.   /2 3 2 3 ↑/ (circumflex) for /2 3 ↑/.

_____C.   /2 3 2 3 ↑/ (circumflex) for /2 3 2 →/.

_____D.   *Other Intonation Problems.*

IV.   CLARITY

Place a check next to the category that best describes the reason for the student's lack of clarity. Use the additional space for needed comments.

_____A.   *Mispronunciation.*

_____B.   *Extremely Rapid and Choppy Rhythm.*

_____C. *Inadequate Projection.*

_____D. *Slurred or Slushy Pronunciation.*

_____E. *Clenched or Tight Jaw.*

Index

Index
of Consonants, Vowels
and Diphthongs

VOWELS

DIPHTHONGS